Famous First Papers for the Neurointensivist

Eelco F.M. Wijdicks

Famous First Papers for the Neurointensivist

Springer

Eelco F.M. Wijdicks, MD, PhD, FACP
Division of Critical Care Neurology
Mayo Clinic
Rochester, Minnesota
USA

ISBN 978-1-4614-3181-7 ISBN 978-1-4614-3182-4 (eBook)
DOI 10.1007/978-1-4614-3182-4
Springer New York Heidelberg Dordrecht London

Library of Congress Control Number: 2012938368

Printed on acid-free paper

Springer is part of Springer Science+Business Media (www.springer.com)

Preface

History in neurology has always focused on exceptional neurologists, grandees in the research laboratory and chronic—often degenerative—neurologic disorders. There has been little historical work in acute neurologic conditions, precisely because neurology is not perceived through this perspective. This book is an attempt to mine the early descriptions of clinical signs—now used to alert to a serious neurologic illness—and to present the development of treatment of these acute disorders.

Standard clinical practice in neurology takes time to mature. Once accepted, physicians rarely know where diagnostic signs and syndromes originated. Few have actually seen or read the original manuscript. This proclivity of physicians applies to a certain extent to the acute neurosciences. Terms such as *Cushing ulcer*, *cerebral T waves*, *cerebral salt wasting syndrome*, and other designations or eponyms have rarely been explored historically, and this book attempts to do that.

Why do we want to know? One could argue that sufficient knowledge of a topic is only acquired through historical probing. Going back to the primary source is part of a comprehensive learning process and when scrutinizing these papers one may find not only the challenges of the discovery, but also the uncertainties of the first conclusions. Sometimes eponyms have become folklore (e.g., Biot breathing) or are rarely used.

This book has many first papers and—using a standard format—are discussed in 60 short historical notes. The original title page with, in some instances, key tables and figures are shown in clear reproductions. I have cited statements and even paragraphs when I believed it had historical significance, even if it read oddly for today's standards. This is followed by a brief discussion of the findings and its implications. A final comment provides a perspective and later developments. Landmark clinical trials are included that apply to the field of acute neurology and include winners and losers. This book also briefly discusses the birth of intensive care units.

Some of the material has been previously published, but the overwhelming majority is new research and presented here for the first time. There is an unmanageable large quantity of papers that could be useful to this book, and this book is obviously a selection. The chapters are concise and I hope contain the necessary details. All selected papers are clinical observations or clinical trials.

A collection of brief essays on landmark papers in acute neurology is more than just an exercise in curiosity or a "boutique" book to wither away on library shelves. I have tried to go beyond the dry realm of academia and tried to communicate interesting anecdotes. It is also an attempt to organize important clinical discoveries, structure the specialty, and honor the investigators and study groups. Some techniques in the Neurosciences Intensive Care unit are still in development (i.e., electrophysiologic and metabolic monitoring), others have not lasted very long (i.e., evoked potentials). Some areas—albeit revolutionary discoveries—are predominantly in the domains of neurosurgery (intracranial pressure monitors) or interventional neuroradiology (endovascular coil embolization) and are best covered in other works.

This book truly focuses on the descriptions of acute and critically ill neurologic patients. When these observations were made, the field of neurocritical care did not exist as it is today. The title is therefore not famous first papers *by* neurointensivists, and I would hope that book will be written one day.

The title also implies the book is solely for neurointensivists but—of course—I hope it will be worthwhile for all physicians regularly involved with critically ill neurologic and neurosurgical patients. I suspect any physician with a historical inclination would want to look through it. It should be of interest to neurologists, neurosurgeons, intensivists, emergency physicians, and fellows in these specialties. It may even be a resource for journal clubs. In the end, I would think that understanding the beginnings of acute neurology serves physicians better and allows them to look into the future.

Eelco F.M. Wijdicks

Acknowledgments

Writing a medical history book requires a considerable effort, and librarian support is indispensable. I am very grateful to Wanda Elkharwily who found the original sources and pointed me to others I probably would have missed. To find these works was labor intensive, but also riveting. The photography of the manuscripts title pages and other relevant figures were expertly made by Peggy Chihak. I again thank my devoted secretaries Tammy Drees and Donna Larkin for typing, formatting, seeking permissions, and other essential support needed to finish this book.

I thank the editorial staff of Springer Publishing and in particular Richard Lansing, who not only suggested the project but also kept reminding me just to do it. This book is what I wanted to write someday, and I am glad it is here. I thank Robin Weisberg for expert editing of the manuscript.

The last word of gratitude as always is to the light of my life, my lovely wife Barbara and our children Coen and Marilou. I am very fortunate to have their unbridled enthusiasm for what I do.

Contents

1 First and Famous: Criteria and Qualifiers

E.F.M. Wijdicks, *Famous First Papers for the Neurointensivist*,
DOI 10.1007/978-1-4614-3182-4_1,

In science the credit goes to the man who convinces the world, not to the man to whom the idea first occurred.

—Sir William Osler

The need for this book may need further justification and its title may generate some questions. What are the objective criteria for "famous" and how does one determine whether a place in the pantheon is assured? Is there such a thing as a pantheon? When is a paper uncompromisingly the first one and is there not some arbitrariness? Is the clinical trial the first paper, or is it the first case report or cohort that prompted the clinical trial? This book will answer these questions in some detail, but we all would agree that these papers changed everything what came later. Some observations became eponyms, others modified or altered practice, and many brought about further search for a cause and treatment.

In a few instances, the first observation has been recognized as a well-known reference. However, most of the time identifying these papers required searching through multiple references and finally settling on a reference that appeared as the first observation.

Any research of this kind will uncover surprises. Not uncommonly, the first description may have been prompted by an earlier observation. Such an earlier observation often had little detail, but the subsequent corroborating paper—using more patient examples—may have cemented the clinical finding.

In some instances, the label "first" may not be justified, and similar papers exist. Occasionally, multiple abstracts on the same topic were published before a peer reviewed paper appeared.

So how can we best select these works? Total number of citations may be indicative, but every prolific author knows that some of the least earth-shaking manuscripts may get the most citations. At the minimum, five criteria for a credible contribution could be considered: First, at the very least, it is a novel observation, technique, or clinical trial. Second, it is referenced in papers that follow. Third, it may have caused a paradigm shift or close to it. Fourth, it has been accepted in clinical practice and there are followers, and finally, it has survived the test of time. Readers of this book will immediately notice that some of the eponyms and classic observations were quite recent and may not have been appropriately vetted.

There never will be an answer to the question—who is first?—and the originality of the observation may remain open to debate. There may never be an answer to the question of what makes it famous, and academics are not immune to self-promotion, exaggeration, and other attempts to create a legacy. Strong voices may win; work horses may not get noticed. We all may want a piece of the celebrity pie (Fig. 1.1).

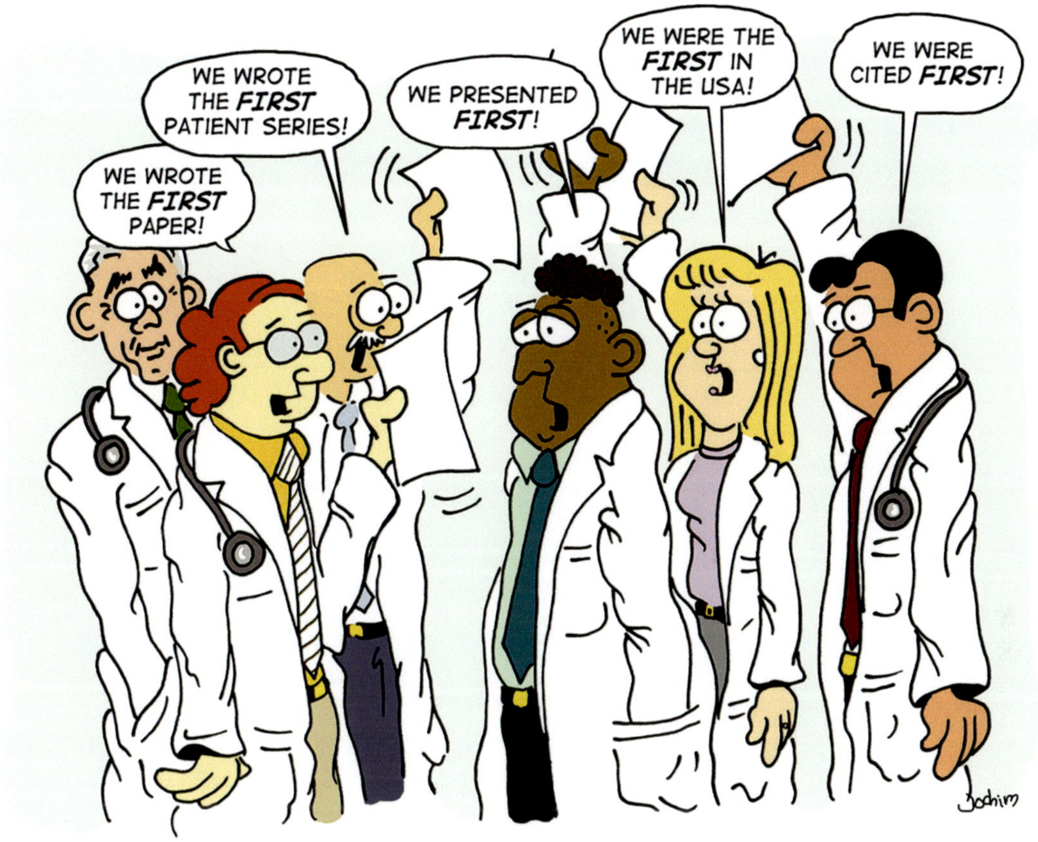
WE WROTE THE FIRST PAPER!
WE WROTE THE FIRST PATIENT SERIES!
WE PRESENTED FIRST!
WE WERE THE FIRST IN THE USA!
WE WERE CITED FIRST!
Jochim

Fig. 1.1 Who was first?

2 The First Neurointensive Care Units

E.F.M. Wijdicks, *Famous First Papers for the Neurointensivist*,
DOI 10.1007/978-1-4614-3182-4_2, © Springer Science+Business Media New York 2013

The idea of a separate hospital space designed to care for sicker patients evolved gradually over several decades mostly because surgery became more complex. There would be one defining event in the 1950s.

Intensive care units (ICUs) started as "specialized care units" or "respiratory care units." These units sprung up as a result of a sudden demand for ventilatory support during large scale poliomyelitis epidemics around the world [2, 3, 10]. Expectedly, these epidemics also led to improvement in mechanical ventilation. In the 1950s, Bendixen and Pontoppidan—both anesthesiologists—used their expertise in management of patients with poliomyelitis in Denmark to create a respiratory care unit in Boston's Massachusetts General Hospital [12].

This reality—being confronted with overwhelming numbers of patients—led to the decision to maintain a unit in the hospital that could care for patients with comparable illnesses.

The Early Days of the Intensive Care Unit

Innovative medical care associated with ICUs has been well chronicled [4, 6, 7, 12, 13, 16]. In the early 1970s, the vast majority of large medical institutions had ICUs constructed in their hospitals. These early ICUs were replaced by multidisciplinary ICUs, trauma units, transplant units, and postoperative care units. Once these specialized areas within a large hospital were established, further development of technology, treatments and standards followed [1]. Some of these were introduced anew (Swann–Ganz catheter), some were developed in the unit (e.g., positioning of the patient during ventilation, nutrition adjusted for critical illness, surveillance of ICU infections). Each unit may have had a different path of development. Hilberman summarized the development of ICUs simply as outgrowths of more demanding care [7]. Thus, surgical recovery units needed for more complex surgeries would become surgical ICUs. Advances in resuscitation techniques and the need to monitor treatable cardiac arrhythmias after myocardial infarction would lead to coronary care units [8]. Further specialization came with burn and transplant units. Therefore, the history of ICUs can be approached from different angles. There is a history of units, history of ICU technology, history of understanding and refinements of specific critical illnesses, history of critical care treatments, and even a history of ICU ethics [16].

The role of nursing care has been underappreciated by physicians who wrote the histories. Generally, there is no mention of nursing involvement in historical reviews and more typically historical reviews focus on technological innovations, and a celebration of pioneers in the field. However, nurses were the ones who saw the patient deteriorate and took action, and intensive care and neurosciences intensive care could not have progressed without specialization in nursing care. Critical care nurses started with the establishment of the American Association of Cardiovascular Nurses in 1969, changing to American Association of Critical Care Nurses and specialty certification became necessary. In the United States and Canada, the respiratory therapy specialty emerged and defined its role in overseeing mechanical ventilation and weaning. Other specialty care involved ICU pharmacists, nutritionists, and social work.

The Society of Critical Care Medicine catapulted the specialty into existence and soon training program guidelines appeared in the United States and abroad [5, 14, 15].

The Early Days of the Neurosciences ICU

The history of neurocritical care as a specialty cannot yet be written and, perhaps even the history of intensive care is far too premature. (One master historian remarked recently that the time finally has come to write the history of the French Revolution.) Some important developments, however, should be recognized.

As alluded to earlier, the history of neurosciences ICUs undoubtedly started with neurosurgeons performing more extensive surgeries. The beginnings of the neurosciences ICU—defining it as a

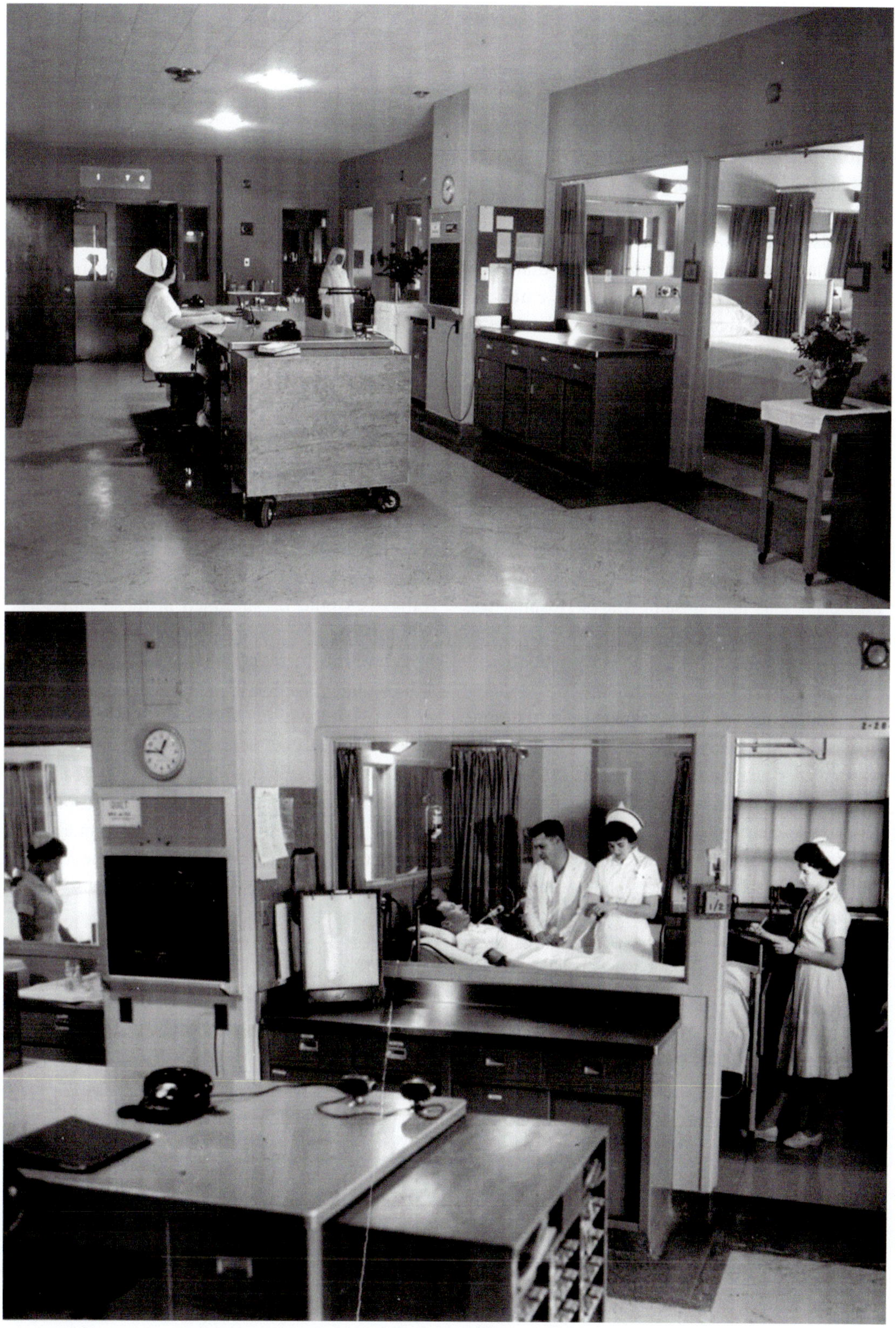

Fig. 2.1 Layout of Mayo Neurosciences Intensive Care Unit (opened in 1958)

combined neurology and neurosurgery ICU—are largely unknown and difficult to tease out. Many of these first units were either for neurosurgical or neurologic patients. In a broader sense, little is known about the triage of patients with acute neurologic conditions in those days.

Historically, neurosurgeon Dandy has been credited with opening the first neurosurgical ICU at Johns Hopkins Hospital in 1932. Indeed, Dandy had the fortitude to understand that some neurosurgical patients needed special care, and he chose a ward that he dedicated to the care of the sicker postoperative neurosurgical patients. In London, the Batten Respiratory Unit at the Institute of Neurology and National Hospital for Nervous Diseases opened in 1954 to treat mostly patients with acute neuromuscular disease, as well as those with stroke and spinal cord disorders who required mechanical ventilation [11].

The development of the neurosciences ICU at Mayo Clinic recently has been reported [18] (Fig. 2.1). This unit at Saint Marys Hospital was one of the first newly built combined neurosciences ICUs in the United States. It started as a unit with predominantly neurosurgical patients, and most of the expertise was developed in the care of these patients. Soon, acutely ill neurologic patients were admitted. A new culture of neurosciences was nurtured with specific attention to the care of the neediest patient. Teaching of nursing staff and the beginnings of administration became part of the neurosciences ICU responsibilities. The development of the neurosciences ICU also can be seen clearly as an outgrowth of nursing ingenuity. Moreover, neurosciences ICU nursing became an accepted subspecialty, and annual meetings were held.

In the United States, most neurosciences ICUs combined neurosurgical and neurologic patients. This would seem logical because acutely ill neurologic patients could need neurosurgical intervention (e.g., cerebral hematoma), and acutely ill neurosurgical patients could benefit from neurologic expertise (e.g., seizure management). Because of the open nature of the neurosciences ICU, physicians from multiple disciplines would closely cooperate in patient management. Often, a close cooperation between neurology and neurosurgery consultants in the neurosciences ICU was needed. There was a renewed interest in closely studying and treating acute neurologic and neurosurgical conditions and this led to a better understanding of the risks for deterioration.

Several other landmark developments should be noted. First, neurologists became interested in acute neurologic conditions (i.e., coma) after patients survived as a result of more advanced resuscitation. Neurologists often were asked to judge the severity of injury and to prognosticate. Neurologists Fred Plum, Raymond Adams, and C. Miller Fisher were the first to describe causes of coma and other acute conditions (i.e., brain death, locked-in syndrome, anoxic-ischemic encephalopathy). A better understanding of neurologic complications of critical illness soon followed, and consultations in ICUs increased.

Second, with the emergence of neurosciences ICUs, coverage was needed. In the 1980s, neurologists would be stationed in these units. The presence of a neurologist in the neurosciences ICU provided a major benefit to neurosurgeons who would not always have the opportunity to immediately go to the bedside (e.g., during a long and complex neurosurgical procedure). Neurologists became more knowledgeable in management of acute neuromuscular respiratory failure, treatment of increased intracranial pressure, and systemic complications specific for acute neurologic disease. Neurologists would join intensivists (mostly anesthesiologists) and developed sufficient hands-on training that would allow them to fully manage these complicated patients.

Third, a flurry of scientific publications followed that would further define the field and its boundaries. Better understanding of causes of deterioration and recognition of opportunities of early intervention would lead to more complex and specialized care.

Finally, in 2004, a Society was founded and with it a journal [17]. Accreditation was sought through the American Academy of Neurology (United Council of Neurologic Specialties).

Those who practiced neurocritical care noted similar deficiencies and concerns as physicians in the general ICUs. These were open ICUs with different physicians with different specialties, lack of leadership, lack of protocols, lack of effective communication, lack of experienced care in emergency conditions, and lack of organized multi-institutional research. All this is changing rapidly due to a new cadre of dedicated neurointensivists. The physical presence of a neurointensivist in a neurosciences ICU should improve care and outcome. Multiple—albeit retrospective—studies have shown that outcome in certain conditions can be improved with an attending neurointensivist [9]. Benchmarks can be defined (mortality, morbidity, length of stay, number of consultations, and actual costs), but evidence may be hard to obtain. Obviously prospective randomization of patients with life-threatening neurologic disease into a general medical or surgical ICU versus neurosciences ICU will be considered unethical and problematic.

Neurocritical care as a specialty is finally established and has been enthusiastically welcomed by many physicians and other health care providers. This fascinating story continues…

References

1. Aitkenhead AR, Booij LH, Dhainaut JF, et al. International standards for safety in the intensive care unit. Intensive Care Med. 1993;19:178–81.
2. Anderson EW, Ibsen B. The anesthetic management of patients with poliomyelitis and respiratory paralysis. BMJ. 1954;2:786–8.
3. Berthelsen PG, Cronqvist M. The first intensive care unit in the world: Copenhagen 1953. Acta Anaesthesiol Scand. 2003;47:1190–5.
4. Calvin J, Habet K, Parrillo JE. Critical care in the United States. Crit Care Clin. 1997;13:363–76.
5. Grenvik A, Leonard JJ, Arens JF, et al. Critical care medicine. Certification as a multidisciplinary subspecialty. Crit Care Med. 1981;9:117–25.
6. Grenvik A, Pinsky MR. Evolution of the intensive care unit as a clinical center and critical care medicine as a discipline. Crit Care Clin. 2009;25:239–50.
7. Hilberman M. The evolution of the intensive care unit. Crit Care Med. 1975;3:159–65.
8. Julian DG. Treatment of cardiac arrest in acute myocardial ischemia and infarction. Lancet 1961;2: 840–44
9. Kramer AH, Zygun DA. Do neurocritical care units save lives? Measuring the impact of specialized ICUs. Neurocrit Care. 2011;14:329–33.
10. Lassen HC. A preliminary report on the 1952 epidemic of poliomyelitis in Copenhagen with special reference to the treatment of acute respiratory insufficiency. Lancet. 1953;1:37–41.
11. Marshall J. The work of a respiratory unit in a neurologic hospital. Postgrad Med J. 1961;37:26–30.
12. Pontoppidan H, Wilson R, Rie MA, et al. Respiratory intensive care. Anesthesiology. 1977;47:96–116.
13. Rosengart MR. Critical care medicine: landmarks and legends. Surg Clin North Am. 2006;86:1305–21.
14. Thijs LG, Baltopoulous G, Bihari D, et al. Guidelines for a training program in intensive care medicine. Intensive Care Med. 1996;22:166–72.
15. Vincent JL, Artigas A, Bihari D, et al. Guidelines for the utilization of intensive care units. Intensive Care Med. 1994;20:163–4.
16. Weil MH. The Society of Critical Care Medicine, its history and its destiny. Crit Care Med. 1973;1:1–4.
17. Wijdicks EFM. A new journal, a new step, a new energy. Neurocrit Care. 2004;1:1–2.
18. Wijdicks EFM, Worden W, Miers A, et al. The early days of the neurosciences intensive care unit. Mayo Clin Proc. 2011;86:903–6.

3 The First Descriptions of Clinical Signs

E.F.M. Wijdicks, *Famous First Papers for the Neurointensivist*,
DOI 10.1007/978-1-4614-3182-4_3, © Springer Science+Business Media New York 2013

Short Historical Note 1

FIXED DILATED PUPIL

The Title of the Paper

Holman E, Scott WMJ. Significance of unilateral dilatation and fixation of pupil in severe skull injuries. JAMA. 1925;84:1329–32.

The Paper and the Times

A "fixed pupil" in a comatose patient is an alarming sign, as everybody knows. It is such a staple of acute neurology that it will be hard to trace back the origin of the observation.

As early as the 1800s, abnormal pupillary reaction to light was noted in papers concerning traumatic brain injury, and one may assume most likely the first observation came with patients who had an acute subdural hematoma. One such description is by Richard Bright in his seminal textbook of Medicine co-written with Thomas Addison (*Elements of the Practice of Medicine*) in 1839. Bright noted a dilated pupil in a patient with epidural hematoma. The pupil became dilated on the second day after head injury. The patient became much less responsive and also developed a slow pulse. However, this clinical observation was not explained nor did any of the investigators that followed explain the association with compression or stretch of the third nerve.

Experimental studies already pointed out the importance of the dilated pupil. Ernst von Bergmann, a German surgeon, provided information in his 1880 classic book on head injuries. He mentioned fixed dilated pupils, but he was unable to clearly localize the lesion. In fact, von Bergmann—as many before him—believed strongly that the lesion was located in the cortex. In fact, his book has illustrations with possible cortical localizations of the oculomotor nerve [243]. Most noticeable was the experimental study by Leyden in 1866 who summarized the changes he found in increased intracranial pressure as follows: change in consciousness was followed by pupil enlargements at least temporarily, most often also in coma and often bilaterally, followed by circulatory symptoms that included abnormal pulse frequency, deep respiration, and later slow respiration. He clearly noted that with increased intracranial pressure, the pupils first became narrow, then dilated, but also noted that they were not always symmetric [245]. Other experiments followed and correlated pupil dilatation to increasing blood pressure waves and constriction with decrease. No further explanations were forthcoming.

Jonathan Hutchinson has been credited with describing, for the first time, a dilated pupil after a traumatic brain injury. In 1867, he documented a clinical pathologic correlation in two cases and noted that the third nerve was compressed, explaining the dilatation of the pupil [109].

Hutchinson described it in patients with "hemorrhage from the middle meningeal artery" and due to gravitation of blood toward the base. Jacobson later suggested it be named the *Hutchinson's pupil.*

In 1887, however, Macewen provided more details, and his description is telling:

> Many instances have been observed of dilatation and fixity of one pupil, while its fellow, perhaps with the exception of a little sluggishness of movement, remained normal. These were all cases of fracture of the middle fossa of the skull, and in comparatively few of them was the diagnosis verified by postmortem examination. … In those cases in which postmortem examination were obtained, the basal fracture was continued into or toward the vertex, and the clot in most instances occupied the whole of the middle fossa from the petrous portion of the temporal to the vertex, the convolutions, especially the ascending, being considerably compressed. … In those that recovered, the dilatation gave way slowly, and was followed by a degree of contraction, along with sluggishness of movement which ultimately passed off, though in one case it still remained small and sluggish at the termination of the fifth month from the date of the accident [144].

The fixed dilated pupil only became recognized as a key neurologic sign in the early twentieth century.

The Details of the Paper

Holman and Scott were perhaps the first researchers to point out the clinical significance of pupillary enlargement—the operation should be on the side of the fixed pupil (Fig. 3.1). They cited several previous observations ignoring this symptom and pointed out the paucity of descriptions of

SIGNIFICANCE OF UNILATERAL DILATATION AND FIXATION OF PUPIL IN SEVERE SKULL INJURIES *

EMILE HOLMAN, M.D.
AND
W. M. J. SCOTT, M.D.
CLEVELAND

No problem in emergency surgery presents greater difficulties of decision than the care of patients who are unconscious following fractures and injuries of the skull. The reasons for these difficulties are many. The occurrence of contralateral brain injury by "contrecoup," the fallacy of interpreting external damage (or absence of it) as an indication of the extent and location of the internal injury, the wide varieties of internal damage that may occur, and the relative greater or lesser importance of such damage according to its location, all combine to make standardization of the procedure to be followed quite impossible. On occasions, rare but nevertheless of sufficient frequency that their occurrence must be constantly borne in mind, the slightest delay in surgical intervention may place the patient beyond relief. One such experience stands out with particular vividness.

Case 1.—A young baseball player was hit on the side of the head by a pitched ball. He walked to the bench, but soon complained of headache of increasing severity. A physician was called; there was some delay in transporting the player to the hospital, and before his arrival there he had become unconscious. Further delay was encountered, and the patient died within two hours of the injury, undoubtedly a victim of intracranial hemorrhage.

Any sign that may enable one more definitely to recognize the presence of increasing pressure and to localize the injury more accurately is a welcome aid. We present, therefore, a number of experiences that have prompted us to place considerable reliance on the appearance of a unilateral dilatation and fixation of the pupil as an indication of unilateral cerebral compression, due more particularly to hemorrhage.

It is uniformly recognized that fractures at the base of the skull, with edema and hemorrhage compressing and involving the medulla, are not in the least benefited by an anterior decompressive operation. In striking contrast to the inefficacy of surgery in the treatment of these basal fractures is the benefit that may be gained in those cases in which the injury is limited more or less to the anterior chamber, and often to one of the two cerebral hemispheres. This injury may be a contusion or a laceration of the brain with a subdural hemorrhage, or a rupture of the middle meningeal artery or of its branches, with an extradural hemorrhage. Each of these injuries may, through a slowly progressive localized pressure, due to edema or hemorrhage, produce the general effect of unconsciousness. Surgical intervention directed toward a decompression, or toward the control of hemorrhage at its site, will, in many instances, relieve the general effect, with probable recovery of the patient. Such recovery depends, of course, on the extent of the cortical damage, and on the absence of an associated basal injury.

It is generally agreed that the history of an interval of consciousness after the injury, followed by uncon-

---

* From the Surgical Service of the Lakeside Hospital.
* Read before the Clinical and Pathological Section of the Cleveland Academy of Medicine, Jan. 2, 1925.

Fig. 3.1 Title page

patients who deteriorated and lapsed into coma in the literature.

Holman and Scott found that anisocoria of the pupils may be transitory but that it was quickly followed by bilaterally widely dilated pupils. They suggested that "the mechanism of its appearance is not obvious, but it is assumed that the intracranial course of the third nerve, as it lies against the bony wall of the cranium, lends itself peculiarly well to compression from a pressure applied lateral and superior to it."

The authors emphasized that "unilateral dilatation and fixation of the pupil is a valuable aid in determining the location of the intracranial injury and hemorrhage following head injuries."

The Message and Acceptance

Papers followed that pointed toward the possible mechanism of a fixed pupil. These papers described experiments that noted stretch of the third nerve, compression against the clivus, and compression of the uncus of the temporal lobe, all possibly explaining how a third nerve palsy could mechanically occur [187, 227].

Holman and Scott's observation was specifically cited by Rand who emphasized that an enlarged dilated pupil could indicate the site of the lesion [187]. This remained a fairly consistent finding when patients were examined. Rand concluded:

> It's believed that the hemorrhage is usually greatest on the side of the dilated pupil. … In cases in which hemiplegia and the dilated pupil were homolateral, intracranial hemorrhage was found on the same side. … In some cases one is unable to assign any cause for the homolateral hemiplegia and other extensive damage to the opposite cerebral hemisphere has been found at autopsy. This may account for the contralateral hemiplegia.

Reid and Cone, who performed animal experiments documenting the appearance of a dilated pupil in a monkey, eventually cemented the origin of fixed dilated pupils. They rapidly infused Ringers solution through a burr hole and found compressed oculomotor nerves from displaced hippocampal gyrus [189].

The clinical sign rapidly became mentioned in neurology and neurosurgery textbooks, and additional observations were added over time. Currently, we know that a unilateral fixed dilated pupil is seen early and can be followed by bilateral fixed pupils in a patient with an acute hemispheric mass. The shape of the pupil may change and become irregular, "football," or oval-shaped. An oval-shaped pupil ipsilateral to the mass is most frequently seen but transitory, quickly becoming round, midsized, or dilated and fixed to light. Increased intracranial pressure is commonly associated with an oval-shaped pupil [154]. The shape may be explained by differences in parasympathetic tone in various segments and thus could imply midbrain involvement rather than peripheral fibers.

The presence of a unilaterally fixed pupil is now considered by many neurologists and neurosurgeons a result of an oculomotor lesion from direct compression, compression of the midbrain oculomotor complex, or traction of the oculomotor nerve against the clivus. There is surprisingly little proof of any of these theories, and it has been made clear that clinicopathologic correlation—due to time passed between both observations—is unreliable [193, 194].

Short Historical Note 2

DECEREBRATE RIGIDITY

The Title of the Paper

Bricolo A, Turazzi S, Alexandre A, Rizzuto N. Decerebrate rigidity in acute head injury. J Neurosurg. 1977;47: 680–98.

The Paper and the Times

Decerebrate rigidity—a term originally coined by Sir Charles Sherrington [16, 207, 208] is a classic neurologic sign. Sherrington famously described decerebrate rigidity in his transection experiments in cats and demonstrated the existence of a transverse plane at the level of the corpora mammillaria, red nucleus, and between anterior and posterior colliculi. Transection at that level would produce decerebrate rigidity. Rigidity disappeared when a transection was performed caudal to that plane at the level of the vestibular nuclei. When after a mesencephalic section the cerebellum was removed, the signs of decerebrate rigidity did not disappear.

The counterpart in man had been described in multiple earlier observations, but its meaning—in physiologic sense—remained elusive [114, 198, 247, 260]. The clinical features of decerebrate rigidity were a sudden yielding with stretching of the muscle ("clasp-knife" phenomenon) and invariable presence of clonus or subclonus tendon reflexes. Extensor rigidity with head retraction had been noted by clinicians in comatose patients and was mostly apparent in patients with cerebral hemorrhage extending into the ventricles [198].

Kinnier Wilson found decerebrate rigidity in cases of cerebral hemorrhages, meningitis, and intracranial tumors [260]. He described three groups: patients with decerebrate rigidity and tonic fits combined, patients with a decerebrate posture without tonic fits, and patients with tonic fits without persisting decerebrate posture.

Hughlings Jackson reported similar observations in patients with cerebellar tumors. He likened them to "tetanus-like seizures" and described patients with opisthotonus, extension of the lower extremities, and flexion of the upper extremities.

In 1923, Walshe noted the following:

> The patient lay motionless and unconscious on her back with the head in a median position. There was no trace of head retraction. The arms lay across the chest semi-flexed at the elbows with the forearms slightly pronated in the wrist and digit flexed. The legs lay extended and abducted with the feet plantar flexed. There was spasticity of moderate degree in all four limbs, definitely more pronounced in the arms than the legs [248].

Walshe also noted that there was clear evidence of further progressive functions of the "vital medullary centers."

Mollaret and Bertrand's 1945 monograph is equally of interest, and the authors again emphasized that what is seen clinically may be different from what was observed in animal experiments [164].

In their 1966 classic text, Plum and Posner stated that decerebrate rigidity was seen in four clinical circumstances: massive and bilateral forebrain lesions, rostrocaudal deterioration, destructive or expanding posterior fossa lesions compressing the midbrain and rostral pons, severe metabolic disorders and intoxications depressing the diencephalon and forebrain [180].

Most observations were case series until a comprehensive description by Bricolo and associates. The aim of this manuscript was to report in more detail the postural patterns and their association with other neurologic signs and to assess its significance.

The Details of the Paper

This study includes 800 patients with severe head injuries admitted to the Department of Neurosurgery of Verona Hospital (Fig. 3.2). More than two-thirds of patients required mechanical ventilation. Decerebrate rigidity developed in 317 of 800 patients (40%) and mostly early after admission. The authors divided decerebrate rigidity into several types: full, unilateral, alternating, combined and mixed decerebrate rigidity, and decorticate rigidity (Fig. 3.3). Full decerebrate rigidity was observed in 35% of the patients. "The symptoms consisted of clenching of the jaw and extension of the four limbs, the upper limbs more than the lower; the arms were also adducted and internally rotated, the shoulders lifted, and the feet

Decerebrate rigidity in acute head injury

Albino Bricolo, M.D., Sergio Turazzi, M.D., Alberto Alexandre, M.D., and Nicola Rizzuto, M.D.

Department of Neurosurgery, City Hospital of Verona and Department of Neurology, University of Padua in Verona, Verona, Italy

✔ A comprehensive study of the motor patterns, usually grouped under the heading "decerebrate rigidity," was carried out in a series of 800 patients with severe head injuries. The incidence of these manifestations was 39.6%, and when they were present chances of survival were reduced from 79.4% to 28.1%. Clinical and electromyographic investigations revealed heterogeneous and unstable motor manifestations that did not fit into the classical groups of experimental models of decerebrate rigidity. Combinations of extensor and flexor attitudes and/or responses were frequently found in the same patient, but could be separated into homogeneous groups. Each recognized postural pattern had its own distinct neurological signs and prognosis. Age did not significantly affect the outcome; however, intracranial expanding lesions (73.5%), impairment of the brain-stem oculomotor system (49.8%), and deep coma (88.9%) all contributed to an unfavorable course. Surgical treatment was effective when performed for intracranial hematomas and in patients with incomplete extensor rigidity. Good recovery was achieved in 16% of decerebrate patients, while 12.1% survived in prolonged coma or with severe disabilities.

All clinical and neuropathological data suggest that extensor motor abnormalities in the acute phase of cerebral traumatic disease do not always conclusively indicate structural brain-stem damage. A critical analysis of so-called "decerebrate rigidity" (rejecting in some instances its Sherringtonian implications) may allow for a more accurate clinical assessment of the severity of head injury.

Key Words · decerebrate rigidity · head injury · neuropathology · brain-stem lesions · coma · prognosis · electropolygraphy ·

Fig. 3.2 Title page

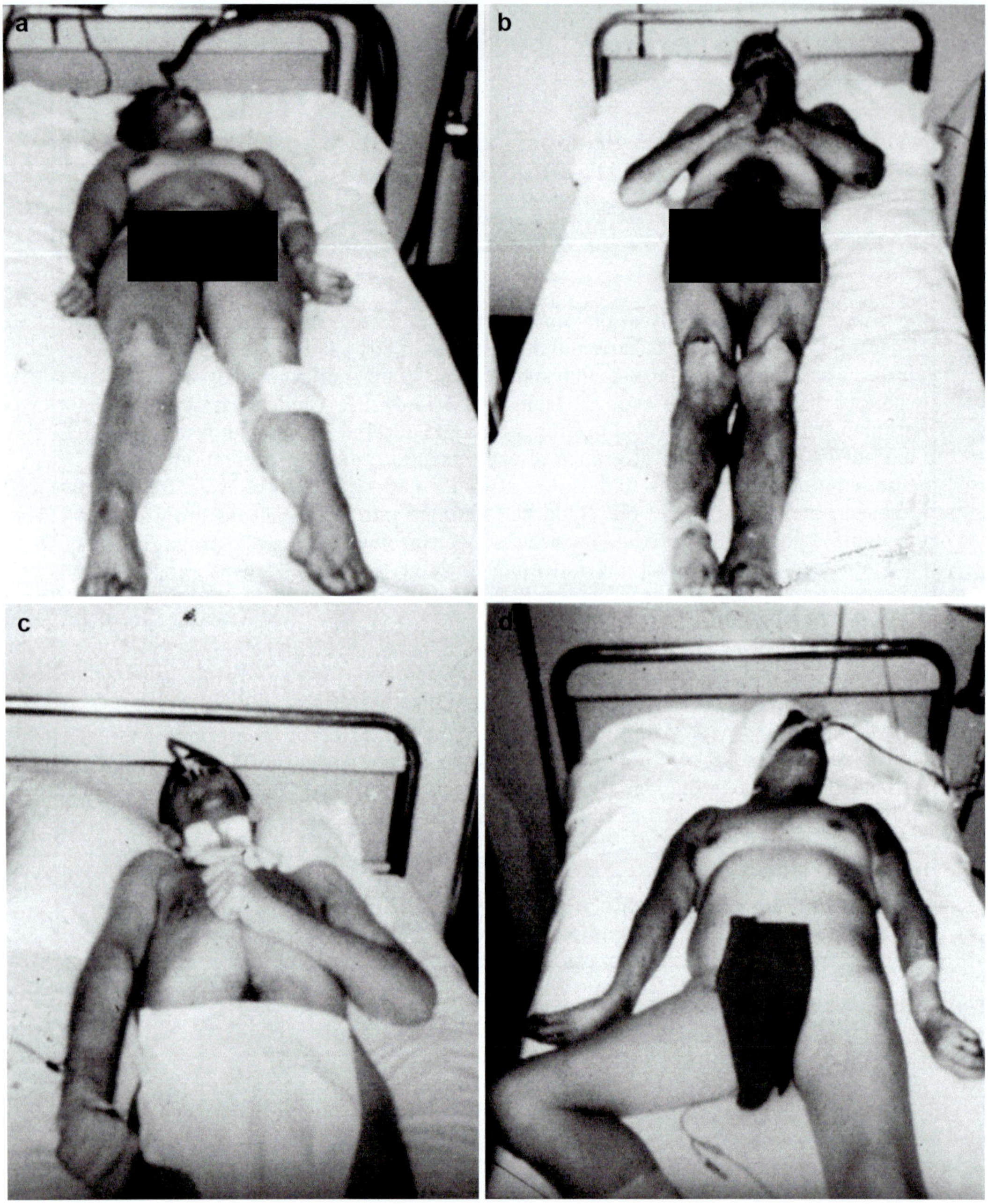

Fig. 3.3 Types of decerebrate rigidity (see text)

in plantar flexion." Unilateral decerebrate rigidity was observed in 12% of patients "who developed extensor motor activity of the limbs on one side." Only 7% of the patients showed decorticate rigidity, with "triple flexion of the upper limbs, adduced on the trunk, and clenched fists, while the lower limbs were hyperextended." Twenty patients with severe head injuries developed a more complex posture, consisting of extensor rigidity on one side and a decorticate posture on the other. Only five patients showed mixed decerebrate rigidity described as "flexor rigidity of the lower limbs and hyperextension of the upper limbs." The authors felt it was more commonly seen after a noxious stimulus and therefore could have been easily missed by the observer.

Most notable was the observation that the alternating decerebrate rigidity pattern comprised the largest group (40%), and the patients showed "a greatly variable postural attitude, either spontaneously or evoked, consisting of extensor or flexor rigidity in the same limb." The authors also emphasized the common simultaneous occurrence of dysautonomia with cardiac arrhythmias, increased blood pressure, temperature disturbances, sweating, tachypnea, and periodic or irregular breathing. Mortality in patients with decerebrate rigidity increased to 80% and was twice as frequent than in patients without these motor responses.

The authors concluded:

> The commonly accepted concept that in man decerebrate rigidity is the clinical expression of a physiological-anatomical result of brainstem transection must be rejected. … However, the most important finding from our data is that not all patients with decerebrate rigidity had structural lesions in the brainstem areas that were responsible for regulation of postural tonus. The absence of this close association in five cases provides further proof that, at least during the acute stage of head injury, decerebrate rigidity does not conclusively indicate brainstem structural damage. The localizing value of extensor motor abnormalities in patients with severe head injuries is not proven. … The use of terms such as "decerebration" and "decerebrate state," because of their Sherringtonian implication, should be restricted to define a clinical condition due to severe midbrain dysfunction. This is implied when a stable and complete extensor posture combines with deep coma and brainstem ocular signs.

The Message and Acceptance

Decerebrate posturing has been observed in brain stem lesions and in lesions involving injury to both hemispheres without evidence of brainstem injury or tissue displacement. This motor response is often but not invariably an indicator of a severe structural brain injury [62, 129, 198, 261]. The site of the responsible lesion is both corticospinal and striospinal, and the response can be produced by injuries of all sorts. Precise localization of lesions on computed tomography or magnetic resonance imaging scans have not been possible nor has it been feasible to confirm the exact lesions as demonstrated by Sherrington in his animal experiments. These abnormal motor responses remain an important indication of the degree of brain injury and often are accompanied by other signs of brainstem injury. Decorticate and decerebrate posturing are likely a representation of a more diffuse lesion and can be part of a rostrocaudal deterioration pattern in patients with an expanding mass resulting in flexion, extension, and flaccidity, in that order. Decerebrate postering may persist and when it does-irrespective of its cause-portends a somber outlook. When it disappears recovery is quite likely.

Short Historical Note 3

CUSHING REFLEX

The Title of the Paper

Cushing H. Concerning a definite regulatory mechanism of the vasomotor centre which controls blood pressure during cerebral compression. Bull Johns Hopkins Hosp. 1901;12:290–2.

The Paper and the Times

In 1783, Monro published "*Observations on the Structure and the Function of the Nervous System.*" Monro's basic premise was that the skull was a rigid container filled with brain and blood. In 1846, however, Burrows added cerebrospinal fluid (CSF) to these components and also claimed that any change in any of these three components had to lead to a change in the other components for intracranial volume to remain constant.

At the turn of the nineteenth century, researchers became interested in the effect of increased intracranial pressure (ICP) as a result of increased intracranial volume. Von Bergmann was one of the early pioneers in explaining intracranial pressure following trauma [243, 244]. Von Bergmann's experiments, using high pressure suddenly applied to the brain, described animals with "clonic spasms". Slow heartbeat, deep and snoring respirations, vomiting, and incontinence were other remarkable symptoms. These symptoms were not seen when ICP was slowly increased. Immediately after injury, blood pressure rises and then falls. They interpreted apnea as a "paralysis of the respiratory center," but if mechanical ventilation was applied, the pulse remained strong. Hill suggested that these early effects were due to diminished flow in the bulbar centers. Hill also concluded that death occurs when ICP equals the blood pressure in the carotid arteries [102].

Cushing's physiologic contributions have become legendary, and his name became attached to this phenomenon, which was described in some detail by many before (Fig. 3.4). Increase in blood pressure with brain compression became known as "Cushing's law" or "Cushing's response," or even "Cushing's phenomenon," but a better term is *Cushing reflex* [76].

The Details of the paper

The experimental setup was simple. Cushing used dogs, cats, and monkeys in his experiments [54–57]. The animals were anesthetized with ether. A catheter placed in the femoral artery recorded the blood pressure through a mercury manometer. He also recorded respiration and combined the records to show the changes over time. Subsequently, he made a large midline trephine opening, opened the dura, and placed a glass window ("fenster") in the opening of the skull to expose the venous convolutions and pial arteries in order to observe changes in caliber (Fig. 3.5). Another burr hole was made over the cervical cord with opening of the dura. A metal cannula was screwed into the trephine hole to which an intracranial soft rubber tube was attached. The ICP was raised by filling the rubber bag with saline. Cushing observed blanching of the cortical arteries when the ICP increased and an improvement when blood pressure rose.

Cushing noted that until the ICP ("Hirndruck") exceeds that of the blood pressure and the pressure rises slowly, only mild tachycardia and tachypnea are seen (Fig. 3.6). However, when the ICP rapidly rises, "Kussmaul–Tenner"spasms (extensor rigidity), bladder and bowel incontinence, apnea, and a "prominent vagus effect" meaning bradycardia and asystole were noted. Again the "vagus effects" could be avoided with a much slower rise in blood pressure. Cushing was able to repeat the experiments. "With reasonable limits of compression, however, this compensatory action may be indefinitively prolonged."

Cushing summarized his results as follows:

> As a result of these experiments a simple and definite law may be established, namely, that an increase of intracranial tension occasions a rise of blood pressure which tends to find a level slightly above that of the pressure exerted against the medulla. It is thus seen that there exists a regulatory mechanism on the part of the vasomotor centre which with great accuracy enables the blood pressure to remain at a point just sufficient to prevent the persistence of an anaemic condition of the bulb,

CONCERNING A DEFINITE REGULATORY MECHANISM OF THE VASO-MOTOR CENTRE WHICH CONTROLS BLOOD PRESSURE DURING CEREBRAL COMPRESSION.[1]

By Harvey Cushing, M. D.

During the course of a long series of observations undertaken for Professor Kocher in the Physiological Institute of Bern in an attempt to elucidate certain questions of dispute regarding the circulatory phenomena which are consequent upon cerebral compression, it has been observed that there is a constant tendency on the part of the blood pressure to remain at a level above that of the pressure exerted upon the brain.

The fact that cerebral compression occasions a rise in blood pressure is universally known but it does not seem to have been recognized that the degree of this elevation occurs *pari passu* with the degree of compression (measured in millimetres of mercury) to which the medullary centres are subjected. It is ordinarily stated by the numerous experimentors who have dealt with problems of compression that fatal symptoms originate when the intracranial pressure approaches or reaches the height of the arterial tension. The fact that the arterial tension is a varying quantity which regulates itself so as to overcome the effects of the increased intracranial pressure seems never to have received attention.

In the greater number of my early observations the experimental compression has been made by means of quicksilver which was allowed to enter a thin rubber bag at the end of a metallic canula which was screwed into a trephine opening in the skull. By this method it was impossible to estimate with exactitude the degree of compression exerted against the medulla since the elasticity of the bag, the resistance of the dura in spite of its preliminary liberation from the skull, and the fact that the brain does not transmit the pressure from such a localized foreign body equally in all directions were always elements of uncertainty in the calculation. Nevertheless the method sufficed to call attention to the fact above mentioned, namely, that when the degree of compression was increased so as to exceed that of the blood pressure the latter would in turn almost invariably rise to a level exceeding that of the intracranial tension. In this way the blood pressure could be carried to indefinite heights, occasionally to 250 mm. of mercury or more, and be held there until the centres in the medulla became permanently fatigued.

The suggestion thus offered as to a definite regulatory mechanism which counteracts the compression anæmia by elevation of blood pressure was further strengthened by direct observation, of the cerebral circulation through an accurately fitting glass window inserted in another trephine opening under which the dura had been opened. When the intracranial tension had been carried up to the point of blanching the convolutions and indeed of obliteration of the pial arteries themselves, it could be seen through this fenestra that this condition of anæmia was but a transient one, since in a few seconds the vessels would once more fill and the circulation become reestablished. On some occasions, to be explained later, the circulation could be seen to appear and disappear with rhythmic periodicity, the intracranial tension meanwhile remaining at the same level.

The opportunity of testing the truth of the hypothesis thus suggested has been offered in the *Laboratorio di Fisiologia* of Turin[2] where a simple but more graphic method of

[1] Reprinted from the Archives Italiennes de Biologie for 1901.

[2] I am deeply indebted to Professor Mosso in Turin and to Professor Kronecker in Bern for extending to me the privileges of their laboratories while carrying out these observations.

Fig. 3.4 Title page

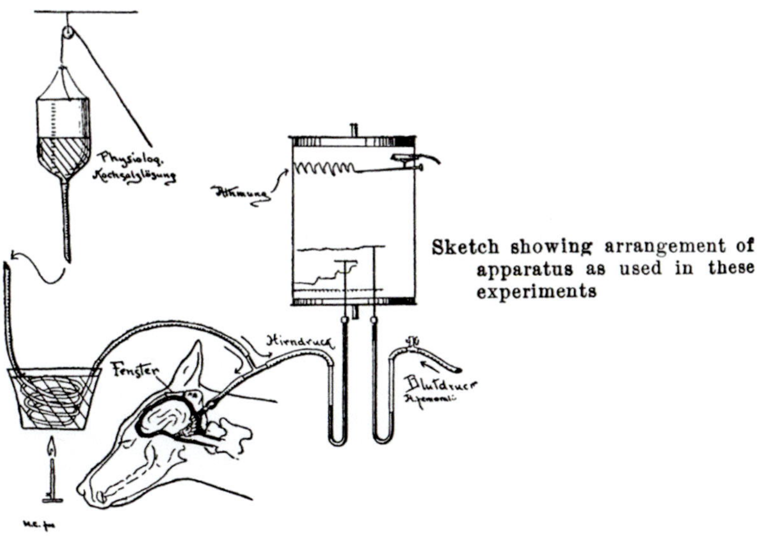

Fig. 3.5 Experimental setup (sketch from original article)

demonstrating that the rise is a conservative act and not one such as is consequent upon a mere reflex sensory irritation.

The Message and Acceptance

Cushing's data found its way into multiple publications. A major historical work on the subject found that the experiments on the vasopressor response were published in five communications in German and English between 1901 and 1903; four papers authored by Cushing and one chapter included in Kocher's book on cerebral concussion [54–57, 76, 124, 125]. Kocher and Cushing advanced the field substantially by proposing the following stages of medullary compression:

Stage 1: Accommodation (*kompensation*). In this stage, the CSF is displaced out of the cranial vault followed by encroachment upon the cerebral venous bed with little change in the systemic circulation.

Stage 2: Early clinical manifestations (*anfangsstadium des manifesten hirndruckes*). In this stage, blood from the capillaries has been expelled; "anoxemia" of the vital bulbar centers results in rise of the systemic blood pressure. The pulse rate is retarded, but the pulse has a full quality. The respiratory rate also is reduced.

Stage 3: Advanced clinical manifestations (*hohe stadium des manifesten hirndruckes*). In this stage, the respirations are more snoring and rhythmic and may become Cheyne–Stokes type. Papilledema is seen, and pupils become irregular.

Stage 4: Medullary collapse (*lahmungs stadium*). In this stage, the "vital centers are exhausted." The blood pressure is decreasing, and patient is in shock with all reflexes abolished, pupils dilated, and irregular respirations with apneic episodes.

In 1928, Heymans further refined Cushing's findings by showing an initial tachycardia associated with hypertension just before the onset of bradycardia [101]. Others described a state of sympathoactivation secondary to medullary hypoxia mediated by depolarization of rostral ventrolateral medulla presynaptic neurons [89, 225, 253].

Changes in breathing patterns became an important cue for increased ICP. In a comparable experiment, Jennet found increased respiratory rate followed by irregularity, depression, and periods of apnea to be reproducible signs of increased ICP [115].

It is well known that many researchers before Cushing did very similar experiments. These included Paul Cramer, Ernst von Bergmann, Ernst von Leyden, Georg Althann, Friedrich Jolly, Friedrich Pagenstecher, Henri Duret, Bernard Naunyn, and Julius Schreiber. Nonetheless, Cushing's experiments and data deduction have been considered far more careful, elaborate, and refined than his rivals [76].

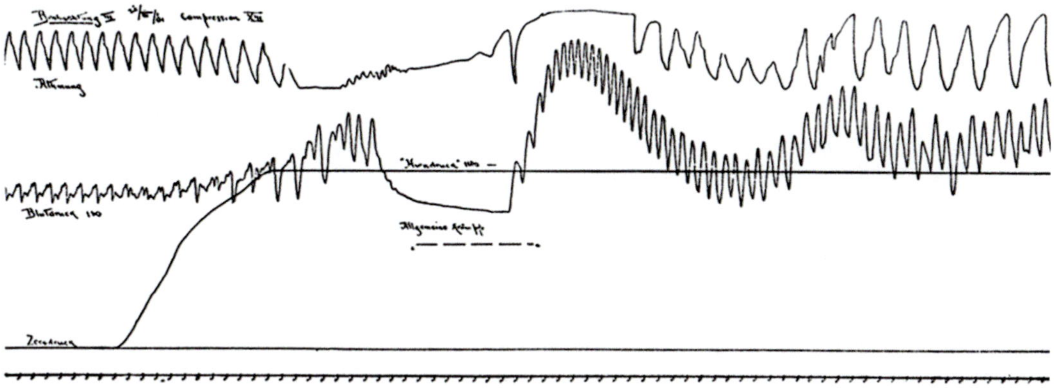

Fig. 3.6 Tracing of Cushing's experiment. The figure shows increased blood pressure (*Blutdruck*), increased intracranial pressure (*Hirndruck*), absent breathing (*Athmung*), and spasms (*Krämpfe*)

Short Historical Note 4

FALSE LOCALIZING SIGNS

The Title of the Paper

Collier J. The false localizing signs of intracranial tumor. Brain. 1904;27:490–508.

The Paper and the Times

Once clinical signs are known, they are traced to a specific location in the brain, and this approach has been axiomatic for both neurologists and neurosurgeons. The explosion of neuroimaging modalities may have challenged the clinical ability, and clinicians have become well aware that not infrequently magnetic resonance imaging scans point toward a different location or even explanation. However, early in the 1900s with a plain skull x-ray as the only imaging test, signs were recognized that could "falsely" point toward another region of the brain than predicted on the basis of anatomical knowledge. The most common "error" made by a neurosurgeon was operating on a presumed infratentorial tumor only to discover no tumor existed [71, 240]. The most commonly reported false localizing signs were lesions of the cranial nerves, particularly palsies of the abducens, trigeminal, and oculomotor nerves [11, 131].

Acute false localizing signs also were relatively common in the acute setting. Neuro-ophthalmologic signs were mostly encountered, such as a sixth nerve palsy associated with increased intracranial pressure and a fixed pupillary dilatation opposite from the actual site of the mass lesion [63, 92, 170, 192, 228]. Hemiparesis at the same site of a hemispheric lesion causing tissue shift also had been recognized but was more common in more slowly expanding tumors [117].

The Details of the Paper

Collier described that "false localizing signs" were mostly attributed to "indirect intracranial results of intracranial new growth" (Fig. 3.7). These signs were found in 13% of the 161 cases. The abducens nerve was affected more than any other cranial nerve, more commonly right-sided, and also equally unilateral or bilateral. The abducens lesion has been traditionally explained by the fact that it has a long course, but Collier suggested that the sixth nerve was the only cranial nerve that pursues a longitudinal rather than oblique or transverse course. Therefore, with backward shifting of the brain stem, the sixth nerve is easily damaged. In his words:

> If the paralysis of these nerves is the result of shifting backwards of the brainstem from supratentorial pressure, the effect being direction upon the nerves attached to the brainstem, in proportion as that direction is more nearly frontal caudal direction, then the shifting backwards of the brainstem would cause paralysis of the sixth nerve first, then of the third nerve, and lastly the seventh and eighth, while the nerves which are transversely directed or with sinuous course would be little affected.

Collier also describes the occurrence of Jacksonian epilepsy, and general convulsions with tumors of the brainstem and cerebellum. These patients had significant ventricular distention but no other lesion that could explain the "local convulsion."

Collier also considered vascular lesions in regions remote from the tumor that could give rise to false localizing signs and a misdiagnosis. Other explanations were locally spreading edema. However both causes were less clearly identified at autopsy.

The Message and Acceptance

Collier introduced the term "false localizing sign", which remains the best description of the phenomenon. Others suggested terms, such as "nonlocalizing signs," particularly for neuro-ophtalmology signs such as divergence paresis and convergency insufficiency with no clear precise localization [137].

The presence of an abducens paresis in supratentorial tumors fascinated many neurosurgeons. Stretching of the nerve due its long course or compression at its exit at the pontomedullary junction, compression by the anterior inferior cerebellar artery, and compression at the clivus exit were alternative explanations, but Collier rejected that notion. The presence of false localizing signs also interested Harvey Cushing. He suggested that abducens palsies may in some cases be attributed to arterial constriction and that also would explain the recovery.

THE FALSE
LOCALISING SIGNS OF INTRACRANIAL TUMOUR.

BY JAMES COLLIER, M.D., B.Sc. F.R.C.P.
Assistant Physician to St. George's Hospital and to the National Hospital, Queen Square.

THIS communication is based upon the results of 161 consecutive cases of intracranial tumour which have been examined in the Pathological Laboratory of the National Hospital during the years 1894-1904. The examinations were made by Dr. Colman, Dr. Risien Russell, Dr. Batten, Dr. Farquhar Buzzard, and by the writer of this paper.

The majority of these cases came under the writer's personal clinical observation. His best thanks are here expressed to his colleagues upon the staff of the National Hospital, to Dr. Colman, and to Dr. Farquhar Buzzard, Pathologist to the Hospital, for their kind permission to make use of the clinical and pathological notes upon these cases.

The object of this paper is to show :—

(1) That local signs appearing late in the course of intracranial tumour, where general signs alone have pre-existed, are often of false portent.

(2) The relative frequency with which local signs have been due in this series of cases to the presence of vascular lesions, meningitis, hydrocephalus, local spreading œdema of the brain, secondary deposits of new growth, and posterior degeneration.

(3) That the absence of usually accepted local signs during the early days of illness in intracranial tumour is in itself a most important localising indication, confining the disease to the supratentorial region.

(4) That true localising signs at one time present may later become concealed or undemonstrable owing to the

Fig. 3.7 Title page

The rarity of false localizing symptoms was noted in one study of 250 cases of intracranial meningioma with no evidence of palsy of the ninth, tenth, eleventh, and twelfth cranial nerves but with false localizing signs in 20 tentorial tumors [83]. Other single cases were reported, for example, a left parietal astrocytoma presenting with a fifth and eighth right cranial nerve palsy [68].

Most mystifying are patients with a fixed pupil opposite to the acute hemispheric lesion [41, 45, 155]. Traditional explanations have been compression of the oculomotor nerve by the herniating uncus of the temporal lobe (the pupiloconstrictor fibers are superficially located and easily injured) [226]. The opposite pupil becomes involved when the brain stem shifts downward, pulling on the opposite oculomotor nerve and causes bilateral fixed and dilated pupils. Thus, dilation of the opposite pupil at onset is hard to explain. Rotation of the brain stem in the axial plane could slacken the ipsilateral oculomotor and stretch the opposite oculomotor. Ischemia of the cranial nerve nucleus is another distinct possibility [45, 89, 195].

False localizing signs also have been described in spinal cord lesions with compressive cervical myelopathy causing a false localizing thoracic sensory level largely explained by ischemia of the medial portion of the spinothalamic tracts [171, 216]. Other false localizing signs pertaining to the practice of neurocritical care are pseudo-internuclear ophthalmoplegia—suggesting a brainstem lesion—in myasthenia gravis. Many other acute signs, such as an acute Horner's syndrome in intracerebral hematoma have never been explained satisfactorily.

Short Historical Note 5

BRAIN HERNIATION

The Title of the Paper

Jefferson G. The tentorial pressure cone. Arch Neurol Psych. 1938;40:857–76.
McNealy DE, Plum F. Brainstem dysfunction with supratentorial mass lesions. Arch Neurol. 1962;7:10–32.

The Paper and the Times

In the early 1930s, most of the reports on neurologic findings in rapidly deteriorating patients involved expanding tumors. It was clearly appreciated at the time that tumors cause clinical signs as a result of invasion, compression, circulatory compromise, or as a result of abnormalities of the cerebrospinal fluid (CSF) circulation causing hydrocephalus. Shift with damage to brain tissue against the dural edge or over taut vessels also had been described.

When brains were examined at autopsy, pathologists noted that the uncus of the hippocampal gyrus was squeezed through the tentorial opening, and in the most severe cases with supratentorial lesions, the cerebellar tonsils had herniated into the foramen magnum. In 1920, Meyer was the first pathologist to describe herniation into the incisura tentorii (less known as Bichat's cistern). Despite suggesting that the lumbar puncture in the presence of herniation could be hazardous, the paper did not present any actual clinical examples.

In those days, lumbar puncture was considered a dangerous procedure for some patients, particularly in lesions of the posterior fossa. It was well known that this diagnostic test in patients with papilledema as a result of increased intracranial pressure (ICP), could cause further rapid worsening, often cessation of respiration. These concerns were addressed in Jefferson's paper, and he described that herniation through the tentorium could cause compression of the brainstem and eventually could squeeze the contents of the posterior fossa through the foramen.

In the early part of the twentieth century, coma was described using several elements of neurologic examination but usually in combination with other physical findings. So, many textbooks would describe changes in breathing (slow, shallow, quiet, slow and noisy, sighing), pulse (weak, fluttering, rapid), odor of breath (urinous odor of uremia and acetone in diabetes), pupils (dilated, irregular, variable, contracted), and temperature (increased, high, subnormal). These were all unsuccessful attempts to grasp the difficulty of neurologic examination of coma. Perhaps as one of the first, DeJong's 1950 textbook *The Neurological Examination*, included details on cranial nerve examination and emphasized the value of eye signs in localization.

In the early 1960s, more emphasis was placed on clinical findings that could help physicians recognize these acute deteriorations from displacement of tissue through the tentorium or through the foramen of magnum. A variety of acute clinical symptoms emerged—a fixed pupil, abnormal motor-responses, irregular or periodic breathing, and acute hypertension—and all of them were identified as indications for neurosurgical intervention [115, 116, 189, 238, 242].

What was unknown, however, was the precise clinical course and subsequent stages in patients who deteriorated. Many earlier publications describing a large variety of neurologic symptoms were difficult to summarize into a pattern and were not categorized in different stages [201, 226, 241]. This changed with the publication of McNealy and Plum's paper. Their observations would introduce the term "rostrocaudal deterioration", which for the first time presented what appeared to be a predictable succession of clinical signs when a patient would spiral down.

Both Jefferson's and McNealy and Plum's papers (Fig. 3.8 and 3.9) introduced the clinical signs of brain herniation to the medical audience, but as expected, it would take some time for these clinical signs to be understood and used consistently.

The Details of the Paper

Jefferson's report includes several cases, and they are described in detail after a brief introduction on regional and anatomical relations and a brief historical overview on the herniation patterns known to neuropathologists.

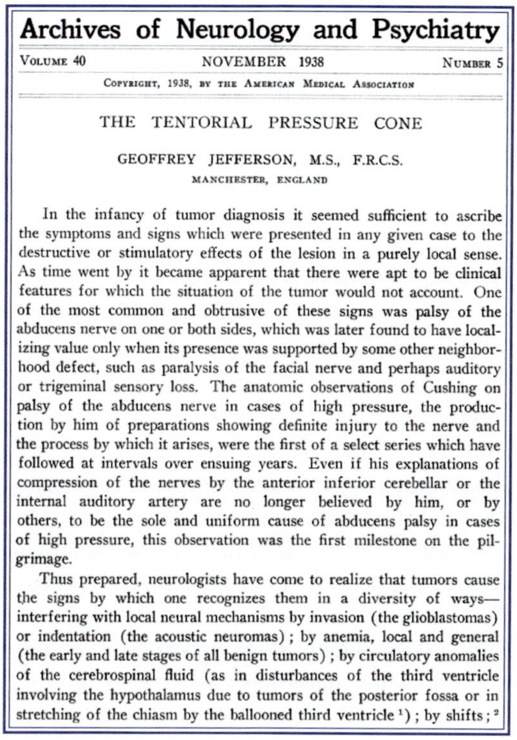

Archives of Neurology and Psychiatry

VOLUME 40 NOVEMBER 1938 NUMBER 5

COPYRIGHT, 1938, BY THE AMERICAN MEDICAL ASSOCIATION

THE TENTORIAL PRESSURE CONE

GEOFFREY JEFFERSON, M.S., F.R.C.S.

MANCHESTER, ENGLAND

In the infancy of tumor diagnosis it seemed sufficient to ascribe the symptoms and signs which were presented in any given case to the destructive or stimulatory effects of the lesion in a purely local sense. As time went by it became apparent that there were apt to be clinical features for which the situation of the tumor would not account. One of the most common and obtrusive of these signs was palsy of the abducens nerve on one or both sides, which was later found to have localizing value only when its presence was supported by some other neighborhood defect, such as paralysis of the facial nerve and perhaps auditory or trigeminal sensory loss. The anatomic observations of Cushing on palsy of the abducens nerve in cases of high pressure, the production by him of preparations showing definite injury to the nerve and the process by which it arises, were the first of a select series which have followed at intervals over ensuing years. Even if his explanations of compression of the nerves by the anterior inferior cerebellar or the internal auditory artery are no longer believed by him, or by others, to be the sole and uniform cause of abducens palsy in cases of high pressure, this observation was the first milestone on the pilgrimage.

Thus prepared, neurologists have come to realize that tumors cause the signs by which one recognizes them in a diversity of ways—interfering with local neural mechanisms by invasion (the glioblastomas) or indentation (the acoustic neuromas); by anemia, local and general (the early and late stages of all benign tumors); by circulatory anomalies of the cerebrospinal fluid (as in disturbances of the third ventricle involving the hypothalamus due to tumors of the posterior fossa or in stretching of the chiasm by the ballooned third ventricle [1]); by shifts; [2]

Fig. 3.8 Title page

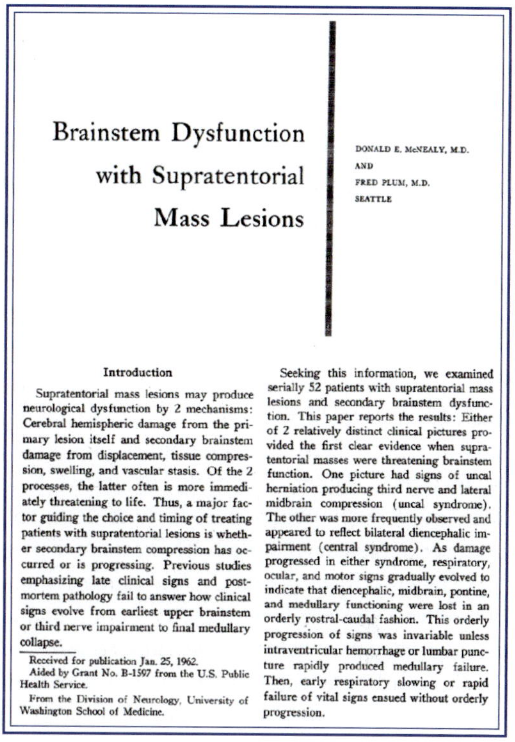

Brainstem Dysfunction with Supratentorial Mass Lesions

DONALD E. McNEALY, M.D.
AND
FRED PLUM, M.D.
SEATTLE

Introduction

Supratentorial mass lesions may produce neurological dysfunction by 2 mechanisms: Cerebral hemispheric damage from the primary lesion itself and secondary brainstem damage from displacement, tissue compression, swelling, and vascular stasis. Of the 2 processes, the latter often is more immediately threatening to life. Thus, a major factor guiding the choice and timing of treating patients with supratentorial lesions is whether secondary brainstem compression has occurred or is progressing. Previous studies emphasizing late clinical signs and postmortem pathology fail to answer how clinical signs evolve from earliest upper brainstem or third nerve impairment to final medullary collapse.

Seeking this information, we examined serially 52 patients with supratentorial mass lesions and secondary brainstem dysfunction. This paper reports the results: Either of 2 relatively distinct clinical pictures provided the first clear evidence when supratentorial masses were threatening brainstem function. One picture had signs of uncal herniation producing third nerve and lateral midbrain compression (uncal syndrome). The other was more frequently observed and appeared to reflect bilateral diencephalic impairment (central syndrome). As damage progressed in either syndrome, respiratory, ocular, and motor signs gradually evolved to indicate that diencephalic, midbrain, pontine, and medullary functioning were lost in an orderly rostral-caudal fashion. This orderly progression of signs was invariable unless intraventricular hemorrhage or lumbar puncture rapidly produced medullary failure. Then, early respiratory slowing or rapid failure of vital signs ensued without orderly progression.

Received for publication Jan. 25, 1962.
Aided by Grant No. B-1597 from the U.S. Public Health Service.
From the Division of Neurology, University of Washington School of Medicine.

Fig. 3.9 Title page

Jefferson's first case was a patient with a parietal astrocytoma who developed a hemiplegia over several years and died suddenly after a lumbar puncture. Within a few hours after CSF removal, the patient developed severe headache and became comatose. His neck and arms were notably rigid, and his legs were in "extreme extensor hypertonus." He also had "decerebrate attacks" with rigidity of the neck and adduction of the arms. At autopsy, marked deformity of the midbrain was noted.

The second case was a patient with a frontal meningioma who deteriorated rapidly on admission and presented with dilation of pupils and papilledema. Again, markedly increased tone was found with hypertonus in both legs and extensor of plantar responses. This patient died in "spontaneous hyperthermia." The increased tendon reflexes and the hypertonicity were found to be suggestive of a "tentorial pressure cone."

The third case was a patient with a meningioma in the temporal fossa who died suddenly during surgery. Pathology showed that there was a "double pressure cone, one into the hiatus tentorii and the other into the foramen magnum."

The fourth case involved a patient with a worsening characterized by bilateral pupillary dilatation, half flexed legs that were very rigid, and extreme neck rigidity suggestive of meningitis. A glioblastoma was found with the temporal lobe pushed into the edge of the incisura tentorii.

Jefferson suggested that the tentorial pressure cone could be recognized by the development of a "decerebrate state linked with pupillary alterations, such as the 'hutchinsonian pupil'." The descriptions, albeit new, lacked neither further neurologic detail nor a comprehensive explanation.

Several decades later, McNealy and Plum's article appeared. The study included 52 patients with a supratentorial mass, who were seen over a 24-month period and who were selected from serial observations in 220 comatose patients admitted to the emergency room at King County Washington Hospital. The patients were selected for examinations when the lesions were inoperable or when they had surgery and continued to deteriorate. Neurologic examination was done by both authors at regular intervals up to 6 h. Clear notice was made of respirations, pupils, oculovestibular reflexes, and motor function. Respiration was observed for pattern and depth and brainstem reflexes, in particular the pupils, were categorized in large, mid-position, or small pupils. The provoked ocular movements were tabulated as hyperactive, dysconjugate, impaired, or absent. The motor responses were described as decorticate rigidity and decerebrate rigidity following noxious stimulation via the trigeminal (deep supraorbital pressure) and spinothalamic (skin pinch, testicular pressure, and Achilles tendon pressure) pathways. The authors were able to identify 27 cases with what they called "central syndrome" and 7 patients with what they called "uncal syndrome". These syndromes progressed, according to the authors, in stages. The central syndrome (Fig. 3.10) progressed from a diencephalic stage, in which respiration was frequently interrupted by sighing or agitation. In this early stage small pupils (1–3 mm), easily elicitable horizontal doll's eye movements, in addition to a unilateral hemiplegia reflecting the primary lesion, were noted. This then progressed to a midbrain upper pons stage in which Cheyne–Stokes respiration changed to sustained hyperventilation, small pupils changed to a fixed mid-position, and doll's head eye movements became progressively more difficult to find. With further progression, a lower pontine upper medullary stage appeared and eventually, the patient progressed to a medullary stage in which the respiration became slow, irregular in rate or depth, and eventually interrupted by deep sighs or gasps. At this time, the pupils dilated widely and no stretch reflex could be obtained.

The manuscript also described in detail the development of third nerve midbrain stage in the setting of uncal herniation and a combination of both central and uncal herniation. The authors found that sudden progression, skipping over stages instead of a predictable rostrocaudal deterioration, was typically found in a patient with a cerebral hemorrhage that ruptured in the ventricle.

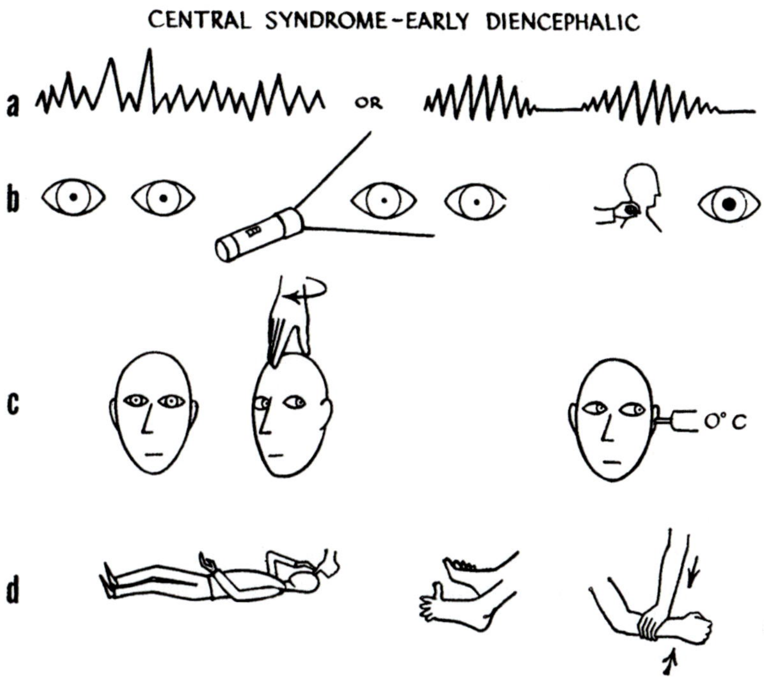

Fig. 3.10 Signs used to define a herniation stage by Plum and Posner (i.e., central syndrome)

The Message and Acceptance

For the first time, Jefferson's paper further elucidated the clinical features of increased ICP and compression of the brainstem through herniation of brain tissue. The herniation could be either through the tentorial opening or through the foramen magnum. The clinical features involved sudden presentation of pupillary changes, neck stiffness, and extensor posturing. Hyperthermia often also was noted indicative of "central hyperthermia." Jefferson referred to "Hutchinsonian pupil," which was related to a unilateral fixed pupil associated with uncal herniation.

Clinical signs of tentorial and tonsillar herniation had been recognized by prominent neurosurgeons. Cushing also considered an increase in ICP to be the main reason for tonsillar herniation, and he felt that medullary compression would eventually cause respiratory failure. In a seminal case, a young boy developed respiratory arrest and Cushing decided not only to do supratentorial surgery but also to-albeit unsuccesfully-perform emergency suboccipital craniotomy to relieve the medullary compression believed to be caused by tonsillar herniation [206]. The author called it "a surgeon's courage in times of despair" but more likely primary brainstem injury from displacement caused the signs rather than compression [206].

The central and tentorial herniation patterns, as described in this paper, became the basis of Plum and Posner's monograph, "The Diagnosis of Stupor and Coma" (McNealy was one of Plum's residents together with Swanson and Posner but McNealy died prematurely) [180].

For many decades since the original description, these patterns remained ingrained in neurologist's minds and provided a teachable template. The didactics of neurologic examination of coma would now refer to these stages. However, the years that followed would find evidence to the contrary [152]. Very few patients—when they worsen—do progress in these stages with all four components—pupils, oculocephalics, motor response, and respiration—changing in a manner that can be exactly predicted.

Coning and herniation are well-accepted terms (and even a codable diagnosis), but the clinical correlates are less clearcut. Magnetic resonance imaging may show massive displacement but not with a perfect clinical correlate. The clinical entity of brain herniation—despite neuropathologic and radiologic findings—has not been fully worked out and in parts has remained quite inexplicable.

Short Historical Note 6

NEUROGENIC HYPERVENTILATION

The Title of the Paper

Plum F, Swanson AG. Central neurogenic hyperventilation in men. Arch Neurol Psych. 1958;81:335–49.

The Paper and the Times

Before respiratory patterns could be linked to specific brain injury, progress was made in the discovery of the morphology of the medullary respiratory center. Most of the early work can be attributed to Legallois' experiments in 1812 in which stimulation of the pneumotaxic center increased the respiratory rate [136].

Abnormal breathing patterns had been recognized as indicative of a primary brain lesion and most commonly known were periodic breathing patterns. In the early papers on acute neurologic disease, the terms stertorous, gasping, or overventilation or hyperpneu were used frequently without further characterization.

There was reluctance to attribute hyperventilation to a brain lesion rather than to a compensatory response in acute illness. Rapid breathing was mostly seen as Kussmaul breathing in patients with a diabetic coma. Alveolar hyperventilation was typically observed as a response to hypoxia or metabolic acidosis or was associated with a specific pulmonary disorder. Hyperventilation with respiratory alkalosis also had been incidentally noted in hepatic encephalopathy and patients in the last stages of deep coma. These descriptions were followed by a series of studies linking brain injury to abnormalities of the rhythm of breathing. In the first half of the twentieth century, hyperventilation as a direct result from an acute brain lesion was not specifically mentioned in leading medical and neurologic textbooks.

The Details of the Paper

Hyperventilation associated with a brain lesion was first carefully described by Plum and Swanson (Fig. 3.11). The paper reports nine patients with acute lesions in the pons mostly caused by embolus to the basilar artery and compared them with 25 patients with brain lesions elsewhere who lacked hyperventilation (The control cases involved bilateral hemispheric lesions and unilateral hemispheric lesions.).

In their original description, the patients all had clinical signs pointing to a pontine lesion. Many patients had constricted pupils with skew deviation of the eyes or disconjugate motion, including internuclear ophthalmoplegia in four patients. Decerebrate rigidity was also noted.

As expected, the patients with central hyperventilation had a marked alkalosis (Fig. 3.12). The authors also reported frequent other respiratory abnormalities with six patients having Cheyne–Stoke type breathing and periodic breathing, usually preceding the central hyperventilation.

The hyperventilation could be reduced or eliminated by oxygen therapy or by carbon dioxide inhalation. The study also carefully eliminated hypoxemia and metabolic acidosis as possible causes of hyperventilation. The authors also found that the arterial pH must fall to approximately 7.2 before respiration is stimulated by acidosis.

Autopsy demonstrated medial pontine destruction. The authors hypothesized that structures in the medial pontine reticular formation were inhibitory to respiration, and thus, a central neurogenic hyperventilation is the result of an uninhibited stimulation of the medullary respiratory centers by the lateral pontine reticular formation. The authors found only one report with disease in the cerebral hemispheres causing neurogenic hyperventilation.

The Message and Acceptance

It has been understood that both respiratory rate and alveolar ventilation are controlled by the respiratory centers in the pons and medulla. Thus, any neural, humoral input, or direct structural injury can lead not only to hyperventilation but also to hypoventilation or apnea.

Central neurogenic hyperventilation has now been well recognized in patients with catastrophic brain injury. Neurogenic hyperventilation can be seen in comatose patients with

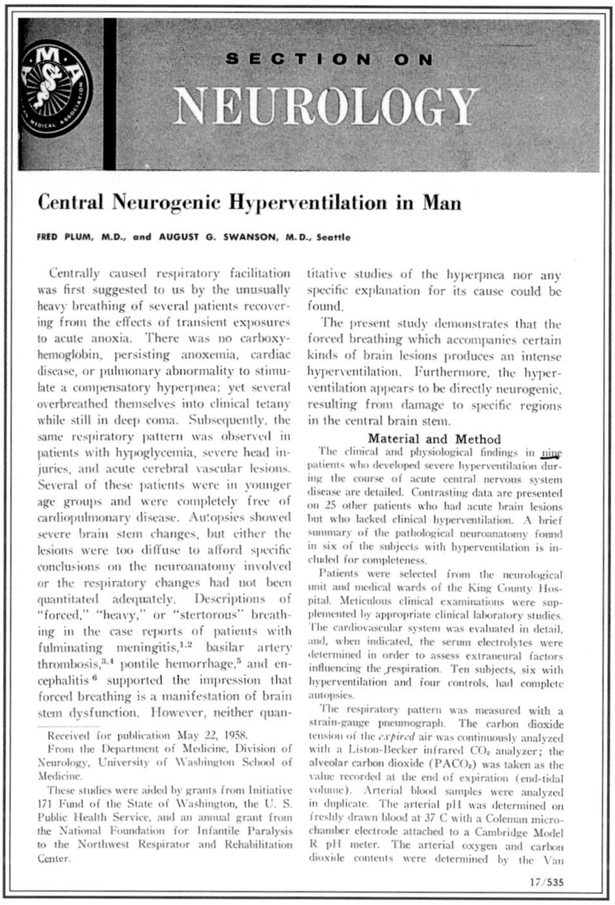

SECTION ON

NEUROLOGY

Central Neurogenic Hyperventilation in Man

FRED PLUM, M.D., and AUGUST G. SWANSON, M.D., Seattle

Centrally caused respiratory facilitation was first suggested to us by the unusually heavy breathing of several patients recovering from the effects of transient exposures to acute anoxia. There was no carboxyhemoglobin, persisting anoxemia, cardiac disease, or pulmonary abnormality to stimulate a compensatory hyperpnea; yet several overbreathed themselves into clinical tetany while still in deep coma. Subsequently, the same respiratory pattern was observed in patients with hypoglycemia, severe head injuries, and acute cerebral vascular lesions. Several of these patients were in younger age groups and were completely free of cardiopulmonary disease. Autopsies showed severe brain stem changes, but either the lesions were too diffuse to afford specific conclusions on the neuroanatomy involved or the respiratory changes had not been quantitated adequately. Descriptions of "forced," "heavy," or "stertorous" breathing in the case reports of patients with fulminating meningitis,[1,2] basilar artery thrombosis,[3,4] pontile hemorrhage,[5] and encephalitis[6] supported the impression that forced breathing is a manifestation of brain stem dysfunction. However, neither quantitative studies of the hyperpnea nor any specific explanation for its cause could be found.

The present study demonstrates that the forced breathing which accompanies certain kinds of brain lesions produces an intense hyperventilation. Furthermore, the hyperventilation appears to be directly neurogenic, resulting from damage to specific regions in the central brain stem.

Received for publication May 22, 1958.

From the Department of Medicine, Division of Neurology, University of Washington School of Medicine.

These studies were aided by grants from Initiative 171 Fund of the State of Washington, the U. S. Public Health Service, and an annual grant from the National Foundation for Infantile Paralysis to the Northwest Respirator and Rehabilitation Center.

Material and Method

The clinical and physiological findings in nine patients who developed severe hyperventilation during the course of acute central nervous system disease are detailed. Contrasting data are presented on 25 other patients who had acute brain lesions but who lacked clinical hyperventilation. A brief summary of the pathological neuroanatomy found in six of the subjects with hyperventilation is included for completeness.

Patients were selected from the neurological unit and medical wards of the King County Hospital. Meticulous clinical examinations were supplemented by appropriate clinical laboratory studies. The cardiovascular system was evaluated in detail, and, when indicated, the serum electrolytes were determined in order to assess extraneural factors influencing the respiration. Ten subjects, six with hyperventilation and four controls, had complete autopsies.

The respiratory pattern was measured with a strain-gauge pneumograph. The carbon dioxide tension of the *expired* air was continuously analyzed with a Liston-Becker infrared CO_2 analyzer; the alveolar carbon dioxide ($PACO_2$) was taken as the value recorded at the end of expiration (end-tidal volume). Arterial blood samples were analyzed in duplicate. The arterial pH was determined on freshly drawn blood at 37 C with a Coleman microchamber electrode attached to a Cambridge Model R pH meter. The arterial oxygen and carbon dioxide contents were determined by the Van

17/535

Fig. 3.11 Title page

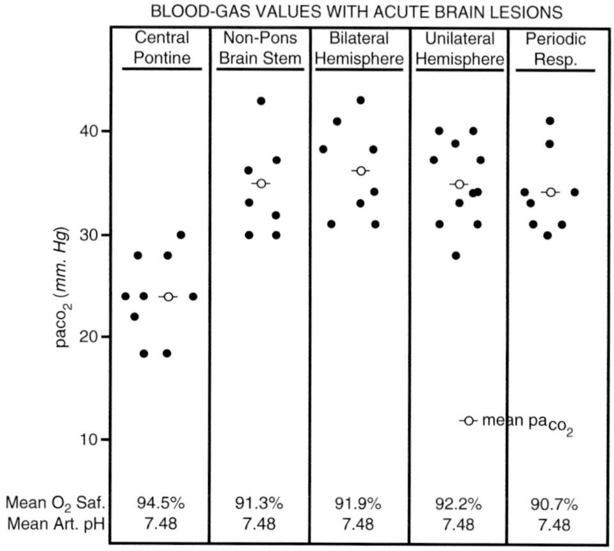

Fig. 3.12 Blood gas values in central neurogenic hyperventilation

anoxic-ischemic encephalopathy and patients with upper brainstem compression and shift from a new hemispheric lesion [113, 234]. If neurogenic hyperventilation is present, the disorder is a consequence of a midbrain or pontine lesion and can be associated with pontine hemorrhages, embolus to the basilar artery, and progressive signs of brainstem compression from a hemispheric lesion [84, 100, 169, 234]. Later case reports found a correlation with brainstem tumors [84, 174, 209, 210]. Other signs localizing the lesion to the brainstem are often present. For unknown reasons, the incidence of primary brainstem lymphoma or astrocytoma in patients with central neurogenic hyperventilation is high, but it also has been reported in multiple sclerosis [231] and brainstem encephalitis [169], but again the responsible lesion is in the pons. The patient cannot inhibit respiratory drive; carbon dioxide rebreathing augments the patient's need to breathe and increases the respiratory rate. Infiltration of tumor, whether lymphoma or astrocytoma, presumably destroys the inhibiting descending neurons from the pons to the medullary respiratory center. Lactate production from the tumor, another possibility, has been discounted by several studies as a major trigger.

In traumatic brain injury, periodic hyperventilation may occur with tachycardia, fever, and sweating and is related to sympathetic hyperactivity syndrome. It may be the most commonly underrecognized manifestation of acute brain injury and often the most commonly undertreated. Central neurogenic hyperventilation usually is continuously present and seemingly wearing out the patient. Hyperventilation in this setting also can be more erratic and may result in difficulty ventilating patients due to asynchrony with the ventilator. In sustained neurogenic hyperventilation, respiratory alkalosis is considerable with pH values greater than 7.6. This type of breathing disorder is best muted with infusion of potent respiratory depressants such as fentanyl.

Short Historical Note 7

BIOT BREATHING

The Title of the Paper

Biot MC. Étude Clinique et Expérimentale sur la Respiration de Cheyne-Stokes. New York: Harper & Brothers; 1878.

The Paper and the Times

Several classic central periodic breathing patterns have been described. Biot breathing is a breathing pattern in patients with acute neurologic disease—also perhaps better known as ataxic breathing. Biot breathing can be contrasted with Cheyne–Stokes breathing (periodic stereotypical crescendo–decrescendo hyperpnoea followed by apnea) and apneustic breathing (periodic prolonged inspiratory hold). The breathing pattern Biot described is irregular and rapid, with intermittent pauses. Biot breathing is not commonly mentioned in the neurologic literature but surfaces occasionally in the anesthesia literature.

The Details of the Paper

Camille Biot made his seminal observations early in his career in the Hôtel Dieu Hospital in Lyon [22]. Biot wrote two main articles on breathing patterns. One large exploratory work focused on his observations on Cheyne–Stokes breathing [20, 21]. In each paper, he described patients who were admitted to the Hôtel Dieu Hospital with Cheyne–Stokes respiration, his major interest. In his first article, he described a patient who had respiratory movements that gradually decreased and increased but were irregular, and he was one of the first to publish recordings of this type of respiration in a 16-year-old patient with tuberculous meningitis [20].

The breathing pattern Biot described is irregular and rapid, with rhythmical pauses lasting 10–30 seconds but sometimes with alternating periods of apnea and tachypnea. This breathing pattern lacked the crescendo–decrescendo cycles attributed to Cheyne–Stokes breathing and was completely irregular with varying periods of apnea. He named it *rhythme méningitique*.

In 1878, a larger thesis was published entitled *Étude de Clinique et Expérimentale sur la Respiration de Cheyne-Stokes* [21] (Fig. 3.13). This paper described theories of the origins of Cheyne–Stokes breathing. Biot argued that Cheyne–Stokes breathing included an increase in pulse during the pause and reduction of blood pressure during apnea. In this now discounted theory, the accumulation of carbon dioxide would increase the activity of the vasomotor center, and vasoconstriction would cause progressive ischemia of the respiration center resulting in deep breaths.

Biot added a section on earlier observations of the breathing pattern [14, 21] (Fig. 3.14 and 3.15). This respiration had been described as slow and with accelerating periods increasing to 10–20/min with unequal chest expansion: some short and incomplete, others long, deep, and often interrupted by gasps. The unevenness of breathing was not related to the heart rate. In another report, vomiting, constipation, and high fever along with short, incomplete, intermittent, and gasping breathing were considered characteristics of meningitis. He also recognized that similar patterns had been described in Trousseau's textbook [239]. Sigismond Jaccoud thought this breathing pattern was an agonal phenomenon. In his description, the pulse slows down, and the breathing changes and becomes irregular and interrupted with deep sighs that are easy to recognize [112]. Biot concluded that a big sigh comes before the pause, and the periods are irregular. These were the two main characteristics that were always seen in meningitis and, thus, should be considered characteristic but different from the regular crescendo and decrescendo cycles of Cheyne–Stokes breathing. Biot concluded that this breathing pattern should be considered separately and not as a variant of Cheyne–Stokes breathing.

The Message and Acceptance

Many publications have inappropriately described Biot breathing as "periodic and consisting of groups of full respiratory effort" [5]. Biot breathing often is confused with cluster breathing, regular cycles of deep breaths with variable periodicity.

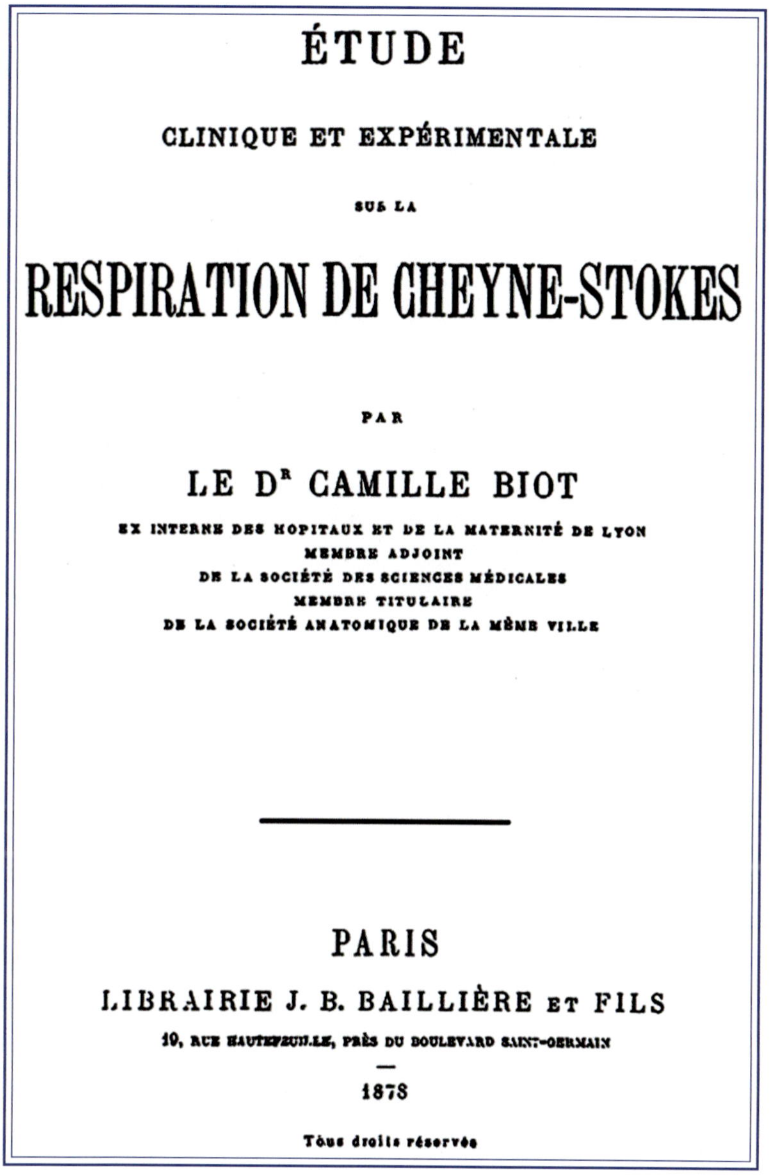

ÉTUDE

CLINIQUE ET EXPÉRIMENTALE

SUR LA

RESPIRATION DE CHEYNE-STOKES

PAR

LE DR CAMILLE BIOT

EX INTERNE DES HOPITAUX ET DE LA MATERNITÉ DE LYON
MEMBRE ADJOINT
DE LA SOCIÉTÉ DES SCIENCES MÉDICALES
MEMBRE TITULAIRE
DE LA SOCIÉTÉ ANATOMIQUE DE LA MÊME VILLE

PARIS
LIBRAIRIE J. B. BAILLIÈRE ET FILS
19, RUE HAUTEFEUILLE, PRÈS DU BOULEVARD SAINT-GERMAIN
—
1878

Tous droits réservés

Fig. 3.13 Title page

An experimental study on Biot periodic breathing in cats created more confusion, and Biot breathing was called cluster breathing. Lesions in the pneumotaxic system of the rostral pons resulted in a breathing pattern that the authors explained as possible cyclic hypoxemia [252].

There is very little mention of Biot breathing in clinical papers, in particular those on meningitis. There are very few citations on clinical studies accurately documenting Biot breathing, confusing it again with cluster breathing. Plum and Posner, mentioned Biot in their description of ataxic breathing seen in the bulbar form of poliomyelitis [182]. It will remain unclear if Biot breathing had the same characteristics. Miller Fisher, in his work on neurologic examination of the comatose patient, correctly identified the main characteristics of Biot breathing and separated it from (regular) cluster breathing [74].

In the German literature, the eponym appeared first in Hofbauer's 1904 book, *Das Biotische Atmen*, on the differential diagnosis of shortness of breath, but the author also stated he had not observed this type of breathing and in each case the breathing pattern was more likely Cheyne–Stokes breathing [105]. In the English literature, it appeared in the title of a 1911 review article by Connor, who observed seven patients, six of whom had meningitis [49]. Biot breathing may have become less obvious as a consequence of intensive care. One would expect that patients with this type of irregular breathing and poor oxygenation will likely be intubated as soon as they are seen and have their breathing assisted by mechanical ventilation.

P. S. Nous avons dit dans les pages précédentes que les différents auteurs, qui ont écrit sur la respiration de Cheyne-Stokes, l'avaient signalée dans les méningites tuberculeuses. L'occasion s'est présentée à nous, ces jours-ci, d'en observer un cas chez un jeune homme de seize ans. Nous avons relevé plusieurs tracés pneumographiques (V. *Planche IV*, p. 523). Or, ces tracés diffèrent notablement de ceux qu'on a pu voir planche I, surtout en ce que avant et après la pause il n'y a pas ces mouvements respiratoires graduellement diminués et graduellement augmentés; mais une respiration le plus souvent profonde, dyspnéique, répondant à un *gros soupir* poussé par le malade à ces moments. Or, d'autre part, Trousseau, dont le génie observateur ne peut être mis en doute, donne dans sa *Clinique* (tome II, page 240), comme signe de la méningite tuberculeuse une irrégularité plus ou moins périodique de la respiration; mais la lecture de ce passage fait voir que ce n'est pas le type de Cheyne-Stokes.

Sans vouloir d'un seul fait tirer des conclusions définitives, il semblerait néanmoins que dans les méningites ce n'est pas le vrai type respiratoire de Cheyne-Stokes qui existe, mais un type plus ou moins voisin, plus ou moins régulier. C'est d'ailleurs un point que nous nous proposons d'étudier dans des recherches ultérieures.

Fig. 3.14 The first description of Biot's breathing different from Cheyne–Stokes breathing
Translation: "We stated in the previous pages that the various authors who wrote about Cheyne-Stokes respiration had mentioned it in tuberculous meningitis. We have observed the case of a 16-year-old young man. We collected several pneumographic graphs. These graphs are conspicuously different from those that we saw in fig I, especially in that before and after the pause there is no respiratory movement that gradually decrease and increase; but, a respiration that is deep, dyspnoeic, like a big sigh from the patient during those moments. On the other hand Trousseau, which undoubtedly astute observation, noted in his Clinique (part II, page 240), that periodic irregularity of breathing is a sign of tuberculous meningitis; but the reading of this paragraph shows that it is not Cheyne-Stokes. Without wanting to come to a definitive conclusion, it seems that in meningitis it is not really the true type of Cheyne-Stokes respiration, but close to this type and more regular. It is an issue that should be the subject of future study."

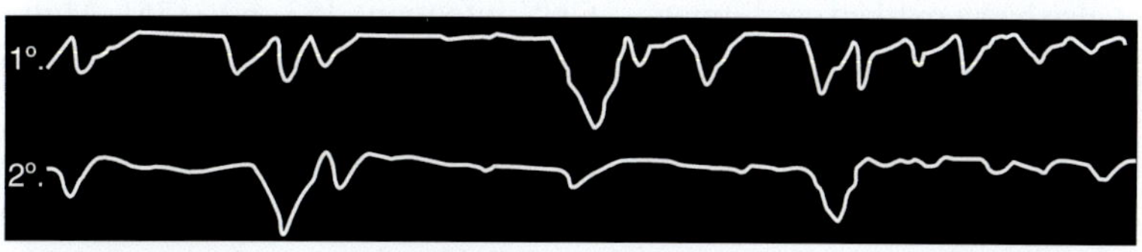

Fig. 3.15 The recorded periodic breathing pattern described by Biot

Short Historical Note 8

CHEYNE–STOKES BREATHING

The Title of the Paper

Cheyne J. A case of apoplexy in which the fleshy part of the heart was converted into fat. Dublin Hosp Rep. 1818;2:216–23.

The Paper and the Times

Of all "neurogenic" breathing patterns, Cheyne–Stokes breathing (CSR) is the most known but also most unrecognized. Not infrequently, physicians are called at the bedside for apneic periods only to discover it is part of a periodic breathing pattern. As early as antiquity, abnormal respiration has been noted in "apoplexy" and described often nonspecifically as infrequent and deep.

In the 1800s, studies appeared that periodically linked brain injury to abnormalities of the rhythm of breathing. Many physicians in the earlier days were able to describe abnormal breathing patterns, but it was John Cheyne and later William Stokes who described the ascending and descending waxing and waning pattern [175].

CSR often is related to changes in alertness and therefore should be part of assessing acutely ill neurologic patients [40]. Its appearance in a patient with a previously regular breathing pattern may be a valuable "neurologic" sign.

The Details of the Paper

Cheyne published his observation in *Dublin Hospital Reports*, a journal he had founded several years before (Fig. 3.16). In 1818, he described a 60-year-old man who was diagnosed with apoplexy and at autopsy was found to have a cerebral infarct. The patient also had a marked cardiomegaly and Cheyne found an "extremely irregular and unequal pulse." His description is legendary:

> The respiration is a first slow and heaving then irregular and sometimes convulsive and lastly, interrupted. The patient from relaxation of the palate, snores loudly during inspiration, and sometimes during expiration the upper lip, from relaxation or palsy is loudly blown up from the teeth, as we often see it upon great exhaustion, as in the subsiding of an epileptic fit. Sometimes the breathing is soft. Immediately before death the respiration is irregular and is performed perhaps not more than three of four times in the minute. the irritability of the heart survives the respiration sting with my finger over the artery of a person who died of apoplexy. I distinctly felt the pulse beat after the last expiration. Interrupted respiration is justly considered as the most dangerous symptom. … For several days his breathing was irregular; it would entirely cease for a quarter of a minute, then it would become perceptible, though very low, then by degrees it became heaving and quick, and then it would gradually cease again: this revolution in the state of his breathing occupied about a minute, during which there were about thirty acts of respiration [43].

Stokes felt the breathing pattern was pathognomonic, a fatty degeneration of the heart.

> The symptom in question was observed by Dr. Cheyne, although he did not connect it with the specialties of the heart. … It consisted of the occurrence of a series of inspirations increasing to a maximum then declining in force and length, until a state of apparent apnea is established. In this condition, the patient may remain for such a length of time as to make his attendants believe that he is dead and a low inspiration followed by one more decided marks the commencement of a new ascending and then descending series of inspiration. This symptom as occurring in its highest degree I have only seen in the first weeks previous to the death of the patient [220].

Stokes' recognition of this breathing pattern in congestive heart failure was equally important, and he recognized that its appearance had prognostic impact. This seminal observation is still true today despite marked improvement in medical management of congestive heart failure.

The Message and Acceptance

The periodic pattern was recognized but was frequently mentioned as a common symptom in CNS infections [53, 69, 175]. Multiple authors described the symptoms in tuberculous meningitis, often blurring the boundaries with Biot breathing. Others observed CSR with patients who had a hemorrhage into the medulla oblongata, linking it to an abnormality of the respiratory centers. The neurologic diseases that associated itself with CSR were meningitis, encephalitis, cerebral hemorrhage, cerebral infarcts, cerebellar hemorrhage, and ruptured

A CASE

OF

APOPLEXY,

IN WHICH THE

FLESHY PART OF THE HEART WAS CONVERTED INTO FAT.

BY J. CHEYNE, M. D. &c.

DOUBTS having been entertained of the conversion of the fleshy part of the heart into fat, and only one dissection, * in as far as I know, having been published illustrative of that very curious morbid alteration, the following case and dissection have been thought of sufficient importance to meet the public eye.

In this dissection, although no chemical experiment was made in proof of the matter into which the heart was converted being fatty, I have no doubt that it was

* See a dissection, illustrative of this morbid change, in an elaborate paper on inflammation of the heart, by Dr. Duncan, jun. *See Edin. Med. and Surgical Journal, Jan.* 1816.

Fig. 3.16 Title page

intracranial aneurysm [175, 250]. Many authors recognized two separate types: one associated with intracranial lesions and the other with cardiac disease. Attempts to distinguish the two were many, but none were accepted. Hughlings Jackson, in 1895, emphasized the neurologic origin of Cheyne–Stokes breathing after he examined a patient deteriorating with a brain tumor: "The respiratory centers in cases of Cheyne-Stokes respiration due to a grave cerebral lesion will be left more than is normal to their own inherent automatism, and will presumably be more susceptible to the state of the blood, and perhaps to the influence of the vagi" [106]. In addition, he mentioned "In the cases of Cheyne–Stokes breathing the supposition I am considering is that higher level inhibition is taken off both medulla respiratory centers, whereupon, respiration proper being greater, apnea occurs, and the respiratory movements cease."

Plum et al. hypothesized that CSR resulted from inappropriate periods of hyperventilation alternating with posthyperventilation apnea and found cortical dysfunction in all his patients, suggesting a preferential neurogenic cause.

CSR most often is seen in sleep. Later studies found that apnea duration bears no relation to circulation time or cardiac output [44, 119, 160, 167]. Current views include instability of respiratory control due to hyperventilation, prolonged circulation time, and reduced blood gas buffering capacity. More recent studies in patients with cardiac disease and stroke are confirming strikingly high prevalence of central sleep apnea with respiration. In central sleep apnea, there are cyclic apneas caused by transient lack of respiratory effort and not upper airway obstruction [104, 262]. CSR is often associated with impairments in sleep and are more common in patients with heart disease. Nonetheless, continuous positive airway pressure ventilation improved CSR in only 50%.

Miller Fisher's observations in comatose patients are also noteworthy [74]. He identified several variations of CSR. There may be only waxing and waning without an apneic period. The respiration may be slow or rapid, and a combination of CSR and hyperpnea may occur. Miller Fisher also observed that high fever tends to abolish CSR. A short-cycle CSR with short apneic and hyperpneic phases of only a few breaths was seen in neurologic patients with intracranial disease. He eloquently concluded "when the comatose patient is breathing quietly, regularly and slowly as in sleep one usually can be sure that the neurologic state is not desperate" [74].

Short Historical Note 9

ONDINE'S CURSE

The Title of the Paper

Severinghaus JW, Mitchell RA. Ondine's curse – failure of respiratory center automaticity while awake. J Clin Res. 1962;10:122.

The Paper and the Times

There has been significant interest in discovering breathing patterns that could be highly specific for neurologic disease, naming them and setting them apart from the classic Cheyne–Stokes breathing pattern. Bulbar poliomyelitis had been traditionally associated with hypoventilation, but the mechanism here was different. Before applying the term Ondine's curse to central hypoventilation by Severinghaus and Mitchell, a single case was described by Ratto et al with loss of automaticity of breathing after a brainstem stroke [188].

Severinghaus and Mitchell used a clever name for primary alveolar hypoventilation syndrome. Ondine's curse now refers to patients with long episodes of apnea while asleep but who can breathe on command. They referred to the original German fable "the sleep of Ondine" by Giraudoux. The curse was a punishment for unfaithfulness and Ondine took away her husband automatic functions. It included loss of all automatic functions—seeing, hearing, moving, and breathing.

The Details of the Paper

The paper that coined the term was an abstract with little details (Fig. 3.17). Three patients with apnea after high cervical cord or brainstem surgery and may have had bilateral spinothalamic tract cordotomies for pain relief. In cervical tractomy for intractable pain, the reticulospinal tracts activate phrenic nerve motor neurons and ascending spinoreticular fibers.

The Message and Acceptance

The term *Ondine's curse* has become entrenched in medical literature, but it remains a very rare form of sleep apnea [223]. The term has been used freely and not entirely correctly. It is now used for sleep apnea, hypoventilation syndrome, and loss of automatic ventilation [97]. Pulmonary pathology should be excluded, and typically, there is a rise in partial pressure of carbon dioxide with no response in ventilation. The condition can be mimicked by high doses of opioids. It has been described in congenital central hypoventilation associated with mutation of the *PHOX2B* gene, but in this condition, there is also a defect in cardiac control [46]. Acquired forms of Ondine's curse always have involved lesions in the respiratory centers of the medulla oblongata. Multiple cases of central hypoventilation have been described with acute stroke, tumors, infections, multiple sclerosis, and cervical cordotomy [6, 25, 46, 47, 85, 151, 157]. Lesions are bilateral in the ventrolateral brainstem between the trigeminal nerve nucleus and the upper cervical level [218]. The disorder is of interest to critical care physicians but will likely be rarely diagnosed in its pure form and may be difficult to demonstrate [221]. Diaphragmatic pacing has been successful.

ONDINE'S CURSE - FAILURE OF RESPIRATORY CENTER AUTOMATICITY WHILE AWAKE. J.W. Severinghaus and R.A. Mitchell*. Cardiovascular Research Institute, University of California Medical School, San Francisco.

We have studied three patients who exhibited long periods of apnea even when awake, but breathed on command. All three became apneic during surgery involving the high cervical cord or brain stem. Postoperatively, they were awake and apprehensive, sometimes hyperventilating with irregular rate and depth. They required artificial respiration when asleep and became apneic when sleep was induced with 70% N_2O or with 75-100 mg. thiopental. CO_2 response curves showed very low sensitivity and an erratic threshold. P_{ACO_2} over 70 did increase restlessness and sweating normally, and respiratory rate and depth became more regular at high P_{ACO_2}. One patient had no cough and gag reflexes, no carotid body response to lobeline, and convulsed from anoxia with several apneic periods. One had a vigorous hyperpnea after lobeline (10 mg I.V.) and usually had Cheyne-Stokes respiration when asleep; she also convulsed on several occasions when apnea persisted too long. One died in apnea; two improved over a week's time. The syndrome was first described in German legend. The water nymph, Ondine, having been jilted by her mortal husband, took from him all automatic functions, requiring him to remember to breathe. When he finally fell asleep, he died. Similar cases have been reported with bulbar poliomyelitis. It is proposed that the syndrome results from damage of the medullary CO_2 chemoreceptor.

Fig. 3.17 Title page

Short Historical Note 10

ASTERIXIS

The Title of the Paper

Adams RD, Foley JM. The neurologic disorder associated with liver disease. Res Proc Assoc Nerve Ment Dis. 1953;32:198–237.

The Paper and the Times

The early literature on coma specifically concentrated on how organ failure affects the brain. Well known are the descriptions of British physician Richard Bright leading to the triad "arterial hypertension," "albuminuric retinitis," and "manifestations involving the central nervous system." Bright noted that patients in the earlier stages of renal failure developed "myoclonus" and could evolve into a more serious state with seizures.

Another challenge for physicians was to distinguish a set of clinical signs that would be characteristic for liver failure. The "mental" changes were often nonspecifically described as stupor. Frerichs' description of liver disease involved two stages: excitement (delirium and convulsions) and depression (progressive stupor and coma). Frerichs emphasized a transitional phase of "gloomy, irritable temper and restlessness" but also "quiet, harmless wandering" [80]. The emergence of jaundice marked the development of delirium, convulsions, and coma.

Abnormal motor movements were noted, but the descriptions were far from distinct and without understanding of its physiology. Descriptions often included "muscular tremors," "rigors," "partial twitching or convulsions," or "jactitations." Others observed "choreiform movements" or "tonic spasms."

Parallel to better understanding of these clinical manifestations were the neuropathologic descriptions of the consequences of the organ disease. Earlier observations included enlargement of nuclei of the protoplasmic astrocytes with similarities to Wilson's hepatolenticular degenerations [1–3]. Adams and Foley would publish a major treatise that would "define more precisely the clinical neurologic syndrome presented by patients with different types of liver disease."

The Details of the Paper

The material came from observations made by the neurologic and medical services and the Mallory Institute of Pathology of the Boston City Hospital and data obtained through assistance of collaborators from Massachusetts General Hospital (Fig. 3.18). Clinical observations were made on 60 patients who developed hepatic coma most from "Laennec's cirrhosis of alcoholic type." All patients admitted to the wards were examined carefully by the authors, and after an initial comprehensive neurologic examination, patients were examined daily after the first signs of hepatic coma. Special attention was given to testing of concentration (speed, subtraction) and the presence of abnormal movements. Adams and Foley noted "a peculiar intermittency of sustained muscle contraction that presents as a irregular flapping movement when the arm and legs are held outstretched, a fluctuating rigidity of the limbs grimacing, sucking and grasp reflexes and at times convulsions completing the clinical picture."

Adams and Foley described it even more clearly in the following observation and confirmed using an oscillographic record of the outstretched arm that showed a brief succession of two to five beats of rhythmic discharge with a frequency of 8–16 seconds followed by a silent interval of 0.2–0.5 seconds that correspond with a lapse of posture (Fig. 3.19):

> It is most consistently and most effectively demonstrated by having the patient hold his arms and hands outstretched with the fingers spread apart. Depending on the severity of the process, as this posture was maintained there appeared at irregular intervals of a fraction of a second to seven seconds, a series of movements consisting usually of lateral deviations of the fingers, flexion-extension of the fingers at the metacarpophalangeal joint and flexion-extension at the wrist. The movements were rapid and arrhythmic and one phase, i.e flexion when the arms were outstretched in a pronated position, was always more rapid that the other. They tended to occur in bursts, at a rate of one every second or two. … In the legs the abnormality of movement would be demonstrated most easily by having the recumbent patient elevate his leg and

CHAPTER XI

THE NEUROLOGICAL DISORDER ASSOCIATED WITH LIVER DISEASE[1]

RAYMOND D. ADAMS AND JOSEPH M. FOLEY

INTRODUCTION

The adverse effect of deranged liver function on the brain is exemplified in two classes of disease, hepato-lenticular degeneration (Wilson's disease) and hepatic coma. Hepato-lenticular degeneration, the subject of the preceding chapter, has been a discovery of the present century and, although rare, has excited much interest owing to the prominence of the neurological symptoms. Hepatic coma, the topic of the present discussion, has been known since ancient times, and although a frequent complication of all types of liver disease has not attracted the attention that it deserves.

Fig. 3.18 Title page

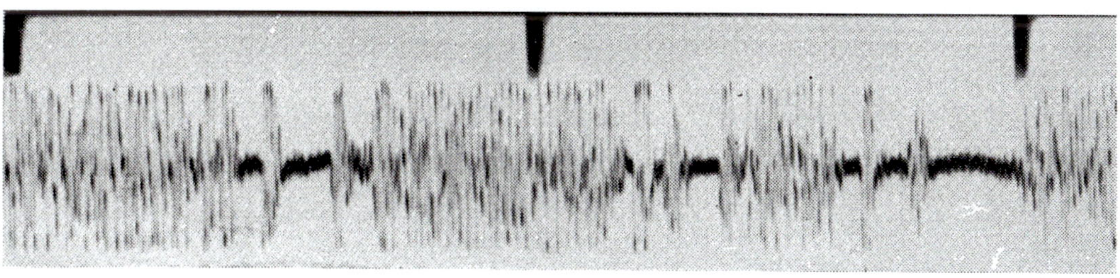

Fig. 3.19 Recording of asterixis

> dorsiflex his foot. Then, at irregular intervals there would be a sudden flexion at ankle knee or hip followed by a slower extension. In the face strong closure of the eyelids strong retraction of the corners of the mouth or pursing of the lips were required to demonstrate this peculiarity of movement. It was also seen in the protruded tongue.

Adams also described for the first time a "paratonic rigidity" of the plastic type persisting throughout both passive flexion and extension of any joint. Repeated grimacing, together with motor restlessness, also was noted to be common.

Adams and Foley also described "a blunt spike and wave" activity that later was named "triphasic wave" by Bickford and Butt [19].

The Message and Acceptance

The term *asterixis* was not mentioned in the paper or in the attached discussion that concentrated on the neuropathologist findings. According to Laureno's biography of Raymond Adams, the term was coined by Foley [132] Adams recalled that Foley, over a bottle of Metaxa in a Greek café, discussed a possible term with a classic scholar from Boston College, and they were searching for a word that indicated lack of steadiness. The term *asterixis* denoted inability to maintain posture (a-privative, sterixis-support).

Asterixis was considered "one of the most characteristic features of hepatic coma." However, Adams and Foley pointed out in their original paper that the sign had been seen in uremia, polycythemia, and heart failure and hypokalemic stupors.

Other causes for asterixis would be reported over the ensuing years, and the sign is now part of the neurologist's catalogue of clinical signs. Terms such as negative myoclonus seem confusing and have been discouraged [39]. A very good video clip of asterixis recently has been published [162].

Asterixis cannot be accurately localized in the brain, but it has been suggested that it is caused by abnormal function of diencephalic motor centers that regulate the tone of the agonist and antagonist muscles [162]. Unilateral asterixis has been seen in acute thalamic or putaminal lesions, but also in pontine and medulla oblongata lesions. Therefore, its pathophysiology and localization remain unclear [120, 122, 178].

Asterixis most commonly is seen in dialysis units and guide nephrologists as to whether dialysis is indicated. This hallmark clinical sign, however, is not commonly recognized by non-neurologists because it requires a certain positioning of hands and fingers.

Short Historical Note 11

NEUROGENIC PULMONARY EDEMA

The Title of the Paper

Weisman SJ. Edema and congestion of the lungs resulting from intracranial hemorrhage. Surgery. 1939;6:722–9.

The Paper and the Times

Moutier can be credited by suggesting in 1918—as one of the first—that pulmonary edema may have an origin in an acute lesion in the central nervous system [166]. Earlier reported cases, however, were confounded by other potential triggers of the autonomic nervous system and included seizures. For many years, pulmonary injury was seen in combat injury and appeared a major factor in early mortality [18, 211]. Gunshot wounds to the head also were associated with severe pulmonary edema soon after presentation, and in all of these instances, a central sympathetic discharge has been considered the major driver [48, 99, 145]. It was also known in poliomyelitis [10].

In the laboratory, several—each differently designed—experimental studies could produce neurogenic pulmonary edema [26, 30, 42, 190]. This included bilateral cervical vagotomy, blunt trauma to the head, simulated sudden increases in intracranial pressure, and injection of intercisternal fibrinogen and thrombin and could all result in a sympathetic storm. Other experiments produced lesions in the dorsal nuclei of the vagal nerve and medial reticular nuclei, pre-optic region, and the rostral hypothalamus, and much of this effort was to identify an "edemagenic" region [81].

However, pathologists were unable to consistently demonstrate hypothalamic lesions. Richards in his seminal study of 88 patients with pulmonary edema and acute intracranial disease found none [191].

Clinicians also noted that a decrease of consciousness was always present, superficially suggesting that the reticular activating system had to be affected. Others simply explained the phenomenon away as patients predisposed to cardiac failure or that stupor led to aspiration and chemical pneumonitis.

Pulmonary edema also could be prevented by stellate gangliotomy but not after bilateral vagotomy [150]. Some investigators suggested that the main problem was in the systemic circulation with "hyperepinephrinism", causing systemic hypertension; however, there also were investigators who suggested exactly the opposite, namely, hypotension, hemoconcentration, and injury to the lung capillaries. Clinical approaches evolved and included endotracheal intubation, positive pressure ventilation, digitalis, or α- or β-adrenergic blocking agents.

The Details of the Paper

Weisman's frequently cited study was remarkably simple but at some level informative (Fig. 3.20). The autopsy study consisted of spontaneous and traumatic hemorrhages compared with controls with no cranial, cardiac, or pulmonary disease. The purpose also was to determine whether congestion of the lungs was more often seen in fatal traumatic hemorrhages as compared with spontaneous hemorrhages. Marked differences between the weights of the lungs after a hemorrhage were found when compared with controls, but no difference in absolute weight was found between the spontaneous and traumatic hemorrhages. Most importantly, the data included information about the rapidity of the lung edema, and the data showed that edema and congestion developed in most cases within 30–60 min after the injury. Figure 3.21 shows that 57% of the traumatic hemorrhages had lungs weighing more than 900 g, but pulmonary edema was found in only 2% of controls.

Weisman's observation confirmed early pulmonary edema but did not attempt to examine the brain pathology in detail.

The Message and Acceptance

The topic remained of little clinical interest, but in 1975, an influential paper appeared in the *Lancet*. Theodore and Robin proposed a new explanation and summarized their hypothesis in a flowchart (Fig. 3.22). The basic premise was that a massive α-adrenergic discharge would cause systemic vasoconstriction that would then lead to a transiently increased pulmonary blood volume

EDEMA AND CONGESTION OF THE LUNGS RESULTING FROM INTRACRANIAL HEMORRHAGE

SYDNEY J. WEISMAN, B.S., MINNEAPOLIS, MINN.

(From the Department of Pathology, University of Minnesota Medical School)

PATHOLOGISTS have observed at the autopsy table that in cases of intracranial hemorrhage there is often a marked pulmonary edema and congestion. Many theories have been advanced, but as yet there is no unanimity of opinion concerning the basic cause. The purpose of this study is to record the condition of the lungs in 686 cases in which death was due to intracranial hemorrhage.

HISTORICAL REVIEW

Hess[1] found pulmonary edema in cases of brain tumor, epilepsy with death during a convulsion, various diseases of the medulla, and diseases of the peripheral vagus. Of special interest is his observation that pulmonary edema results from injuries to the central nervous system. He reports that Moutier in 1918 was the first to notice edema of the lungs after gunshot wounds of the head, the edema occurring within one hour after the accident, with a slow pulse and a rising blood pressure. Hess concluded that the cause of the edema of the lungs was related to both the vagus and the sympathetic innervation of the lung.

Brunn[2] produced edema of the lungs in dogs by section of the vagi followed by an intravenous injection of 1 per cent NaCl. He also noted that, if he ligatured the pedicles of the kidneys before cutting the vagi and giving intravenous NaCl, edema of the lungs did not develop.

Fig. 3.20 Title page

TABLE VI

COMBINED WEIGHTS OF THE LUNGS IN CASES OF TRAUMATIC INTRACRANIAL HEMORRHAGE IN WHICH DEATH OCCURRED WITHIN 1 HOUR

COMBINED WEIGHT OF THE LUNGS	TRAUMATIC		CONTROL	
	NUMBER	%	NUMBER	%
100-200	0	0	0	0
200-300	0	0	1	0.5
300-400	0	0	16	8.0
400-500	1	1.7	48	24.0
500-600	4	6.7	56	28.0
600-700	4	6.7	38	19.0
700-800	6	10.0	28	14.0
800-900	11	18.3	9	4.5
900-1,000	5	8.3	4	2.0
1,000-1,100	9	15.0	0	0
1,100-1,200	6	10.0	0	0
1,200-1,300	4	6.7	0	0
1,300-1,400	3	5.0	0	0
1,400-1,500	3	5.0		
1,500-1,600	3	5.0		
1,600-1,700	0	0		
1,700-1,800	0	0		
1,800-1,900	0	0		
1,900-2,000	0	0		
2,000-2,100	1	1.7		
	60	100.0	200	100.0

Fig. 3.21 Lung weights in brain injury and controls

through two mechanisms [236, 237]. One mechanism was shift of blood from the systemic to pulmonary circulation, and the other was increased aortic and systemic arterial pressure that would decrease left ventricular compliance and increase left atrial pressure. This would displace pulmonary blood volume into low pressure areas, resulting in structural pulmonary vascular injury ending up in pulmonary edema and pulmonary hemorrhages. The authors also confidently stated that there would be very little cardiac injury contributing to the entire picture. They reasoned that acute cardiac failure rarely leads to instantaneous development of pulmonary edema. Later studies, however, documented associated cardiac injury with often severe apical ballooning in patients with acute brain injury [9]. Apical ballooning also was described in patients with ruptured aneurysms and status epilepticus [79]. In these patients, the ventricular ejection fraction suddenly declined to 10–20%.

Therefore, there is increasing evidence that pulmonary edema in subarachnoid hemorrhage may have a cardiogenic origin or at least a cardiac contribution. Structural damage to the myocardium has been described with contraction bands and subendocardial myocardial injury as characteristic histologic features.

The treatment of neurogenic pulmonary edema is basically trying to improve oxygenation in a fluid-filled lung [32]. In many patients, alveoli are flooded, and there is very little aeration. Treatment is positive expiratory pressure ventilation with oxygen insufflation to the trachea, inhaled nitric oxide, and use of vasopressures and inotropes.

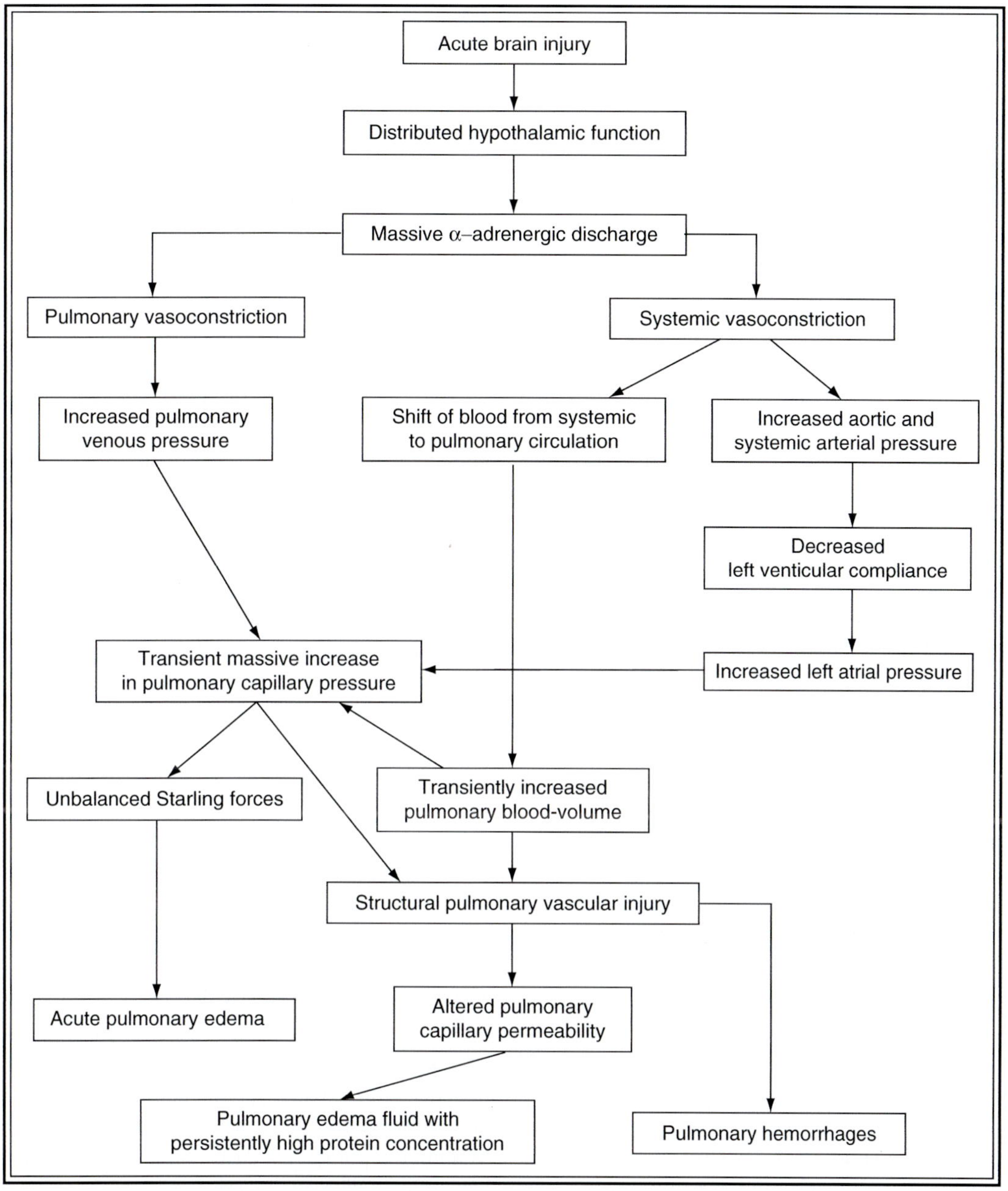

Fig. 3.22 A concept to explain neurogenic pulmonary edema

Short Historical Note 12

CEREBRAL T WAVES

The Title of the Paper

Burch GE, Meyers R, Abildskov JA. A new electrocardiographic pattern observed in cerebrovascular accidents. Circulation. 1954;9:719–23.

The Paper and the Times

Experimental studies in cats have long demonstrated that extrasystoles could be produced after stimulation of the posterior hypothalamus and nodal or ventricular rhythms after stimulation of the posterior corpora quadrigemina or even posterior portions of the cerebellum. Most interestingly, these extrasystoles could be abolished when cats' brainstems were lesioned at the "Sherrington's level of decerebration," suggesting a center above that level. A study in head injured mice found repolarization abnormalities likely as a result of vagal stimulation but not in animals pretreated with atropine [111]. Others found that electrocardiographic irregularities remained after bilateral vagal section and suggested a mechanism more likely through sympathetic pathways [65]. Intraventricular injections of caffeine citrate in cats produced a rise in blood pressure and marked cardiac arrhythmias. Therefore, most of the electrocardiographic (EKG) changes were observed in the laboratory and not in hospitals. Textbooks or papers on coronary artery disease only incidentally suggested that the changes on EKGs could be the result of acute brain injury, but none were considered "characteristic."

In 1947, Byer reported on large T waves and prolonged QT intervals, but many patients had severe hypertension, neurogenic pulmonary edema, or eclampsia, making the connection with acute brain injury less clear [28].

In 1953, Levine reported a patient with an autopsy-proven subarachnoid hemorrhage and nonspecific T-wave abnormalities but no evidence of a myocardial infarction [139].

Burch's brief report has been credited as one of the first studies in patients with recent stroke; he claimed to have described a new EKG pattern (Fig. 3.23).

The Details of the Paper

Burch described large amplitude T waves and large U waves in patients with "cerebrovascular accidents." The typical T wave had the same configuration as in myocardial ischemia and was usually negative in the standard and chest leads. Positive large T waves were found in the chest leads recorded from the right of the transition zone in lead V3. In this study of 17 patients, seven had a cerebral hemorrhage, seven had a subarachnoid hemorrhage, and three had an ischemic stroke. Most EKGs were performed within 24–48 h after the onset of symptoms but in two patients 4–7 days after the ictus. Most pronounced changes were seen in patients with subarachnoid hemorrhage. In some instances, the T waves were very large, occupying the entire interval between the R and P complexes (Fig. 3.24). In some cases, large U waves were seen in proximity to the T waves, but distinct enough to be noticed as marked deflections. The electrographic pattern was maintained for at least 9 days in three patients and more than 11 days in one patient. Additionally, 5 of the 17 described patients had bradycardia. Interestingly, several patients had hyperglycemia. The authors could not explain the mechanism, and surprisingly, there were no measurements of electrolytes or acid–base balance presented that might have caused alterations in T waves.

The Message and Acceptance

After the Burch et al. paper, two case series appeared. Wasserman [251] described 12 patients with mostly subarachnoid hemorrhage and intracerebral hemorrhage, and Cropp and Manning reported 29 cases with subarachnoid hemorrhage with five autopsies of the heart that were unrevealing [52]. Later papers described electrographic changes in traumatic brain injuries, and EKG changes also were noted during brain operations, pneumoencephalography, cerebral tumors, poliomyelitis, and cerebral hemorrhage. Hersch claimed that an increased QT interval and increased voltage of the P wave was far more characteristic in traumatic brain injury [98].

T-wave abnormalities usually cannot be considered without close observation of the QRS

A New Electrocardiographic Pattern Observed in Cerebrovascular Accidents

By G. E. Burch, M.D., Robert Meyers, M.D., and J. A. Abildskov, M.D.

An electrocardiographic pattern was encountered in patients with cerebrovascular accidents which consisted primarily of T waves of large amplitude and duration. Large U waves were often present which may fuse in part or entirely within the T wave. Because of the presence and fusion of the T and U waves, the prolonged Q-T interval associated with the pattern was most probably a Q-U interval.

During the past several years a distinctive electrocardiographic pattern has been observed in some patients with cerebrovascular accidents at the Charity Hospital at New Orleans. No reference to this association was found in the literature, although others have observed changes in the electrocardiograms of patients with cerebrovascular accidents.[1, 2, 3] Since no detailed description of the electrocardiographic pattern has been published, it is not possible to compare the pattern reported here with the isolated electrocardiographic changes noted by others.

In its most characteristic form, the pattern consists essentially of T waves of considerable amplitude and width and a long Q-T interval. Prolongation of the Q-T interval has been mentioned in association with cerebrovascular accidents,[3] but there has been no detailed description of the configuration of the associated T wave.

A review of the case histories of patients with a diagnosis of cerebral hemorrhage, subarachnoid hemorrhage or unclassified cerebrovascular accidents at Charity Hospital during the year 1950 revealed 10 electrocardiograms with the syndrome. In addition, tracings with this pattern from one private patient,* two patients observed in 1949, one in 1951 and three in 1952 were included, making a total of 17 electrocardiograms included in this report.

Table 1 summarizes certain clinical data concerning the patients whose electrocardiograms were studied. In most instances the diagnosis of cerebrovascular accident was established by clinical study alone. Hemorrhage was demonstrated by spinal puncture in 14 of the 17 patients, and in the remaining three parenchymal hemorrhage or arterial thrombosis (classified as C.V.A. in table 1) was diagnosed on the basis of neurologic manifestations.

Results

Results are summarized in table 1 and figures 1, 2 and 3.

Q-T Interval. The Q-T interval was pro-

Fig. 3.23 Title page

and ST segments. T waves become abnormal in ventricular hypertrophy, left bundle branch block, hyperkalemia, and pericarditis [139], but the predominant theory in "cerebral" T waves is a surge of catecholamines. Experimental studies also found a right sided dominance of the insular cortex, but this association has not been consistently found in clinical studies [103, 173, 235].

The origin of these T waves was further questioned by Koskelo et al., who felt that subendocardial hemorrhages could explain cerebral T waves and other transient EKG abnormalities [127]. Persistently high levels of calcium would explain the hypercontracted state followed by cell membrane destruction. Hyperkalemia would explain the peaked T waves on the EKG.

In current practice, most of the EKG abnormalities are seen after massive cerebral hemorrhage and aneurysmal subarachnoid hemorrhage. Most are QT prolongation, ST-segment changes, and either large, flattened, or inverted T waves [38].

Prolonged QT interval has been noted after ischemic stroke, and a correlation with poor outcome has been identified [4, 133]. A recent retrospective study found ST- and T-wave abnormalities, most commonly T-wave inversions and ST elevations, in 27% of patients with EKG readings. None of these abnormalities predicted fatal arrhythmias. Echocardiographic studies have repeatedly shown ventricular dysfunction in these patients. One study found corresponding regional wall motion abnormalities in patients with transient ST-segment elevation. Another study found that inverted T waves and QT segment prolongation were significantly correlated with left ventricular function [265].

Nonetheless, the cerebral T waves remain quite common in the spectrum of EKG abnormalities associated with acute major brain injury. Cardiologists are rarely thrilled when these T waves are found and virtually always suppose a "cerebral" cause.

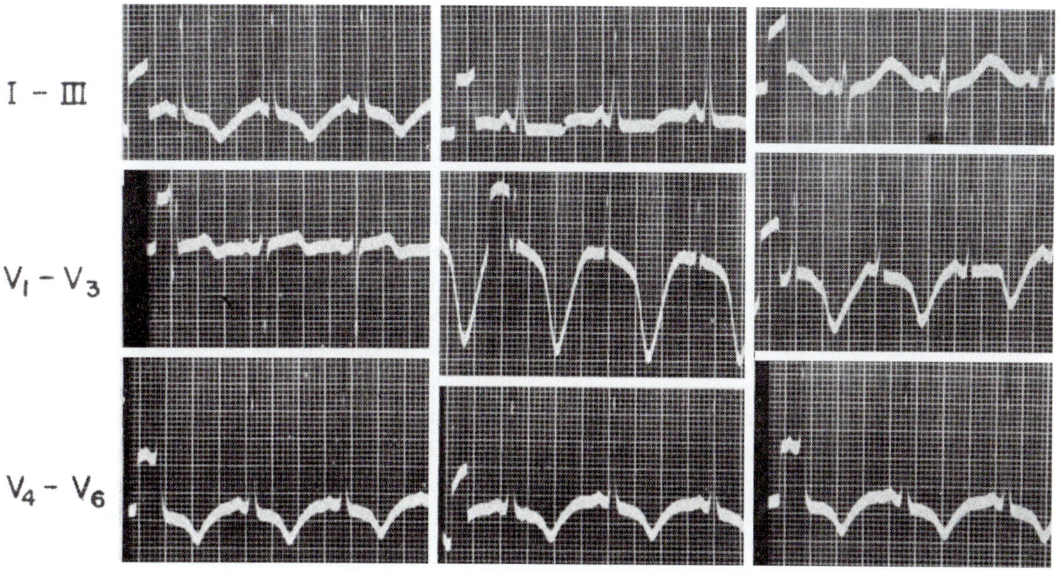

Fig. 3.24 Patient with ischemic stroke and electrocardiogram 72 h after ictus with typical (negative) T waves

Short Historical Note 13

NEUROGENIC CARDIAC INJURY

The Title of the Paper

Koskelo P, Punsar S, Sipilä W. Subarachnoid hemorrhage and ECG changes in intracranial bleeding. BMJ. 1964; 1:1479–80.

Doshi R, Neil-Dwyer G. Hypothalamic and myocardial lesions after subarachnoid hemorrhage. J Neurol Neurosurg Psychiatry. 1977;40:824–26.

The Paper and the Times

For many years, electrocardiographic (EKG) changes after acute brain injury were mistaken for acute myocardial infarction. Surgery was postponed or patients were subjected to coronary angiography, only to find normal anatomy. Earlier, autopsy studies of the heart found no abnormalities, but careful microscopic review of the myocardium under these circumstances was uncommon. Most concerning clinical scenarios were patients presumably presenting with chest and head pain, EKG changes suggesting myocardial injury, admission to a coronary care unit, anticoagulation treatment, and rerupture of a cerebral aneurysm later but with normal myocardium and coronary arteries at autopsy [17, 254]. In contrast, some authors found "gross excess of coronary occlusion" in middle aged men who died from ruptured aneurysms [197].

Cardiac lesions from experimental brain lesions had been reproduced multiple times in different species such as dogs, baboons, and mice [95, 196]. Subendocardial hemorrhage could be produced by stellate ganglion stimulation [123]. Proof that the central nervous system was involved came with Melville studies [161]. Stimulation of the anterior hypothalamus resulting in ST-segment depression on EKG could—after repeated stimulation—produce cytoplasmic eosinophilia, loss of cross striations (the alternating segments of thick and thin protein filaments), and hemorrhage. Hall would later reproduce this "myocardial cell degeneration" already several hours after hypothalamic stimulation [91].

Norepinephrine infusion could produce similar findings, and this phenomenon was called "L-norepinephrine myocarditis" [230]. Jacob et al. also reported myocardial changes, as well as suggesting a pathway to explain these injuries after experimentally causing subarachnoid hemorrhage. Hypertension occurred with a variety of severe cardiac arrhythmias and ultrastructure abnormalities with close resemblance to norepinephrine injections [110].

The question remained whether these changes could be found in humans. In 1954, Smith and Fomlinson published an autopsy study of 235 patients with fatal intracranial disease and found 29 patients with subendocardial hemorrhage [213]. (In contrast, there were only three patients with subendocardial hemorrhage in 607 autopsies without intracranial pathology). Studies had not combined EKG changes with myocardial pathology in acute brain injury.

The Details of the Paper

Three patients with a ruptured intracranial aneurysm were reported 10 years after the first clinical description of EKG abnormalities by Burch et al. These cases were then compared with a fourth case with a typical recent anteroseptal infarction, but no intracranial disease and striking similarities in EKG changes were found. The autopsy in these three patients with deep negative T-waves or positive T-U fusion waves showed subendocardial hemorrhages (Fig. 3.25).

Macroscopically, the hearts were normal except for left ventricular hypertrophy and coronary arteries were atherosclerotic but not occluded. The findings included "numerous small and confluent spots of subendocardial hemorrhages at the left ventricular side of the interventricular septum." In case 2, hemorrhages were found in the papillary muscles. They concluded "contrary to earlier explanations, we believe then that ECG changes found in connection with intracranial bleeding are caused by cardiac lesions and that they do not simulate myocardial ischemia or injury but are in fact signs of them."

Although hypothalamic lesions had been found after subarachnoid hemorrhage [51], a major work appeared in 1977 by Doshi et al., (Fig. 3.26) linking the cardiac pathology to hypothalamic lesions. Twelve patients with subarach-

Fig. 3.25 Title paper

Subendocardial Haemorrhage and E.C.G. Changes in Intracranial Bleeding

PENTTI KOSKELO,* M.D.; SVEN PUNSAR,† M.D.; WALTER SIPILÄ,‡ M.D.

Brit. med. J., 1964, **1**, 1479–1480

E.C.G. changes in connexion with intracranial (especially subarachnoidal) bleeding resembling those in myocardial infarction were first described by Burch *et al.* in 1954. The most typical change is a deep and broad T-U fusion wave in several leads. The explanation of the changes observed remains obscure (Effert *et al.*, 1961).

The purpose of this paper is to discuss the genesis of these E.C.G. changes on the basis of three cases in which both the typical E.C.G. changes and subendocardial haemorrhages were found.

Case Reports

Case 1

A 54-year-old housewife who had previously been in good health was admitted on 29 November 1959. For the last three years she had gone swimming in winter-time in a hole cut in the ice—a type of winter sport not uncommon in Finland. After one such swim she suddenly collapsed and was brought to the hospital. Examination on admission showed a well-nourished woman with severe pulmonary oedema. The heart sounds were distant and there were no murmurs. Blood-pressure was 185/105 mm. Hg. Consciousness was clear and there were no signs of pareses. The E.C.G. on admission showed slightly negative T-waves in leads I, II, and V_4 through V_6. A myocardial infarction was suspected.

She recovered quickly from the pulmonary oedema and felt better, except for increasing headache. On the following morning a slight stiffness of the neck was noticed and a lumbar puncture revealed bloody spinal fluid. A subarachnoidal haemorrhage was diagnosed. An E.C.G. now showed deep and wide negative T-U fusion waves in all leads except lead III, aVR, and V_1, in which the fusion wave was positive (see Fig.). S.G.O.T. was normal on two successive days.

During the days that followed the headache gradually diminished, the blood content of the spinal fluid decreased, and the E.C.G. changes became less severe. On the eighth day in hospital she had a second intracranial haemorrhage and died two days later.

Necropsy revealed a ruptured aneurysm of the left internal carotid artery at the junction of the posterior communicating and middle cerebral arteries. The left temporal lobe showed some oedema and a few petechiae. The heart weighed 375 g. The coronary arteries were fully open and devoid of any atherosclerosis. The myocardium and the heart valves were macroscopically normal. Numerous small and confluent spots of subendocardial haemorrhages were seen at the left ventricular side

arachnoid haemorrhage was made. An E.C.G. taken on the first day in hospital showed biphasic or negative T-U fusion waves in leads I, II, aVL, and V_2 through V_6 and a positive T-U fusion wave in lead aVR. QRS was somewhat notched in leads I, II, aVR, and aVL. The E.C.G. changes were more marked two days later (see Fig.) and thereafter began to show some improvement.

The patient became subjectively symptomless in a few days. On the seventeenth day in the hospital she suddenly developed pulmonary oedema, lost consciousness, and died in a few hours.

Necropsy revealed a ruptured aneurysm of the right middle cerebral artery at its first major division and a haematoma 5 cm. in diameter in the right cerebral hemisphere. The heart weighed 500 g. The left ventricle was slightly hypertrophied. The myocardium and the heart valves were macroscopically normal. The coronary arteries were fully open and they were only slightly atheromatous. Several petechial haemorrhages were seen under the left ventricular endocardium, mainly at the septum and the papillary muscles.

Case 3

A 65-year-old married woman was admitted on 2 July 1960 because of a left-sided hemiparesis and loss of consciousness. Her blood-pressure had been raised for several years. Examination showed a well-nourished woman. Heart and lungs were normal on auscultation. Blood-pressure was 235/130 mm. Hg. The liver was palpable three fingerbreadths below the costal margin. There was no oedema. Spinal fluid was clear on admission but later contained blood. Serum potassium was normal. An E.C.G. on admission (see Fig.) revealed flat T-waves in leads I, II, aVR, aVL, and V_6. Deep negative T-waves were present in leads V_1 through V_5. High R-waves suggested the presence of left ventricular hypertrophy. The T changes were much less pronounced three days later.

She died on the fifth day in hospital without gaining consciousness. At necropsy a massive haemorrhage was found in the right cerebral hemisphere. The heart weighed 310 g. The coronary arteries were moderately atheromatous but not obstructed. The myocardium and the valves were macroscopically normal. Several small subendocardial haemorrhages were seen at the left side of the interventricular septum and at the anterior wall of the left ventricle.

To sum up, the three cases presented above showed changes in the E.C.G. typical of those described in intracranial bleeding, and at necropsy subendocardial haemorrhages in the left chamber of the heart.

Hypothalamic and myocardial lesions after subarachnoid haemorrhage

R. DOSHI AND G. NEIL-DWYER

From the Departments of Neuropathology and Neurological Surgery, Brook General Hospital, London

SUMMARY The hypothalamus and myocardium of 12 patients who had died after a subarachnoid haemorrhage, and of six patients who had died from other intracranial pathology were examined. Only in the patients who had died from subarachnoid haemorrhage were histological lesions found in both the hypothalamus and myocardium. The possible significance of these findings is discussed with particular reference to the sympathetic nervous system.

Increased and prolonged sympathetic activity in patients after subarachnoid haemorrhage (Tomomatsu *et al.*, 1964; Iliynsky and Astrakhantseva, 1967; Neil-Dwyer *et al.*, 1974) has been strongly linked with a variety of electrocardiographic (ECG) abnormalities occurring in this disorder (Cruickshank *et al.*, 1974). Although there is substantial indirect evidence to support this statement, direct evidence is scanty. Myocardial lesions associated with a subarachnoid haemorrhage have been well documented (Conor, 1969), and similar lesions have been produced in animals either by stimulation of the hypothalamus (Melville *et al.*, 1963; Zavodskaya *et al.*, 1972), or with the parenteral administration of catecholamines (Reichenbach and Benditt, 1970).

Hypothalamic damage in patients after subarachnoid haemorrhage has been well described (Crompton, 1963; Smith, 1963) while a variety of animal experimental work has shown that abnormal hypothalamic function can lead to myocardial damage and cardiovascular disturbances (Melville *et al.*, 1963; Greenhoot and Reichenbach, 1969; Zavodskaya *et al.*, 1972). As yet there has been no clinicopathological study establishing whether there is a correlation between hypothalamic and myocardial lesions occurring in subarachnoid haemorrhage, a requisite if the pathophysiology of this condition is to be understood.

Patients and methods

All patients were admitted into the Neurosurgical Unit at the Brook General Hospital between January and September 1975. The patients were divided into two groups, group 1 containing 12 patients who had died after a subarachnoid haemorrhage, and group 2, a control group of six patients who died from a variety of causes, all of which produced raised intracranial pressure. The necropsies in group 1 were consecutive.

Of the 12 patients in group 1, eight were female and four male, the age range was 21–66 years, and the clinical details are given in Table 1; in group 2 there were four female patients and two male, and the age range was 20–62 years. The majority of patients in the subarachnoid haemorrhage group followed a fairly typical clinical course with a fluctuating but deteriorating level of consciousness, varying blood pressures and pulse rates (Table 1). Electrocardiograms (ECG) were recorded in six cases (Table 1), and in five of these were considered to be abnormal.

Fig. 3.26 Title paper

noid hemorrhage were described, and in six cases, perivascular hemorrhages and periventricular edema that included the paraventricular nucleus and supraoptic nucleus were reported. In one comatose patient with short PR interval, long QTc, and inverted T-wave abnormalities, a complete infarction of the hypothalamus was discovered. Sections of the medulla oblongata were normal. The cardiac histology showed necrosis of muscle fibers with interstitial infiltration by polymorphonuclear leucocytes and macrophages. Myocardial fibers were mangled and separated. The authors felt the myofibrillar degeneration with the ventricular injury was reminiscent of pheochromocytoma.

The Message and Acceptance

These papers were followed by multiple publications showing similar EKG changes but none with descriptions of subendocardial hemorrhages [72, 108, 128, 163, 217].

In 1984, a major autopsy study by Kolin and Norris appeared. The presence of myocardial damage was specifically studied in a series of 58 patients and compared with a control group. The underlying disorders were ischemic stroke, brain tumor, subarachnoid hemorrhage, and meningitis in that order. Transmurally scattered foci of myocardial injury were found in 62% but also in 26% of controls. All patients who died from intracranial causes had presumed increased intracranial pressure. The authors did conclude that these lesions could represent "a harmless epiphenomenon of acute intracranial lesions" [126].

Over time, it became clear that many cardiac abnormalities were reversible with EKG abnormalities normalizing after showing dramatic initial reduction in ejection fraction [135]. In some patients, cardiac injury was associated with underlying coronary artery disease and abnormalities could remain permanent.

Acute brain injury can cause cardiogenic shock—similar to what is seen in "broken heart syndrome" (a reversible but potentially fatal condition brought on by sudden overwhelming stress). The relation between middle aged women in broken heart syndrome, and common occurrence of aneurysmal subarachnoid hemorrhage in middle aged women is fascinating and suggests a common mechanism.

Short Historical Note 14

CUSHING ULCER

The Title of the Paper

Cushing H. Peptic ulcer and the interbrain. Surg Gynec Obst. 1932;55:1–34.

The Paper and the Times

Around the turn of the nineteenth century, "stress" became a research topic, and the science of what stress could do to the body has been credited to Hans Seyle. He proposed a physiologic explanation of stress implicating the hypothalamic–pituitary–adrenal axis and eventually leading to the identification of a corticotrophin-releasing factor. Seyle also has been credited with finding gastric ulcers in rats exposed to stress. Unimaginable today, in these experiments, stress was recreated using randomly applied electric shocks to the rat's tail. Seyle described the so-called stress triad: adrenal hypertrophy, gastrointestinal ulcers, and thymolymphatic atrophy. This concept was further supported by pathologists who recognized that adrenal lesions were associated with gastric ulcers.

The link between the stomach and the brain has been recognized for some time, especially by pathologists. Carl Rokitansky, who published the text *Handbuch Der Pathologischen Anatomie* (1883), described in considerable detail examples of patients with acute perforating ulcers after an acute brain injury Rokitansky was one of the first physicians pointing out such a link and according to Harvey Cushing, Rokitansky was responsible for the following fact:

> There survives in Vienna once it has spread into many pathological laboratories throughout the world, a tradition of the dead house, in effect that ulcerative destruction of the stomach is most often found in the bodies of persons who while digesting have died from a intracranial disorder particularly when it was associated with a terminal fever of high degree.

Although multiple other pathologists had commented on the association before, Rokitansky assumed that the ulcer was created through vagal nerve activity. Mogilnitzkie, from the University of Moscow, published an experimental study showing that stimulation of diencephalon—and in particular, the corpus luysii—resulted in hemorrhages and erosions and perforations in the stomach and duodenum.

Before Cushing's observation, there were no detailed clinical descriptions of stress ulcers after a major acute brain injury.

The Details of the Paper

The basis of this eponym is a paper published in *Surgery, Gynecology and Obstetrics* in 1932 (Fig. 3.27) in which Harvey Cushing describes patients who died unexpectedly from perforated peptic ulcers soon after surgery. Cushing described a series of patients with pathologically proven perforations of the stomach and esophagus:

> What has incited my interest in the subject has been the disturbing experience of having lost three patients from acute perforations of the upper alimentary canal soon after what appeared to be successful operations for the removal of intracranial tumors, and that each of these tumors happen to be situated in a cerebellum could not it seems to me be other than some significance.

All three patients with large cerebellar tumors developed what appeared to be clinical signs of a general peritonitis with widespread submucosal hemorrhages and perforations in the cardia found at autopsy (Fig. 3.28). The perforative peritonitis was completely unexpected as a postoperative complication in all three cases. In one patient, the abdomen became distended and sensitive. Another patient experienced a "sudden violent epigastric pain which spread over the abdomen and into the shoulders." In another case, there was "copious vomiting of brownish black fluid." As befitted Cushing, he then describes a review of his surgical cases of patients with cerebellar astrocytoma, and he identified several more cases in retrospect. Cushing advanced several theories [58, 59]. One included the bile-vomiting theory suggesting that hemorrhagic ulceration could be produced by a combination of bile and acid in a patient who had postoperative vomiting after recovering from the anesthetic. Another theory was the association of

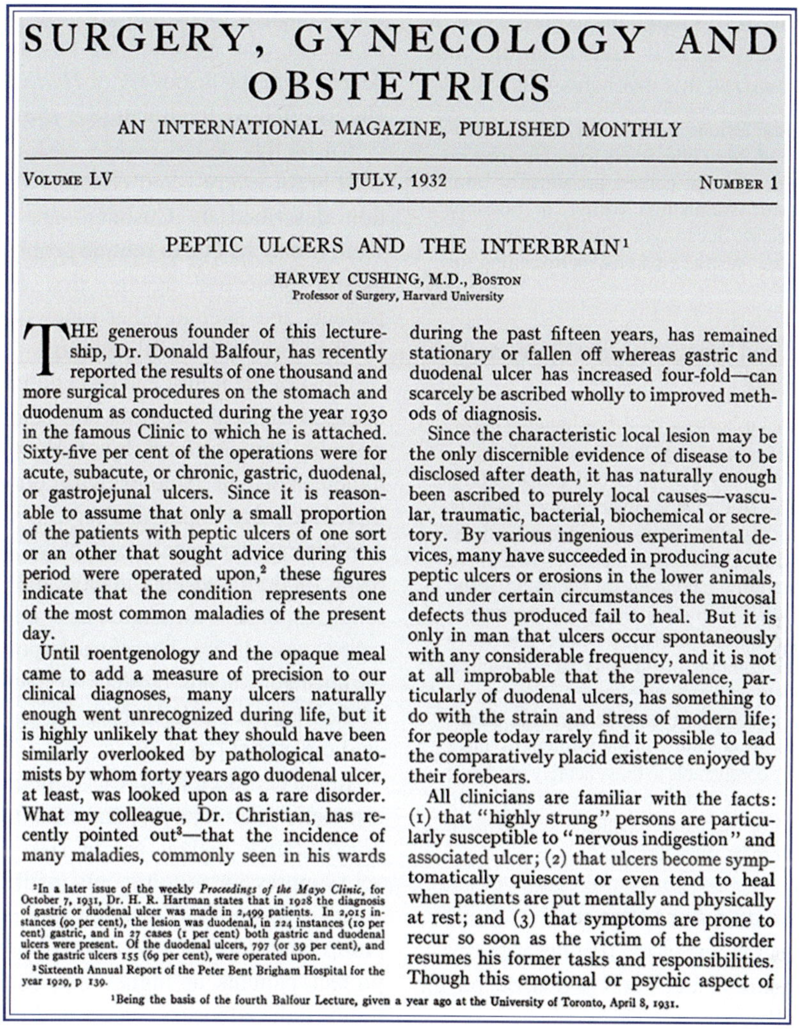

SURGERY, GYNECOLOGY AND OBSTETRICS

AN INTERNATIONAL MAGAZINE, PUBLISHED MONTHLY

VOLUME LV JULY, 1932 NUMBER 1

PEPTIC ULCERS AND THE INTERBRAIN[1]

HARVEY CUSHING, M.D., BOSTON
Professor of Surgery, Harvard University

THE generous founder of this lectureship, Dr. Donald Balfour, has recently reported the results of one thousand and more surgical procedures on the stomach and duodenum as conducted during the year 1930 in the famous Clinic to which he is attached. Sixty-five per cent of the operations were for acute, subacute, or chronic, gastric, duodenal, or gastrojejunal ulcers. Since it is reasonable to assume that only a small proportion of the patients with peptic ulcers of one sort or an other that sought advice during this period were operated upon,[2] these figures indicate that the condition represents one of the most common maladies of the present day.

Until roentgenology and the opaque meal came to add a measure of precision to our clinical diagnoses, many ulcers naturally enough went unrecognized during life, but it is highly unlikely that they should have been similarly overlooked by pathological anatomists by whom forty years ago duodenal ulcer, at least, was looked upon as a rare disorder. What my colleague, Dr. Christian, has recently pointed out[3]—that the incidence of many maladies, commonly seen in his wards during the past fifteen years, has remained stationary or fallen off whereas gastric and duodenal ulcer has increased four-fold—can scarcely be ascribed wholly to improved methods of diagnosis.

Since the characteristic local lesion may be the only discernible evidence of disease to be disclosed after death, it has naturally enough been ascribed to purely local causes—vascular, traumatic, bacterial, biochemical or secretory. By various ingenious experimental devices, many have succeeded in producing acute peptic ulcers or erosions in the lower animals, and under certain circumstances the mucosal defects thus produced fail to heal. But it is only in man that ulcers occur spontaneously with any considerable frequency, and it is not at all improbable that the prevalence, particularly of duodenal ulcers, has something to do with the strain and stress of modern life; for people today rarely find it possible to lead the comparatively placid existence enjoyed by their forebears.

All clinicians are familiar with the facts: (1) that "highly strung" persons are particularly susceptible to "nervous indigestion" and associated ulcer; (2) that ulcers become symptomatically quiescent or even tend to heal when patients are put mentally and physically at rest; and (3) that symptoms are prone to recur so soon as the victim of the disorder resumes his former tasks and responsibilities. Though this emotional or psychic aspect of

[2] In a later issue of the weekly *Proceedings of the Mayo Clinic*, for October 7, 1931, Dr. H. R. Hartman states that in 1928 the diagnosis of gastric or duodenal ulcer was made in 2,499 patients. In 2,015 instances (90 per cent), the lesion was duodenal, in 224 instances (10 per cent) gastric, and in 27 cases (1 per cent) both gastric and duodenal ulcers were present. Of the duodenal ulcers, 797 (or 39 per cent), and of the gastric ulcers 155 (69 per cent), were operated upon.

[3] Sixteenth Annual Report of the Peter Bent Brigham Hospital for the year 1929, p 139.

[1] Being the basis of the fourth Balfour Lecture, given a year ago at the University of Toronto, April 8, 1931.

Fig. 3.27 Title page

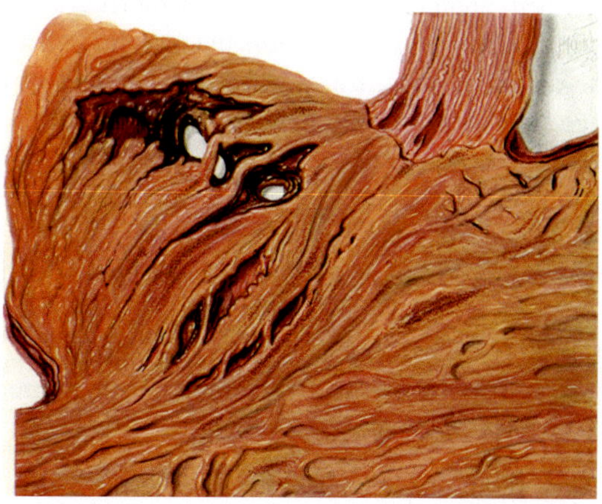

Fig. 3.28 Gross appearance of mucosal surface of stomach and lower esophagus showing hemorrhages and three large perforations

gastric erosions with malignant hypertension, an association that was well known at the time. Cushing summarized this mechanism as follows:

> Extrapyramidal lesions anywhere from the intracranial course of these fiber tracts from the anterior hypothalamus to vagal center, presumably from parasympathetic stimulation within, or possibly from vagal release due to sympathetic paralysis are prone to cause gastric erosions, perforations, or ulcers.

He continued and speculated that there might be an ulcer propensity:

> It is reasonable to believe, therefore, that the perforations following the cerebellar operations forming the base of this study were produced in like fashion by an irritative disturbance either of fiber tracts or vagal centers in the brainstem. … so it may easily be that highly strung persons who incline to the form of nervous instability classified as parasympathetic (vagotonic), through emotion or repressed emotion, incidental to continued worry and anxiety and heavy responsibility, combined with other factors such as irregular meals and excessive use of tobacco, are particularly prone to have chronic digestion disturbances with hyperacidity often leading to ulcer effects wholly comparable to those acutely produced by irritative lesions experimentally made anywhere in the course of the parasympathetic system from tuberal center to its vagal terminals.

The Message and Acceptance

Cushing's paper is one of the first descriptions of a neurogenic stress ulcer and a treatise on the brain–stomach connection [255].

Two years later, Masten (neuropsychiatrist) and Bunts (pathologist) from the University of Wisconsin, Madison, described another eight comatose patients ("each of the patients … could not have felt the pain of the rupture") with meningitis, cerebral hemorrhage, and brain tumors confirming Cushing's observations [156]. The authors agreed with "Cushing's hypothesis of a parasympathetic center in the diencephalon."

Cushing would believe that his own ulcer, which he developed later in life, was caused by things that would upset him [255]. But the psychosomatic theory of the ulcer personality (the tendency to pentup frustrations leading to increased acid production) has largely disappeared with the discovery of *Helicobacter pylori* and its effective treatment [87, 158].

Currently, acute gastric lesions associated with brain injury—and certainly of the proportion described by Cushing—are uncommonly seen. It may be due to routine prophylactic use of gastric protective agents, first used in burn patients and later in other types of critically ill mechanically ventilated patients.

Most of the injury can be explained by a combination of local ischemia and acid. Blood flow may be compromised by marked episodes of hypotension. In patients with polytrauma and increased parasympathetic nervous system activation through the vagal nerve plays a crucial role. More modern concepts involve the sympathoadrenal response with angiotensin constricting the gastric vasculature. Therefore, hypoperfusion and diminished mucous production and compromise of the mucous barrier expose the gastric lining to acidic material [263].

In the neurosciences ICU, patients with severe traumatic brain injury, spinal cord injury, and any postoperative patient are at risk. Prophylactic acid suppression is commonly instituted and after an era of histamine-2 receptor antagonists, proton pump inhibitors became a preferred treatment to protect patients at higher risk for acute brain injury induced gastric ulcers and gastric hemorrhage. It is clear that many patients will have to be treated to prevent one vtransfusion-required gastric hemorrhage and estimates may indicate a less than 1% incidence of significant gastric hemorrhages. The role of *H. pylori* in stress-related ulcers also is unclear, although increased incidence was found in one ICU study. Whether treatment with antibiotics is justified remains unresolved [143, 199, 229]

Mortality in critically ill patients with gastric hemorrhage is substantial, but it is a reflection of the underlying illness. The risks in critically ill neurologic patients are less well known.

Short Historical Note 15

CEREBRAL SALT-WASTING SYNDROME

The Title of the Paper

Peters JP, Welt LG, Sims EAH, Orloff J, Needham J. A salt-wasting syndrome associated with cerebral disease. Trans Assoc Am Physicians. 1950;63:57–64.

The Paper and the Times

As early as 1858, Claude Bernard discovered that a unilateral lesion of the reticular formation produced chlorine diuresis without excretion of glucose [60]. Bilateral lesions further accentuated the chlorine loss, but the response was not inhibited by renal denervation. Others suggested that some connection between the hypothalamus and the proximal tubule of the kidney could exist. The experiments of Jungmann and Meyer (1913) and Hume (1949) found that lesions in the medulla and anterior hypothalamus could produce polyuria and increased sodium excretion in the urine [107, 118].

Hyponatremia, however, became recognized after the wide availability of the flame photometer [82]. Clinicians during this time epoch noted hyponatremia most commonly in patients with tuberculous meningitis but also in those with Guillain-Barré syndrome, extending the link of sodium dysregulation to involvement of the peripheral nervous system.

The first observations of hyponatremia in brain disorders came from Yale University Medical Center, first by Peters in 1950 and later by Cort in 1952 [50]. Peters et al.'s paper spurred a series of case reports on cerebral salt wasting (CSW) in traumatic brain injury, encephalitis, and brain tumors.

The Details of the Paper

In 1950, Peters and associates described three patients (one with encephalitis, one with stroke, and one with a brain stem tumor) with severe hyponatremia in whom balance studies revealed excessive sodium loss in the urine during severe hyponatremia (Fig. 3.29). Hyponatremia could not be corrected by high salt intake or mineralocorticoid administration, and urinary secretion of sodium remained high. Adrenal and pituitary function tests were normal. Clinically, these patients exhibited dehydration, and after volume expansion, the loss of sodium in urine increased.

Because the central nervous system disease was diffuse, the authors could not find a probable site that was responsible for this excessive salt wasting. They offered two hypotheses. The first explanation was excitation of the pituitary gland. Such a lesion may "disorganize an automatic sequence that normally leads to the secretion of adrenocorticotropic hormone and in turn of salt retaining hormone from the adrenal cortex." Peters and associates also speculated that there could be a direct influence off the brain on the kidney, which in turn could modify the tubular salt reabsorption. Abnormality in the nerves supplied to the kidneys could lead to this change in renal hemodynamics.

Why this salt wasting existed in acute brain lesions was further elaborated on in an additional discussion, with one of the contributors suggesting that perhaps CSW might be a compensatory mechanism of the brain to reduce brain swelling. The argument against this concept was that these patients had significant hyponatremias, and with the correction of hyponatremia, the patients' level of consciousness improved.

The clinical implications of CSW syndrome were well understood. Peters noted:

> I tried to bring out the point that this reduction of serum electrolytes is not a reaction that can be neglected, but that it has very serious implications that are manifested not only in systemic symptoms, but also in cerebral symptoms. In the first patient, for example, when we raised his sodium to normal and restored his electrolytes, he became alert for the first time, and the mental improvement after that was striking. I do not believe, therefore, that this is a protective mechanism, because reversing it seems to benefit the cerebrum.

In the three cases, the sodium levels declined to 124, 118, and 117 mEq/L, respectively. An increase in salt intake led all patients to respond with an increase in plasma sodium. Eventually, the discussants decided that the most probable explanation for urinary sodium loss was decreased proximal tubular reabsorption of sodium.

A SALT-WASTING SYNDROME ASSOCIATED WITH CEREBRAL DISEASE

By JOHN P. PETERS

AND (By Invitation)

L. G. WELT, E. A. H. SIMS, J. ORLOFF, and J. NEEDHAM

NEW HAVEN, CONN.

There is evidence that intracranial structures other than the supra-optico-hypophyseal system and the anterior lobe of the pituitary are involved in the regulation of the volume and tonicity of the body fluids. Certain lesions of the cerebrum[1,2] may be associated with a primary polydipsia. Recently it has been demonstrated[3] that lesions in the ventromedian nucleus of the hypothalamus of the rat which are usually associated with hyperphagia are also accompanied by an apparent inability to recognize the need for an adequate intake of water. This has been termed "hypothalamic hypodipsia" and is accompanied by evidences of chronic dehydration. Jungmann and Meyer[4] reported a polyuria with increased excretion of salt in the urine following experimentally induced lesions in the medulla. The polyuria was not abolished by restricting water intake, and salt excretion continued despite a salt-poor diet. They concluded that these effects were mediated by the kidneys in response to a direct nervous stimulus from the site of the lesion. Hume[5] has reported the absence of a normal eosinopenic response to stress in the dog in the presence of a destructive lesion in the anterior hypothalamus. Hilden[6] has reported the association of hypochloremia with hypertensive encephalopathy in five patients. Although reports from two groups of investigators[7,8] provide evidence that direct nervous and vascular connections between the hypothalamus and the anterior pituitary are not essential for the discharge of adrenocorticotrophic hormone in acute stress, it is conceivable that some degree of adrenal cortical insufficiency might be related to an extra-pituitary lesion of the central nervous system.

Depressed concentrations of chloride in the cerebrospinal fluid have been reported in cases of tuberculous meningitis, cerebellar tumors, encephalitis, and poliomyelitis.[9,10] Since the concentration of chloride in cerebrospinal fluid parallels the concentration of this ion in the water of serum, such patients would be expected to have low concentrations

(From the Department of Internal Medicine, Yale University School of Medicine. New Haven, Connecticut)

Fig. 3.29 Title page

The Message and Acceptance

After this first report, Cort in a follow-up paper named the condition "cerebral salt wasting" while reporting a markedly dehydrated patient with a thalamic tumor [50]. This location also suggested a possible connection between the hypothalamus and the proximal tubule of the kidney involved with sodium reabsorption.

CSW became less frequently described and was replaced by the so-called inappropriate antidiuretic hormone syndrome (SIADH). In 1957, Schwartz and co-workers described two patients with bronchogenic carcinoma who presented with such a syndrome [200]. In this disorder, continuous secretions of ADH—not appropriate to changes in plasma osmolality—result in expansion of intervascular volume and dilutional hyponatremia [15].

Since this first description, many other CNS disorders became associated with SIADH, including herpes simplex encephalitis, tuberculous meningitis, brain abscess, cerebral infarction, and brain tumors. Sterns and Silver noted "for over 20 years, the term CSW virtually vanished from the literature" [219].

However, later researchers felt that SIADH was diagnosed too often without a valid basis. In several patients, plasma ADH levels were normal. The term CSW resurfaced and is now again considered the main mechanism of hyponatremia after acute brain injury. Therefore, over the years, hyponatremia after acute brain injury became CSW, SIADH, and CSW again [67, 264]. Some even believe both disorders are present at the same time.

Where did the challenge start? Paul Nelson, a neurosurgeon, studied hyponatremia (using isotope studies) after aneurysmal subarachnoid hemorrhage and found contracted blood volumes [168]. Later studies documented increased natriuretic peptides, negative sodium balance, and reduced central venous pressure [257, 258, 259]. Other studies corroborated these findings and documented hypovolemia in virtually all hyponatremic patients [148].

Current thinking is that CSW is truly a renal salt wasting (RSW) syndrome. One possible clinical way to differentiate between RSW and SIADH in intracranial disease is the determination of serum urate (markedly decreased in RSW) and fractional urate excretion [146, 147, 149].

The fascination with the cause of hyponatremia after acute brain injury continues. With considerable manipulation of fluid status in so many patients in the intensive care unit, it has become very difficult to reliably make accurate diagnosis unless the fluid balance is carefully regulated and standardized.

The treatment is the same—an increase in salt intake—leading Sterns and Silver to note that "perhaps cerebral salt wanting syndrome is the name that fits best" [219].

Short Historical Note 16

NEUROLEPTIC MALIGNANT SYNDROME

The Title of the Paper

Delay J, Pichot P, Lempérière T, et al. Un neuroleptique majeur non phénothiazinique et non réserpinique, l'haloperidol, dans le traitement des psychoses. Ann Med Psychol (Paris). 1960;118:145–52.

The Paper and the Times

Psychopharmacology changed the field of psychiatry – and for patients – psychiatrists seemed to have changed from attentive listeners to "wizards of neurotransmitters" or "psychopharmacologists" [31].

The trial and error of drugs to treat anxiety and psychotic breaks transitioned over many years from morphine to potassium bromide to chloral hydrate to barbiturates to insulin to amphetamines to chlorpromazine and to lithium, and so on, until the first neuroleptics, such as thioxanthene and haloperidol appeared [13].

In the early 1950s, haloperidol was a new neuroleptic agent synthesized in Belgium (Janssen Laboratories) that made a significant impact on the treatment of major psychoses. The first results on its effect on patients were reported by Divry, Bobon, and Collard in 1958 [66]. Comprehensive pharmacokinetic studies appeared several years later in 1976 [77]. The rapid action of this agent would treat significant agitation associated with psychoses. Haloperidol was considered a novel approach to treat manic states and schizophrenia with paranoid ideation.

Side effects were noted and included increased risk for QTc prolongation, torsades de pointes, and cardiac standstill in patients with cardiac or electrolyte abnormalities and those taking other QTc-prolonging drugs. Akathisia or extrapyramidal symptoms were not commonly reported.

However, another major side effect would appear that would cross the boundary of neurology and psychiatry. The fields separated in 1948 with the founding of the American Academy of Neurology and separation of the journal *Archives of Neurology and Psychiatry* in 1959.

The Details of the Paper

The paper describes 62 patients with psychiatric disorders treated with haloperidol and largely describes good improvement with treatment of significant "melancholies" or "manies" (Fig. 3.30). A large number of patients were treated for paranoid behavior.

The paper describes excellent tolerance with intramuscular injections. However, in two cases, the authors observed what they called *dereglements vegetatifs*. These patients developed hyperthermia with major and excessive drooling, rapid dehydration, and stupor lasting for several days. Diffuse maculopapular erythema also was noted. Symptoms resolved spontaneously.

The Message and Acceptance

Since this initial description of a neuroleptic malignant syndrome (NMS), several more cases were described. Delay and associates called it *akinetic hypertonic syndrome* or *syndrome malin des neuroleptiques*. The term neuroleptic malignant syndrome thus is merely a translation. NMS became recognized as an "idiosyncratic life-threatening complication." Later, severe muscle rigidity and rhabdomyolysis became apparent with the syndrome's potential danger for acute myoglobinuria and renal failure.

For clinicians, the suspicion of NMS should be considered high in patients presenting with hyperthermia, rigidity, tachycardia, hypertension, diaphoresis and very high serum creatinine kinase levels. Many patients, obviously, had previous psychotic episodes or were schizophrenics [94, 138, 184, 204, 222].

The symptoms usually begin on the day of administration, but presentation may be far more insidious. Many of the signs are seen in sepsis syndrome, and therefore, an infectious source and bacteremia should be excluded in any less than characteristic case.

Patients with more severe forms of NMS may progress to coma, but the nature of that is not clear and could be the result of hypertensive crises or acute uremia. Computed tomography scan of the brain usually has been normal, but

Un neuroleptique majeur non phénothiazinique et non réserpinique, l'halopéridol, dans le traitement des psychoses, par MM. J. Delay, P. Pichot, Mlle T. Lempérière, MM. B. Elissalde et F. Peigne.

Le « R. 1625 », ou Halopéridol, est un neuroleptique nouveau, dont l'introduction en thérapeutique psychiatrique marque une étape très importante dans la chimiothérapie des psychoses. L'halopéridol est le premier corps chimique connu, non phénothiazinique et non réserpinique, possédant les caractéristiques que l'un de nous a proposées pour définir le terme de neuroleptique. La rapidité de son action et son efficacité permettent déjà de le considérer comme un neuroleptique majeur.

Au point de vue clinique, les premiers essais thérapeutiques de l'halopéridol en psychiatrie ont été rapportés en 1958 par Divry, Bobon et Collard. Employé par voie veineuse, chez des sujets pour la plupart psychotiques, en état de grande agitation, l'halopéridol apparut comme un sédatif très puissant, non hypnotique, agissant à dose minime, entraînant chez tous les malades un retour très rapide au calme psychomoteur. Poursuivant l'expérimentation de l'halopéridol par voie orale comme traitement de fond chez des malades psychotiques, ces mêmes auteurs mirent en évidence les propriétés neuroleptiques très puissantes de ce produit. Ces résultats furent confirmés par les travaux de nombreux auteurs, parmi lesquels il faut citer ceux de Jacobs, de Paquay, Arnould et Burton dans la schizophrénie, ces derniers mettant en outre l'accent sur l'efficacité des doses modérées.

Etude pharmacologique

Au point de vue pharmacologique, l'halopéridol est une amine tertiaire nouvelle ; il s'agit de la 4'-fluoro-4-1-(4-hydroxy-4-(4'-chloro)-phényl-pipéridine)-butyrophénone.

Ann. méd.-psych., 118e année, t. I. — Janvier 1960. 10

Fig. 3.30 Title page

magnetic resonance imaging has rarely been performed. The incidence has been placed at 0.01% in patients treated with antipsychotics, and in larger series, recovery time may be approximately 2 weeks [33–36, 214]. Mortality is related to a number of systemic complications such as aspiration pneumonitis and other complications associated with prolonged care in the intensive care unit [203].

Dantrolene is an effective drug. It was originally synthesized by Snyder and associates in 1967 [214]. Dantrolene has a relaxant effect and was mostly used to treat spasticity. Its effect was first demonstrated in a pig model of malignant hyperthermia.

It is unclear if NMS is a primary muscular problem. The current hypothesis, based on studies in the early 1990s, found that the clinical symptoms of the NMS are much more likely explained by hyperactivity of the sympathoadrenergic system [77, 88, 90]. This could lead to an increase in intracellular calcium ion concentrations and contribute to an increase in muscle tone. Dopamine D_2 receptor antagonism of neuroleptic drugs may cause hyperthermia, may block heat loss pathways, or produce heat due muscular rigidity. It is likely that genetic mutations cause changes in calcium regulatory proteins.

In the most severe cases, electroconvulsive therapy might be necessary to treat the severe autonomic dysregulation, such as marked hypertension, tachycardia and rigidity.

Short Historical Note 17

DIENCEPHALIC SEIZURES

The Title of the Paper

Penfield W. Diencephalic autonomic epilepsy. Arch Neurol Psychiatry. 1929;22:358–74.

The Paper and the Times

Restlessness, temperature spikes, sudden rise in blood pressure with diaphoresis, periods of tachypnea, and tachycardia were well known manifestations in comatose patients, especially in those in a persistent vegetative state. These symptoms were attributed to the autonomic nervous system and merely considered part of the catastrophic injury. When these attacks were frequent, they could lead to hypermetabolism and extreme weight loss. Hyperthermia could rapidly lead to dehydration.

The nature of these symptoms was largely unknown, but many observers felt they were caused by some sort of sympathetic overactivity or exaggerated stress response. Founder and first director of the Montreal Neurological Institute, and later a pioneer in epilepsy surgery, neurosurgeon Wilder G. Penfield described the phenomenon in more detail and introduced a new term in neurology: "diencephalic autonomic epilepsy".

The Details of the Paper

The paper describes a patient with a large tumor in the diencephalon (third ventricle cholesteatoma) (Fig. 3.31). The patient presented with episodes of restlessness, vasodilatation of the skin, sudden rise of blood pressure, lacrimation, diaphoresis, salivation, dilatation of the pupils, protrusion of the eyes, increase of pulse rate and pressure, marked "retardation of the respiratory rate," elicitability of the pilomotor reflex, hiccups, transient shivering, and Cheyne–Stokes respiration.

The case described urine incontinence and episodes in which the patient's temperature fell well below normal. At no point was there a movement of the body that suggested convulsions of extremities or trunk. The patient was mostly lying quietly during the attacks and sometimes could simply answer questions in monosyllables.

Penfield speculated these autonomic convulsions were caused by the irritating presence of an immovable tumor in the diencephalon, suggesting that some kind of mechanical irritation could create ganglia activity that would cause manifestations of the vasculature, sweat, and tear glands. Penfield also felt that this focus was analogous to Jacksonian epilepsy. To support this finding, he quoted stimulation experiments showing that electrical stimulation of the hypothalamus produced sweat secretion. Penfield suggested that the anterior nucleus of the thalamus was the main lesion. Simultaneous recording of epileptic activity was not performed. (Electroencephalogram [EEG] was not widely used in the United States or other countries before 1938)

According to Perkes, Penfield published another case with far more characteristic features of sympathetic hyperactivity syndrome 25 years later. The case involved a 19-year-old man following a severe traumatic brain injury whose condition satisfied contemporary descriptions of paroxysmal sympathetic hyperactivity syndrome. The clinical manifestations included paroxysmal heart rate of 180 beats per min, respiration rate of 40 breaths per min, blood pressure of 156 mmHg, neurogenic hyperthermia, and decerebrate posturing. Paroxysms were precipitated by of the patient stimulation [176].

The Message and Acceptance

Soon after this observation, McLean reported what he called autonomic epilepsy in a patient with a tumor infiltrating the floor and the walls of the third ventricle and summarized the autonomic symptoms as follows: "apprehension, anxiety, agitation, precordial oppression, hunger, tachycardia, dyspnea, anisocoria, sweating, pilomotor phenomena, narcolepsy and hypersomnia" [159]. Many other observations appeared and mostly in the setting of advanced brain tumors. In 1987, Bullard described two patients with severe traumatic head injury (TBI) who developed classic signs and episodes of increased temperature, respiration, pulse, and blood pressure, diaphoresis, and extensor posturing. Computed tomography scans revealed no focal lesion and EEGs revealed only severe slowing [27].

This condition usually is seen in comatose patients after severe TBI and after marked anoxic encephalopathy from asphyxia or cardiac arrest

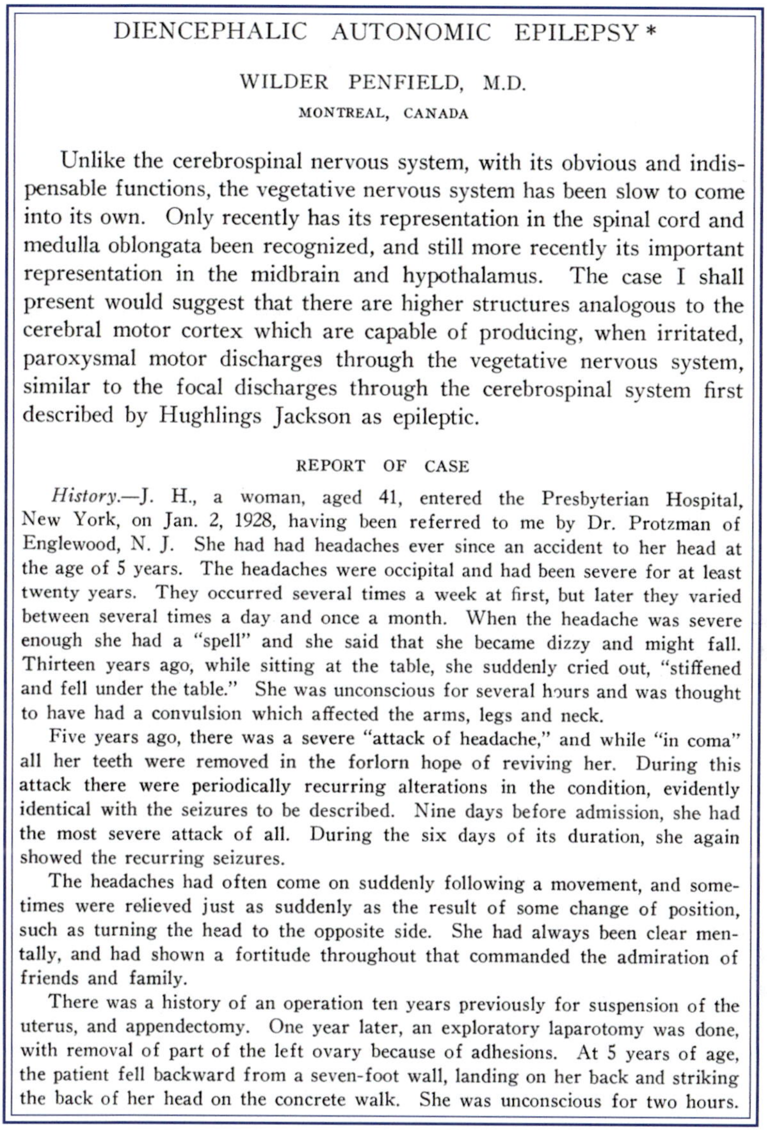

DIENCEPHALIC AUTONOMIC EPILEPSY *

WILDER PENFIELD, M.D.

MONTREAL, CANADA

Unlike the cerebrospinal nervous system, with its obvious and indispensable functions, the vegetative nervous system has been slow to come into its own. Only recently has its representation in the spinal cord and medulla oblongata been recognized, and still more recently its important representation in the midbrain and hypothalamus. The case I shall present would suggest that there are higher structures analogous to the cerebral motor cortex which are capable of producing, when irritated, paroxysmal motor discharges through the vegetative nervous system, similar to the focal discharges through the cerebrospinal system first described by Hughlings Jackson as epileptic.

REPORT OF CASE

History.—J. H., a woman, aged 41, entered the Presbyterian Hospital, New York, on Jan. 2, 1928, having been referred to me by Dr. Protzman of Englewood, N. J. She had had headaches ever since an accident to her head at the age of 5 years. The headaches were occipital and had been severe for at least twenty years. They occurred several times a week at first, but later they varied between several times a day and once a month. When the headache was severe enough she had a "spell" and she said that she became dizzy and might fall. Thirteen years ago, while sitting at the table, she suddenly cried out, "stiffened and fell under the table." She was unconscious for several hours and was thought to have had a convulsion which affected the arms, legs and neck.

Five years ago, there was a severe "attack of headache," and while "in coma" all her teeth were removed in the forlorn hope of reviving her. During this attack there were periodically recurring alterations in the condition, evidently identical with the seizures to be described. Nine days before admission, she had the most severe attack of all. During the six days of its duration, she again showed the recurring seizures.

The headaches had often come on suddenly following a movement, and sometimes were relieved just as suddenly as the result of some change of position, such as turning the head to the opposite side. She had always been clear mentally, and had shown a fortitude throughout that commanded the admiration of friends and family.

There was a history of an operation ten years previously for suspension of the uterus, and appendectomy. One year later, an exploratory laparotomy was done, with removal of part of the left ovary because of adhesions. At 5 years of age, the patient fell backward from a seven-foot wall, landing on her back and striking the back of her head on the concrete walk. She was unconscious for two hours.

Fig. 3.31 Title page

[185, 186]. The terminology is not yet settled, and Perkes identified more than 30 different terms, including diencephalic seizures, tonic decerebrate seizure, acute midbrain syndrome, acute hypothalamic instability, hypothalamic storm, autonomic hyperactivity, hyperpyrexia with sustained muscle contraction, neurostorm, hypermetabolic paroxysmal dysautonomia, and paroxysmal autonomic instability with dystonia [7, 8, 23, 24, 27, 37, 61, 73, 78, 140, 159, 177, 205, 215, 224, 233].

The true nature of these spells, perhaps best termed–*paroxysmal sympathetic hyperactivity syndrome*–remains unknown. This term is preferred because it includes the main characteristics. The spells are paroxysmal manifestations of excessive sympathetic activity. Patients become tachycardic, hypertensive (with increased pulse pressure), tachypneic, febrile, diaphoretic, and often develop markedly increased muscle tone that may result in pseudodystonic postures. In most patients, the excessive sympathetic activity is rapidly overwhelming [232]. The manifestations increase the metabolic demand and risk increase in intracranial pressure.

Effective therapies for this condition are non-cardioselective β-blockers, central α-$_2$-receptor agonists, a dopamine D_2-receptor agonist, a γ-aminobutyric acid $(GABA)_B$ receptor agonist, or $GABA_A$ receptor agonists [176]. Dramatic improvement in the frequency and severity of spells often is seen with combinations of these drugs, but the effect of high dose gabapentin is most impressive.

Short Historical Note 18

THUNDERCLAP HEADACHE

The Title of the Paper

Day JW, Raskin NH. Thunderclap headache: symptom of unruptured cerebral aneurysm. Lancet. 1986;2:1247–8.

The Paper and the Times

Severe unexpected headache of sudden onset has now been associated with aneurysmal rupture, but this distinguishing feature only recently has been recognized. In fact, before widespread use of cerebral angiography, aneurysmal subarachnoid hemorrhage (SAH) was uncommonly diagnosed while the patient was still alive.

In 1956, Walton published a classic series of 312 patients with SAH, which stood out because of its comprehensive description of clinical features. Walton's headache description remains legendary as it describes character and site at onset, variability, and generalized worsening [249]. In this study, 45% of patients had severe headache; 8% intense; 8% mild, but gradually increasing; 6% bursting; and 10% no headache. Less typical descriptions were found in 23%. In nearly 50% of patients, the headache was continuous and only in a third of the patients it was occipitally located.

The notion that headaches—in a less severe form—could precede a major rupture was first suggested in the literature by Gillingham, a neurosurgeon from the Royal Infirmary in Edinburgh. The authors stated "We have become increasingly aware of the significance of the first minor attack of subarachnoid bleeding which is so often missed and only brought out with careful questioning of the patient and his relatives" [86].

Usually, dissection into the wall of the aneurysm with subsequent expansion would, in most instances, cause a painful ophthalmoplegia, but whether headache alone could be the only presentation and accompanied with a normal computed tomography (CT) scan was unknown.

This was not a trivial matter. Neurologists, neurosurgeons, or neurointensivists, after all, would not want to miss a ruptured aneurysm. But they also did not want to subject every patient with a severe headache to a magnetic resonance or cerebral angiogram given the relative paucity of a positive result.

The Details of the Paper

Neurosurgeon John Day and neurologist Neil Rashin describe a 42-year-old woman with an "intense headache of sudden onset, like a hammer hitting my head" (Fig. 3.32). The pain was intense for 12 h, becoming pulsatile accompanied by with nausea and vomiting. Migraine symptoms such as fortification spectra, photophobia, or other visual signs were not noted. A CT scan was normal and a lumbar puncture 12 h after onset was normal with clear cerebrospinal fluid (CSF) and a normal opening pressure. She was discharged but 2 and 5 days later developed similar headaches, accompanied by bilateral throbbing in the temporal areas. CSF was repeated and again was normal. A cerebral angiogram showed diffuse several vasospasm in the anterior and posterior circulation and a large 1-cm carotid aneurysm. During clipping of the aneurysm, the authors noted "No evidence of old or recent hemorrhage was seen despite close inspection of the aneurysm and surrounding structures through the dissecting microscope."

The Message and Acceptance

The term *thunderclap headache*—or as the authors explained it—"like an unexpected clap of thunder" became firmly settled as the best indicator of a SAH [64]. The International Headache Society put forward diagnostic criteria of "primary thunderclap headache" and defined it as a severe headache, sudden in onset, maximum intensity, in less than 1 min, and lasting from 1 h to 10 days [96].

A wide differential diagnosis appeared overtime, and thunderclap headache could be a presenting symptom of cerebral venous thrombosis, cervical arterial dissection, spontaneous intracranial hypotension, pituitary apoplexy, reversible cerebral vasoconstriction syndrome, among other disorders, including posterior reversible encephalopathy syndrome [70, 75, 202, 212].

It is hard to argue that the Day and Raskin's case may have been a reversible cerebral vasoconstriction syndrome with the large aneurysm

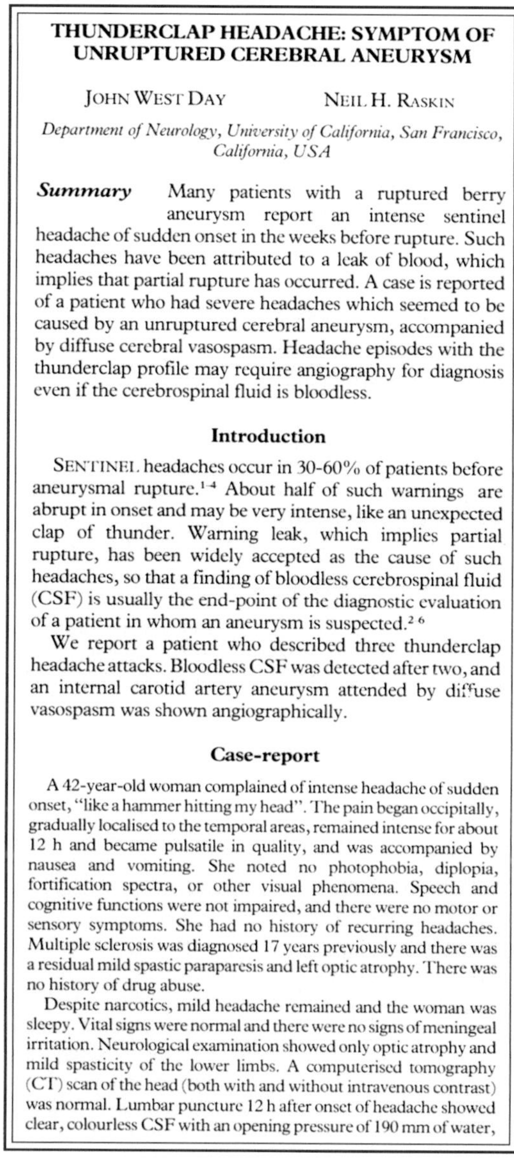

THUNDERCLAP HEADACHE: SYMPTOM OF UNRUPTURED CEREBRAL ANEURYSM

JOHN WEST DAY NEIL H. RASKIN

Department of Neurology, University of California, San Francisco, California, USA

Summary Many patients with a ruptured berry aneurysm report an intense sentinel headache of sudden onset in the weeks before rupture. Such headaches have been attributed to a leak of blood, which implies that partial rupture has occurred. A case is reported of a patient who had severe headaches which seemed to be caused by an unruptured cerebral aneurysm, accompanied by diffuse cerebral vasospasm. Headache episodes with the thunderclap profile may require angiography for diagnosis even if the cerebrospinal fluid is bloodless.

Introduction

SENTINEL headaches occur in 30-60% of patients before aneurysmal rupture.[1-4] About half of such warnings are abrupt in onset and may be very intense, like an unexpected clap of thunder. Warning leak, which implies partial rupture, has been widely accepted as the cause of such headaches, so that a finding of bloodless cerebrospinal fluid (CSF) is usually the end-point of the diagnostic evaluation of a patient in whom an aneurysm is suspected.[2-6]

We report a patient who described three thunderclap headache attacks. Bloodless CSF was detected after two, and an internal carotid artery aneurysm attended by diffuse vasospasm was shown angiographically.

Case-report

A 42-year-old woman complained of intense headache of sudden onset, "like a hammer hitting my head". The pain began occipitally, gradually localised to the temporal areas, remained intense for about 12 h and became pulsatile in quality, and was accompanied by nausea and vomiting. She noted no photophobia, diplopia, fortification spectra, or other visual phenomena. Speech and cognitive functions were not impaired, and there were no motor or sensory symptoms. She had no history of recurring headaches. Multiple sclerosis was diagnosed 17 years previously and there was a residual mild spastic paraparesis and left optic atrophy. There was no history of drug abuse.

Despite narcotics, mild headache remained and the woman was sleepy. Vital signs were normal and there were no signs of meningeal irritation. Neurological examination showed only optic atrophy and mild spasticity of the lower limbs. A computerised tomography (CT) scan of the head (both with and without intravenous contrast) was normal. Lumbar puncture 12 h after onset of headache showed clear, colourless CSF with an opening pressure of 190 mm of water,

Fig. 3.32 Title page

interpreted as an incidental finding, but the issue still remains: Could a thunderclap headache warn physicians that an aneurysm is bound to rupture? [12, 93, 121, 134, 165, 246].

A retrospective study of 71 patients with primary thunderclap headache reported no cases of aneurysmal SAH, with an average follow up of 3.3 years (range, 1–7 years); however, 44% of the patients developed tension headache or migraine after presenting with thunderclap headaches [256]. Prospective studies also confirmed absence of SAH in patients with thunderclap headache and negative neuroimaging and CSF studies [93, 130, 141, 142, 153]. When patients with thunderclap headaches present to a general practitioner, only 25% will have a SAH [142]. Most recently, thunderclap headache without SAH has been associated with recurrence and regrowth of a previously coiled intracranial aneurysm. Again, it remains unknown if these headaches associated with regrowth are a precursor to rebleeding [29].

Alternative terms *warning leaks* or *sentinel headaches* have been proposed but a comprehensible evaluation is needed in any patient with a thunderclap headache [172, 246]. Patients with thunderclap headaches seen in emergency department may have a disorder other than aneurysmal SAH, and in many, after a careful history is taken, the headache is different. Any estimate of its prevalence will likely also be confounded by incomplete evaluations, most notable of which is no lumbar puncture [183].

References

1. Adams RD, Foley JM. The neurologic changes in the more common types of severe liver disease. Trans Am Neurol Assoc. 1949;74:217–9.
2. Adams RD, Foley JM. The disorder of movement in the morecommonvarietiesofliverdisease.Electroencephalogr Clin Neurophysiol Suppl. 1953;3:51.
3. Adams RD, Foley JM. The neurologic disorder associated with liver disease. Res Publ Assoc Res Nerve Ment Dis. 1953;32:198–237.
4. Afsar N, Fak A, Metzger J, et al. Acute stroke increases QT dispersion in patients without known cardiac diseases. Arch Neurol. 2003;60:346–50.
5. Anonymous. "Meningitic" breathing. JAMA. 1957; 165:1568.
6. Auer RN, Rowlands CG, Perry SF, et al. Multiple sclerosis with medullary plaques and fatal sleep apnea (Ondine's curse). Clin Neuropathol. 1996;15:101–5.
7. Baguley IJ, Heriseanu RE, Cameron ID, et al. A critical review of the pathophysiology of dysautonomia following traumatic brain injury. Neurocrit Care. 2008;8:293–300.
8. Baguley IJ, Heriseanu RE, Gurka JA, et al. Gabapentin in the management of dysautonomia following severe traumatic brain injury: a case series. J Neurol Neurosurg Psychiatry. 2007;78:539–41.
9. Bahloul M, Chaari AN, Kallel H, et al. Neurogenic pulmonary edema due to traumatic brain injury: evidence of cardiac dysfunction. Am J Crit Care. 2006;15:462–70.
10. Baker AB. Poliomyelitis, a study of pulmonary edema. Neurology. 1957;7:743–51.
11. Bakheit AMO, Behan PO, Melville ID. Bilateral internuclear ophthalmoplegia as a false localizing sign. J R Soc Med. 1991;84:627.
12. Ball MJ. Pathogenesis of the "sentinel headache" preceding berry aneurysm rupture. Can Med Assoc J. 1975;112:78–9.
13. Ban TA. Pharmacotherapy of mental illness – a historical analysis. Prog Neuropsychopharmacol Biol Psychiatry. 2001;25:709–27.
14. Barrier F. Pratique des maladies de l' enfance fonde sur de nombreuses observations cliniques, Paris, Fortin, Masson et cie, Lyon. Charles Savy Jeune, 2 edit. 1845.
15. Bartter FC, Schwartz WB. The syndrome of inappropriate secretion of antidiuretic hormone. Am J Med. 1967;42:790–806.
16. Bazett HC, Penfield WG. A study of the Sherrington decerebrate animal in the chronic as well as the acute condition. Brain. 1922;45:185–265.
17. Beard EF, Robertson JW, Robertson RC. Spontaneous subarachnoid hemorrhage simulating acute myocardial infarction. Am Heart J. 1959;58:755–9.
18. Benassi G. Cranio-Encephalitic traumatism and pulmonary edema. J Exp Med. 1937;66:405–7.
19. Bickford RG, Butt HR. Hepatic coma; electroencephalographic pattern. J Clin Invest. 1955;34:790–9.
20. Biot MC. Contribution a l'etude du phenomene respiratoire de Cheyne-Stokes. Lyon Med. 1876;23 (517–528):561–7.
21. Biot MC. Etude Clinique et Experimentale Sur la Respiration de Cheyne-Stokes. New York: Harper & Brothers; 1878.
22. Biot MC. Discours prononces aux obseques du docteur. (Camille Biot) 1850–1918. Annales de l' Academie de Macon. tome XXI, 1918–1919: pages 255–271 and plance XII.
23. Blackman JA, Patrick PD, Buck ML, et al. Paroxysmal autonomic instability with dystonia after brain injury. Arch Neurol. 2004;61:321–8.
24. Boeve BF, Wijdicks EFM, Benarroch EE, et al. Paroxysmal sympathetic storms ("diencephalic seizures") after severe diffuse axonal head injury. Mayo Clin Proc. 1998;73:148–52.

25. Bogousslavsky J, Khurana R, Deruaz JP, et al. Respiratory failure and unilateral caudal brainstem infarction. Ann Neurol. 1990;28:668–73.
26. Brunn F. Experimental pulmonary edema. Wien KlinWehnschr. 1932;45:1425–31.
27. Bullard DE. Diencephalic seizures: responsiveness to bromocriptine and morphine. Ann Neurol. 1987;21:609–11.
28. Byer E, Ashman R, Toth LA. Electrocardiograms with large, upright T waves and long Q-T intervals. Am Heart J. 1947;33:796–806.
29. Byrum EP, McGregor JM, Christoforidis GA. Thunderclap headache without subarachnoid hemorrhage associated with regrowth of previously coil-occluded aneurysms. AJNR Am J Neuroradiol. 2009;30:1059–61.
30. Cameron RG, Sheik AH. The experimental production of pulmonary edema with ammonium salts, together with a classification of lung edema. J Pathol Bacteriol. 1951;63:609–17.
31. Carlat D. Unhinged: the trouble with psychiatry – a doctor's revelation about a profession in crises. New York: Free Press; 2010.
32. Carlson RW, Schaeffer Jr RC, Michaels SG, et al. Pulmonary edema following intracranial hemorrhage. Chest. 1979;75:731–4.
33. Caroff SN. Neuroleptic malignant syndrome. J Clin Psychiatry. 1980;41:79–83.
34. Caroff SN, Mann SC. Neuroleptic malignant syndrome. Med Clin North Am. 1993;77:185–202.
35. Caroff SN, Mann SC, Campbell EC. Neuroleptic malignant syndrome. Adverse Drug React Bull. 2001;209:799–802.
36. Caroff SN, Mann SC, Keck Jr PE. Specific treatment of the neuroleptic malignant syndrome. Biol Psychiatry. 1998;44:378–81.
37. Carr-Locke D, Millac P. Diencephalic epilepsy in a patient with agenesis of the corpus callosum confirmed by computerized axial tomography. J Neurol Neurosurg Psychiatry. 1977;40:808–14.
38. Catanzaro JN, Meraj PM, Zheng S, et al. Electrocardiographic T-wave changes underlying acute cardiac and cerebral events. Am J Emerg Med. 2008;26:716–20.
39. Caviness JN, Truong DD. Myoclonus. Handb Clin Neurol. 2011;100:399–420.
40. Chemiack NS, Longobardo G, Evangelista CJ. Causes of Cheyne-Stokes respiration. Neurocrit Care. 2005;3:271–9.
41. Chen R, Sahjpaul R, Del Maestro RF, et al. Initial enlargement of the opposite pupil as a false localizing sign in intraparenchymal frontal hemorrhage. J Neurol Neurosurg Psychiatr. 1994;57:1126–8.
42. Chen HI, Sun SC, Chai CY. Pulmonary edema and hemorrhage resulting from cerebral compression. Am J Physiol. 1973;224:223–9.
43. Cheyne J. Cases of apoplexy and lethargy. London: Underwood; 1812.
44. Cherniack NS, Longobardo GS. Cheyne-Stokes breathing. An instability in physiologic control. N Engl J Med 1973;288:952–7.
45. Chung KH, Nadana Chandran K. Paradoxical fixed dilatation of the contralateral pupil as a false localizing sign in intra parenchymal frontal hemorrhage. Clin Neurol Neurosurg. 2007;109:455–7.
46. Cohen-Cymberknoh M, Shoseyov D, et al. Late-onset central hypoventilation presenting as extubation failure. Isr Med Assoc J. 2010;12:249–50.
47. Cohn JE, Kuida H. Primary alveolar hypoventilation associated with western equine encephalitis. Ann Intern Med. 1962;56:633–44.
48. Colice GL, Matthay MA, Bass E, et al. Neurogenic pulmonary edema. Am Rev Respir Dis. 1984;130:941–8.
49. Connor L. Biot's breathing. Am J Med Sci 1911;141:350–360
50. Cort JH. Cerebral salt wasting. Lancet. 1954;266:752–4.
51. Crompton MR. Hypothalamic lesions following the rupture of berry aneurysms. Brain. 1963;86:301–14.
52. Cropp CJ, Manning GW. Electrocardiographic changes simulating myocardial ischemia and infarction associated with spontaneous intracranial hemorrhage. Circulation. 1960;22:25–38.
53. Crowell JW, Guyton AC, Moore JW. Basic oscillating mechanism of Cheyne-Stokes breathing. Am J Physiol. 1956;187:395–8.
54. Cushing H. Concerning a definite regulatory mechanism of the vasomotor centre which controls blood pressure during cerebral compression. Johns Hopkins Hosp Bull. 1901;12:290–2.
55. Cushing H. Physiologische und anatomische Beobachtungen uber den Einfluss von Hirnkompression auf den intracraniellen Kreislauf und uber einige hiermit verwandte Erscheinungen. Mitt Grenzgeb Med Chir. 1902;9:773–808.
56. Cushing H. Some experimental and clinical observations concerning states of increased intracranial tension. The Mütter lecture for 1901. Am J Med Sci. 1902;124:375–400.
57. Cushing H. The blood pressure reaction of acute cerebral compression illustrated by cases of intracranial hemorrhage: a sequel to the Mütter lecture for 1901. Am J Med Sci. 1903;125:1017–44.
58. Cushing H. The possible relation of the central (vegetative) nervous system to peptic ulcers. N Engl J Med. 1931;205:979.
59. Cushing H. Peptic ulcer and the interbrain. Surg Gynec Obst. 1932;55:1–34.
60. Cushing AR. The secretion of urine. London; 1926.
61. Darnell RB, Arbit E. Reversible diencephalic dysfunction: episodic hyperhidrosis due to a trapped third ventricle. Neurology. 1993;43:579–82.
62. Davis LE. Decerebrate rigidity in man. Arch Neurol Psychiatry. 1925;13:569–79.
63. Davis M, Lucatorto M. The false localizing signs of increased intracranial pressure. J Neurosci Nurs. 1992;5:245–50.
64. Day JW, Raskin NH. Thunderclap headache: symptom of unruptured cerebral aneurysm. Lancet. 1986;2:1247–8.

65. Dikshit BB. The production of cardiac irregularities by excitation of the hypothalamic centers. J Physiol. 1934;81:382–94.
66. Divry P, Bobon J, Collard J. Report on the neuropsychopharmacological activity of haloperidol (R 1625). Acta Neurol Belg. 1960;60:7–19.
67. Doczi T, Bende J, Huszka E. Syndrome of inappropriate secretion of antidiuretic hormone after subarachnoid hemorrhage. Neurosurgery. 1981;9:384–97.
68. Dodge Jr HW, Clark EC, Wagener HP. Certain false localizing signs of intracranial tumor: report of case. Proc Staff Meet Mayo Clin. 1955;30:453–61.
69. Doyle D. Eponymous doctors associated with Edinburgh, part 2 – David Bruce, John Cheyne, William Stokes, Alexander Monro Secundus, Joseph Gamgee. J R Coll Physicians Edinb. 2006;36:374–81.
70. Edlow JA, Caplan LR. Avoiding pitfalls in the diagnosis of subarachnoid hemorrhage. N Engl J Med. 2000;342:29–36.
71. Ehni G. 'False' localizing signs in intracranial tumor; report of a patient with left trigeminal palsy due to right temporal meningioma. AMA Arch Neurol Psychiatry. 1950;64:692–8.
72. Eisalo A, Perasalo J, Holonen PI. Electrocardiographic abnormalities and some laboratory findings in patients with subarachnoid hemorrhage. Br Heart J. 1972;34:217–26.
73. Engle GL, Aring CD. Hypothalamic attacks with thalamic lesion. I. Physiologic and psychologic considerations. II. Anatomic considerations. Arch Neurol Psychiatry. 1945;54:37–44.
74. Fisher CM. The neurological examination of the comatose patient. Acta Neurol Scand. 1969;45 Suppl 36:1–56.
75. Fisher CM. Painful states: a neurological commentary. Clin Neurosurg. 1984;31:32–53.
76. Fodstad H, Kelly PJ, Buchfelder M. History of the Cushing reflex. Neurosurgery. 2006;59:1132–7.
77. Forsman A, Ohman R. Pharmacokinetic studies on haloperidol in man. Curr Ther Res Clin Exp. 1976;20:319–36.
78. Fox RH, Wilkins DC, Bell JA, et al. Spontaneous periodic hypothermia: diencephalic epilepsy. BMJ. 1973;2:693–5.
79. Fredberg U, Botker HE, Romer FK. Acute neurogenic pulmonary edema following generalized tonic clonic seizure. A case report and a review of the literature. Eur Heart J. 1988;9:933–6.
80. Frerichs FT. Clinical treatise on diseases of the liver (translated by Charles Murchison), vol. 1. London: New Sydenham Society; 1861.
81. Gamble JE, Patton HD. Pulmonary edema and hemorrhage from preoptic lesions in rats. Am J Physiol. 1953;172:623–31.
82. Ganong CA, Kappy MS. Cerebral salt wasting in children. The need for recognition and treatment. Am J Dis Child. 1993;47:167–9.
83. Gassel MM. False localizing signs. Arch Neurol. 1961;4:526–54.
84. Gaviani P, Gonzalez RG, Zhu JJ, Batchelor TT, Henson JW. Central neurogenic hyperventilation and lactate production in brainstem glioma. Neurology. 2005;64:166–7.
85. Giangaspero F, Schiavina M, Sturani C, et al. Cirignotta F. Failure of automatic control of ventilation (Ondine's curse) associated with viral encephalitis of the brainstem: a clinicopathologic study of one case. Clin Neuropathol. 1988;7:234–7.
86. Gillingham FJ. The management of ruptured intracranial aneurysms. Ann R Coll Surg. 1958;23:89–117.
87. Grob GN. The rise of peptic ulcer disease 1900–1950. Perspect Biol Med. 2003;46:550–66.
88. Gurrera RJ. Sympathoadrenal hyperactivity and the etiology of neuroleptic malignant syndrome. Am J Psychiatry. 1999;156:169–80.
89. Guyenet PG, Brown DL. Unit activity in nucleus paragigantocellularis lateralis during cerebral ischemia in the rat. Brain Res. 1986;364:301–14.
90. Guzé BH, Baxter Jr LR. Current concepts. Neuroleptic malignant syndrome. N Engl J Med. 1985;313:163–6.
91. Hall R, Sybers H, Greenhoot J, et al. Myocardial changes after hypothalamic stimulation in the intact, conscious dog. Am Heart J. 1974;88:770–6.
92. Halpern JI, Gordon Jr WH. Trochlear nerve palsy as a false localizing sign. Ann Ophthalmol. 1981;13:53–6.
93. Harling DW, Peatfield RC, Van Hille PT, et al. Thunder clap headache: is it migraine? Cephalagia. 1989;9:87–90.
94. Hasan S, Buckley P. Novel antipsychotics and the neuroleptic malignant syndrome: a review and critique. Am J Psychiatry. 1998;155:1113–6.
95. Hawkins WE, Clower BR. Myocardial damage after head trauma and simulated intracranial hemorrhage in mice: the role of the autonomic nervous system. Cardiovasc Res. 1971;4:524–9.
96. Headache Classification Committee of the International Headache Society. The international classification of headache disorders. Cephalagia. 2004;24:1–151.
97. Hermann DM, Bassetti CL. Sleep apnea and other sleep-wake disorders in stroke. Curr Treat Options Neurol. 2003;5:241–9.
98. Hersch C. Electrocardiographic changes in head injuries. Circulation. 1961;23:853–60.
99. Hess L. Lung edema in organic nervous diseases. Wien Med Wehnschr. 1934;84:285–6.
100. Heyman A, Birchfield RI, Sieker HO. Effects of bilateral cerebral infarction on respiratory center sensitivity. Neurology. 1958;8:694–700.
101. Heymans C. The control of heart rate consequent to changes in the cephalic blood pressure and in the intracranial pressure. Am J Physiol. 1928;85:498–505.
102. Hill L. The physiology and pathology of the cerebrospinal circulation. London: J & A Churchill; 1896.
103. Hockman CH, Mauck Jr HP, Hoff EC. EKG changes resulting from cerebral stimulation. II. A spectrum of ventricular arrhythmias of sympathetic origin. Am Heart J. 1966;71:695–700.
104. Hudgel DW, Devadatta P, Quadri M, et al. Mechanism of sleep-induced periodic breathing in convalescing

stroke patients and healthy elderly subjects. Chest. 1993;104:1503–10.
105. Hofbauer L. Semiologie and differential diagnosis der verschiedenen arten von kurzatmigkeit of grund der atemkurve: Verlag von Gustav Fischer in Jena. 1904:25–28
106. Hughlings Jackson J. Neurological abstracts: XV. Superior and subordinate centers of the lowest level. Lancet. 1895;1:476–8.
107. Hume DM. The role of the hypothalamus in the pituitary-adrenal cortical response to stress. Soc Clin Invest. 1949;Abst. 28.
108. Hunt D, McRae C, Zapf P. Electrocardiographic and serum enzyme changes in subarachnoid hemorrhage. Am Heart J. 1969;77:479–88.
109. Hutchinson J. Four lectures on compression of the brain. Clin Lect Reps London Hosp. 1867;4:10–55.
110. Jacob WA, Van Bogaert A, DeGroot-Lasseel MHA. Myocardial ultrastructural and hemodynamic reactions during experimental subarachnoid hemorrhage. J Moll Cell Cardiol. 1972;4:287–98.
111. Jacobson SA, Danufsky P. Marked electrocardiographic changes produced by experimental head trauma. J Neuropathol Exp Neurol. 1954;13: 462–6.
112. Jaccoud S. Traite de Pathologie Interne. 3 volumes. Paris, Adrien Delahaye et Emile Lecrosnier. 1883:1–911, 911–929, 911–975.
113. Jaeckle KA, Digre KB, Jones CR, et al. Central neurogenic hyperventilation: pharmacologic intervention with morphine sulfate and correlative analysis of respiratory, sleep, and ocular motor dysfunction. Neurology. 1990;40:1715–20.
114. Jefferson G. Bilateral rigidity in middle meningeal hemorrhage. Br Med J. 1921;2:683–5.
115. Jennett WB, Stern WE. Tentorial herniation, the midbrain and the pupil. Experimental studies in brain compression. J Neurosurg. 1960;17:598–609.
116. Johnson RT, Yates PO. Clinicopathological aspects of pressure changes at the tentorium. Acta Radiol. 1956;46:242–9.
117. Jones KM, Seeger JF, Yoshino MT. Ipsilateral motor deficit resulting from a subdural hematoma and a Kernohan notch. AJNR Am J Neuroradiol. 1991;12: 1238–9.
118. Jungmann J, Meyer E. Experimentelle Untersuchungen über die Abhängigkeit der Nierenfunktion vom Nervensystem. Arch Exp Path Pharm. 1913;73:49–80.
119. Khoo MC, Kronauer RE, Strohl KP, Slutsky AS. Factors inducing periodic breathing in humans: a general model. J Appl Physiol. 1982;53:644–59.
120. Kim JS. Asterixis after unilateral stroke: lesion location of 30 patients. Neurology. 2001;56:533–6.
121. King RB, Saba MI. Forewarnings of major subarachnoid hemorrhage. NY State J Med. 1974;74:638–9.
122. Klos KJ, Wijdicks EFM. Unilateral asterixis after thalamic hemorrhage. Neurology. 2008;66:E11.
123. Klouda MA, Brynjolfsson G. Cardiotoxic effects of electrical stimulation of the stellate ganglia. Ann N Y Acad Sci. 1969;156:271–80.
124. Kocher ET. Brain concussion, intracranial pressure, and surgical interventions in brain disease. In: Nothnagel H, editor. Special pathology and therapy [in German]. Vienna: Alfred Hölder; 1901.
125. Kocher ET. Hirnerschütterung, Hirndruck und chirurgische Eingriffe bei Hirnkrankheiten. In: Nothnagel H, editors. Specielle Pathologie und Therapie. 9th vol, 3rd part. Vienna: Hölder; 1901.
126. Kolin A, Norris JW. Myocardial damage from acute cerebral lesions. Stroke. 1984;15:990–3.
127. Koskelo P, Punsar S, Sipilae W. Subendocardial hemorrhage and E.C.G. changes in intracranial bleeding. Br Med J. 1964;1:1479–80.
128. Kreus KE, Kemila SJ, Takala JK. Electrocardiographic changes in cerebrovascular accidents. Acta Med Scand. 1969;185:327–34.
129. Landau WM. Spasticity and rigidity. In: Plum F, (ed) Recent Advances in Neurology, Contemporary neurology studies, vol. 6. Philadelphia: FA Davis; 1969. p. 1–32.
130. Landtblom AM, Boivie J, Fridrickson S, et al. Thunderclap headache: final results from a prospective study of consecutive cases. Acta Neurol Scand. 1996;167:23–4.
131. Larner AJ. False localizing signs. J Neurol Neurosurg Psychiatry. 2003;74:415–8.
132. Laureno R. Raymond Adams, a life of mind and muscle. New York: Oxford University Press; 2009.
133. Lazar J, Manzella S, Moonjelly J, et al. The prognostic value of QT dispersion in patients presenting with acute neurological events. J Invasive Cardiol. 2003;15:31–5.
134. Leblanc R, Winfield JA. The warning leak in subarachnoid hemorrhage in the importance of its early diagnosis. Can Med Assoc. 1984;131:1235–6.
135. Lee VH, Oh JK, Mulvagh SL, Wijdicks EFM. Mechanisms in neurogenic stress cardiomyopathy after aneurysmal subarachnoid hemorrhage. Neurocrit Care. 2006;5:243–9.
136. Legallois C. Experiences sur le Principle de la Vie. Paris: Hautel; 1812.
137. Lepore FE. False and non-localizing signs in neuroophthalmology. Curr Opin Ophthalmol. 2002;13: 371–4.
138. Levenson JL. Neuroleptic malignant syndrome. Am J Psychiatry. 1985;142:1137–45.
139. Levine HD. Non-specificity of the electrocardiogram associated with coronary heart disease. Am J Med. 1953;15:344–55.
140. LeWitt PA, Newman RP, Greenberg HS, Rocher LL, Caine DB, Ehrenkranz JR. Episodic hyperhidrosis, hypothermia and agenesis of the corpus callosum. Neurology. 1983;33:1122–9.
141. Linn FHH, Rinkel GJE, Algra A, et al. Follow up of idiopathic thunderclap headache in general practice. J Neurol. 1999;246:946–8.
142. Linn FH, Wijdicks EFM, van der Graaf Y, et al. Prospective study of sentinel headache in aneurysmal subarachnoid hemorrhage. Lancet. 1994;344: 590–3.
143. Lu WY, Rhoney DH, Boling WB, et al. A review of stress ulcer prophylaxis in the neurosurgical intensive care unit. Neurosurgery. 1997;41:416–26.

144. Macewen W. The pupil in its same neurological aspect. Am J Med Sci. 1887;94:123–46.
145. MacKay MM. Experimental pulmonary edema. IV Pulmonary edema accompanying trauma to the brain. Proc Soc Exp Biol Med. 1950;74:695.
146. Maesaka JK, Batuman V, Yudd M, et al. Hyponatremia and hypouricemia: differentiation from the syndrome of inappropriate secretion of antidiuretic hormone. Clin Nephrol. 1990;33:174–8.
147. Maesaka JK, Gupta S, Fishbane S. Cerebral salt wasting syndrome: does it exist? Nephron. 1999;82: 100–9.
148. Maesaka JK, Imbriano LJ, Ali NM, et al. Is it cerebral or renal salt wasting? Kidney Int. 2009;76: 934–8.
149. Maesaka JK, Miyawaki N, Palaia T, et al. Renal salt wasting without cerebral disease: value of determining urate in hyponatremia. Kidney Int. 2007;71:822–6.
150. Maire FW, Patton HD. Role of the splanchnic nerve and the adrenal medulla in the genesis of "preoptic pulmonary edema". Am J Physiol. 1956;172:623–31.
151. Manning HL, Leiter JC. Respiratory control and respiratory sensation in a patient with a ganglioglioma within the dorsocaudal brain stem. Am J Respir Crit Care Med. 2000;161:2100–6.
152. Maramattom BV, Wijdicks EFM. Uncal herniation. Arch Neurol. 2005;62:1932–5.
153. Markus HS. A prospective follow up of thunderclap headache mimicking subarachnoid hemorrhage. J Neurol Neurosurg Psychiatry. 1991;54:1117–8.
154. Marshall L, Barba D, Toole B, et al. The oval pupil: clinical significance and relationship to intracranial hypertension. Neurosurgery. 1983;58:566–8.
155. Marshman LA, Polkey CE, Penney CC. Unilateral fixed dilation of the pupil as a false-localizing sign with intracranial hemorrhage: case report and literature review. Neurosurgery. 2001;49:1251–5.
156. Masten MG, Bunts RC. Neurogenic erosions and perforations of the stomach and esophagus in cerebral lesions: report of six cases. Arch Intern Med. 1934;54:916–30.
157. Matschke J, Laas R. Sudden death due to central alveolar hypoventilation syndrome (Ondine's curse) in a 39-year-old woman with heterotopia of the inferior olive. Am J Forensic Med Pathol. 2007;28:141–4.
158. Maury E, Tankovic J, Ebel A, et al. An observational study of upper gastrointestinal bleeding in intensive care units: is helicobacter pylori the culprit? Crit Care Med. 2005;33:1513–8.
159. McLean AJ. Autonomic epilepsy: report of a case with observation at necropsy. Arch Neurol Psychiatry. 1934;32:189.
160. McNaughton MT. Pathophysiology and treatment of Cheyne-Stokes respiration. Thorax. 1998;53:514–8.
161. Melville KI, Blum B, Shister HE, et al. Cardiac ischemic changes and arrhythmias induced by hypothalamic stimulation. Am J Cardiol. 1963;12:781–91.
162. Mendizabal M, Silva MO. Images in clinical medicine. Asterixis. N Engl J Med. 2010;363:e14.
163. Menon S. Electrocardiographic changes in simulating myocardial infarction in cerebrovascular accident. Lancet. 1964;2:433–4.
164. Mollaret P, Bertrand I. L'Hypertonie de decerebration chez l'homme. Paris: Masson et Cie; 1945.
165. Morgenstern LB, Luna-Gonzales H, Huber Jr JC, et al. Worst headache and subarachnoid hemorrhage: prospective, modern computed tomography and spinal fluid analysis. Ann Emerg Med. 1998;32:297–304.
166. Moutier F. Hypertension et mort par oedème pulmonaire aigu chez les blessés cranio-encephaliques. Press Med. 1918;26:108–9.
167. Naughton MT. Pathophysiology and treatment of Cheyne-Stokes respiration. Thorax. 1998;53:514–8.
168. Nelson PB, Seif SM, Maroon JC, et al. Hyponatremia in intracranial disease: perhaps not the syndrome of inappropriate secretion of antidiuretic hormone (SIADH). J Neurosurg. 1981;55:938–41.
169. Nystad D, Salvesen R, Nielsen E. Brainstem encephalitis with central neurogenic hyperventilation. J Neurol Neurosurg Psychiatry. 2006;78:107–8.
170. O'Connell JE. Trigeminal false localizing signs and their causation. Brain. 1978;101:119–42.
171. Ochiai H, Yamakawa Y, Minato S, et al. Clinical features of the localized girdle sensation of mid-trunk (false localizing sign) appeared in cervical compressive myelopathy patients. J Neurol. 2002;249:549–53.
172. Okawara SH. Warning signs prior to rupture of an intracranial aneurysm. J Neurosurg. 1973;38:575–80.
173. Oppenheimer SM, Cechetto DF, Hachinski VC. Cerebrogenic cardiac arrhythmias. Cerebral electrocardiographic influences and their role in sudden death. Arch Neurol. 1990;47:513–9.
174. Pauzner R, Mouallem M, Sadeh M, et al. High incidence of primary cerebral lymphoma in tumor-induced central neurogenic hyperventilation. Arch Neurol. 1989;46:510–2.
175. Pearce JM. Cheyne-Stokes respiration. J Neurol Neurosurg Psychiatry. 2002;72:595.
176. Penfield W, Jasper H. VIII: Somatic motor seizures, VII: Subcortical seizures (extra-centrencephalic), A: Mesencephalic seizures. In: Penfield W, Jasper H, editors. Epilepsy and the functional anatomy of the human brain. 1st ed. London: McClelland and Stewart Ltd; 1954. p. 378–87.
177. Perkes I, Baguley IJ, Nott MT, et al. A review of paroxysmal sympathetic hyperactivity after acquired brain injury. Ann Neurol. 2010;68:126–35.
178. Peterson DI, Peterson DW. Unilateral asterixis due to ipsilateral lesions in the pons and medulla. Ann Neurol. 1987;22:661–3.
179. Pitts R. Organization of the respiratory center. Physiol Rev. 1946;26:609–30.
180. Plum F, Posner JB. The diagnosis of stupor and coma. Philadelphia: FA Davis Co; 1966.
181. Plum F, Posner JB. The diagnosis of stupor and coma. 2nd ed. Philadelphia: FA Davis Co.; 1972.
182. Plum F, Posner JB. The diagnosis of stupor and coma 3rd ed. Fa Davis Co., Philadelphia, 1982

183. Polmear A. Sentinel headaches in aneurysmal subarachnoid hemorrhage: what is the true incidence? A systematic review. Cephalagia. 2003;23: 935–41.
184. Pope Jr HG, Keck Jr PE, McElroy SL. Frequency and presentation of neuroleptic malignant syndrome in a large psychiatric hospital. Am J Psychiatry. 1986;143:1227–33.
185. Rabinstein AA. Paroxysmal sympathetic hyperactivity in the neurological intensive care unit. Neurol Res. 2007;29:680–2.
186. Rabinstein AA, Benarroch EE. Treatment of paroxysmal sympathetic hyperactivity. Curr Treat Options Neurol. 2008;10:151–7.
187. Rand CW. Significance of dilated pupil on homolateral hemiplegic side in cases of intracranial hemorrhage following head injuries. Report of seven cases. Arch Surg. 1929;18:1176–80.
188. Ratto O, Briscoe WA, Morton JW, et al. Anoxemia secondary to polycythemia and polycythemia secondary to anoxemia. Am J Med. 1955;19:958–65.
189. Reid WL, Cone WV. The mechanism of fixed dilatation of pupil. JAMA. 1939;112:2030–4.
190. Reynolds RW. Pulmonary edema as a consequence of hypothalamic lesions in rats. Science. 1963;141:930–2.
191. Richards P. Pulmonary edema and intracranial lesions. Br Med J. 1963;5349:83–6.
192. Ro LS, Chen ST, Tang LM, Wei KC. Concurrent trigeminal, abducens, and facial nerve palsies presenting as false localizing signs: case report. Neurosurgery. 1995;37:322–4.
193. Ropper AH. Lateral displacement of the brain and level of consciousness in patients with an acute hemispheral mass. N Engl J Med. 1986;314:953–8.
194. Ropper AH. The opposite pupil in herniation. Neurology. 1990;40:1707–9.
195. Ropper AH, Cole D, Louis DN. Clinicopathologic correlation in a case of pupillary dilation from cerebral hemorrhage. Arch Neurol. 1991;48:1166–9.
196. Samuels MA. The brain-heart connection. Circulation. 2007;116:77–84.
197. Sarner M, Crawford MD. Ruptured intracranial aneurysm. Lancet. 1965;2:1251–4.
198. Scarcella G, Fields WS. Recovery from coma and decerebrate rigidity of young patients following head injury. Acta Neurochir. 1962;10:134–44.
199. Schirmer CM, Kornbluth J, Heilman CB, Bhardwaj A. Gastrointestinal prophylaxis in neurocritical care. Neurocrit Care. 2012;16:184–93.
200. Schwartz WB, Bennett W, Curelop S. A syndrome of renal sodium loss and hyponatremia probably resulting from inappropriate secretion of antidiuretic hormone. Am J Med. 1957;23:529–42.
201. Schwarz G, Rosner A. Displacement and herniation of hippocampal gyrus through incisura tentorii: clinicopathologic study. Arch Neurol Psychiatry. 1941; 46:297–321.
202. Schwedt TJ, Matharu MS, Dodick DW. Thunderclap headache. Lancet Neurol. 2006;5:621–31.
203. Shalev A, Hermesh H, Munitz H. Mortality from neuroleptic malignant syndrome. J Clin Psychiatry. 1989;50:18–25.
204. Shalev A, Munitz H. The neuroleptic malignant syndrome: agent and host interaction. Acta Psychiatr Scand. 1986;73:337–47.
205. Shapiro WR, Williams GH, Plum F. Spontaneous recurrent hypothermia accompanying agenesis of the corpus callosum. Brain. 1969;92:423–36.
206. Shelton BA, O'Hara E, Tubbs RS, et al. Emergency suboccipital decompression for respiratory arrest during supratentorial surgery: the untold story of a surgeon's courage in times of despair. J Neurosurg. 2009;110:391–4.
207. Sherrington CS. Decerebrate rigidity and reflex coordination of movement. J Physiol. 1898;22: 319–22.
208. Sherrington CS. The integrative action of the nervous system (Silliman Memorial Lectures). London: Constable and Co., Ltd; 1906. p. xvi. 412pp.
209. Shibata Y, Meguro K, Narushima K, Shibuya F, Doi M, Kikuchi Y. Malignant lymphoma of the central nervous system presenting with central neurogenic hyperventilation. J Neurosurg. 1992;76:696–700.
210. Siderowf AD, Balcer LJ, Kenyon LC, et al. Raps EC, Galetta SL. Central neurogenic hyperventilation in an awake patient with a pontine glioma. Neurology. 1996;46:1160–2.
211. Simmons RL, Heisterkamp 3rd CA, Collins JA, et al. Acute pulmonary edema in battle casualties. J Trauma. 1969;9:760–75.
212. Slivka A, Philbrook B. Clinical and angiographic features of thunderclap headache. Headache. 1995; 35:1–6.
213. Smith RP, Tomlinson BE. Subendocardial hemorrhages associated with intracranial lesions. J Pathol. 1954;68:327–34.
214. Snyder Jr HR, Davis CS, Bickerton RK, Halliday RP. 1-[(5-arylfurfurylidene) amino]-hydantoins. A new class of muscle relaxants. J Med Chem. 1967;10:807–10.
215. Solomon GE. Diencephalic autonomic epilepsy caused by a neoplasm. J Pediatr. 1973;83:277–80.
216. Sonstein WJ, LaSala PA, Michelsen WJ, Onesti ST. False localizing signs in upper cervical spinal cord compression. Neurosurgery. 1996;38:445–8.
217. Srivastava SC, Robson AO. Electrocardiographic abnormalities associated with subarachnoid hemorrhage. Lancet. 1964;2:431–3.
218. Stankiewicz JA, Pazevic JP. Acquired Ondine's curse. Otolarnygol Head Neck Surg. 1989;101:611–3.
219. Sterns RH, Silver SM. Cerebral salt wasting *versus* SIADH: what difference? J Am Soc Nephrol. 2008; 19:194–6.
220. Stokes W. The diseases of the heart and the aorta. Dublin: Hodges and Smith; 1854. p. 323–4.
221. Straus C, Trang H, Becquemin M-H, Touraine P, Similowski T. Chemosensitivity recovery in Ondine's curse syndrome under treatment with desogestrel. Respir Physiol Neurobiol. 2010;171:171–4.

222. Strawn JR, Keck Jr PE, Caroff SN. Neuroleptic malignant syndrome. Am J Psychiatry. 2007;164: 870–6.
223. Sugar O. In search of Ondine's syndrome. JAMA. 1978;240:236–7.
224. Summers GD, Young AC, Little RA, et al. Spontaneous periodic hypothermia with lipoma of the corpus callosum. J Neurol Neurosurg Psychiatry. 1981;44:1094–9.
225. Sun MK, Reis DJ. Differential responses of barosensitive neurons of rostral ventrolateral medulla to hypoxia in rats. Brain Res. 1993;609:333–7.
226. Sunderland S. The tentorial notch and complications produced by herniations of the brain through that aperture. Br J Surg. 1958;45:422–38.
227. Sunderland S, Bradley KC. Disturbances of oculomotor function accompanying extradural hemorrhage. J Neurol Neurosurg Psychiatry. 1953;16:35–46.
228. Suzuki J, Iwabuchi T. Ocular motor disturbances occurring as false localizing signs in ruptured intracranial aneurysms. Acta Neurochir. 1974;30:119–28.
229. Szabo S. Hans Seyle and the development of the stress concept. Special reference to gastroduodenal ulcerogenesis. Ann N Y Acad Sci. 1998;851:19–27.
230. Szakacs JE, Cannon A. L-norepinephrine myocarditis. Am J Clin Pathol. 1958;30:425–38.
231. Takahashi M, Tsunemi T, Miyayosi T,et al. Reversible central neurogenic hyperventilation in an awake patient with multiple sclerosis. J Neurol. 2007; 254:1763–4.
232. Talman WT. Cardiovascular regulation and lesions of the central nervous system. Ann Neurol. 1985;18: 1–13.
233. Talman WT, Florek G, Bullard DE. A hyperthermic syndrome in two subjects with acute hydrocephalus. Arch Neurol. 1988;45:1037–40.
234. Tarulli AW, Lim C, Bui JD, et al. Alexander MP. Central neurogenic hyperventilation: a case report and discussion of pathophysiology. Arch Neurol. 2005;62:1632–4.
235. Tatschl C, Stöllberger C, Matz K, et al. Insular involvement is associated with QT prolongation: ECG abnormalities in patients with acute stroke. Cerebrovasc Dis. 2006;21:47–53.
236. Theodore J, Robin ED. Pathogenesis of neurogenic pulmonary edema. Lancet. 1975;2:749–51.
237. Theodore J, Robin ED. Speculations on neurogenic pulmonary edema (NPE). Am Rev Respir Dis. 1976;113:405–11.
238. Thompson RK, Malina S. Dynamic axial brainstem distortion as a mechanism explaining the cardiorespiratory changes in increased intracranial pressure. J Neurosurg. 1959;16:664–75.
239. Trousseau A. Clinique Medicale de l'Hotel-Dieu de Paris. Vol 3, 2nd Ed. Paris France, JB Balliere. 1865.
240. Turnbull AR. Multiple false localizing signs in intracranial tumor. Case report. J Neurosurg. 1974; 40:264–6.
241. Vaernet K. Caloric vestibular reactions in transtentorial herniation of the brainstem. Neurology. 1957; 7:833–6.
242. Van Gehuchten P. Le mécanisme de la mort dans certains cas de tumeur cerebrale. Encéphale. 1937;2: 113–27.
243. Von Bergmann E. Die Lehre von den Kopfverletzungen. Stuttgart: Enke; 1880.
244. Von Bergmann E. Head injuries: In Billroth E, Pitha F (eds) Handbuch der Allgemeine and Speciellen Chirurgie. Erlangen, Verlag von Ferden and Enke, 1873.
245. Von Leyden E. Beiträge and Untersuchungen zur Physiologie und Pathologie des Gehirns. Virchows Arch. 1866;37:519–59.
246. Waga S, Otitsubo K, Handa H. Warning signs in intracranial aneurysms. Surg Neurol. 1975;3:15–50.
247. Walshe FMR. Decerebrate rigidity in animals and its recognition in man. Proc R Soc Med. 1922;15: 41–7.
248. Walshe FMR. The decerebrate rigidity of Sherrington in man. Its recognition and differentiation from other forms of tonic muscular contraction. Arch Neurol Psychiatry. 1923;10:1–28.
249. Walton JN. Subarachnoid hemorrhage. Edinburgh: ES Livingstone; 1956.
250. Ward M. Periodic respiration. A short historical note. Ann R Coll Surg Engl. 1973;52:330–4.
251. Wasserman F, Choquette G, Cassinelli R, Bellet S. Electrocardiographic observations in patients with cerebrovascular accidents. Report of 12 cases. Am J Med Sci. 1956;231:502–10.
252. Webber CL, Jr., Speck DF. Experimental Biot periodic breathing in cats: effects of changes in PaO_2 and $PaCO_2$. *Respir Physiol* 1981;46:327–344.
253. Weinstein J, Langfitt T, Kassell N. Vasopressor response to increased intracranial pressure. Neurology. 1964;14:1118–31.
254. Weintraub BM, McHenry LC. Cardiac abnormalities in subarachnoid hemorrhage: a resume. Stroke. 1974;5:384–92.
255. Wijdicks EFM. Cushing's ulcer: the eponym and his own. Neurosurgery. 2011;68:1695–8.
256. Wijdicks EFM, Kerkhoff H, Van Gijn J. Long-term follow up of 71 patients with thunderclap headache mimicking subarachnoid hemorrhage. Lancet. 1988; 2:68–70.
257. Wijdicks EFM, Ropper AH, Hunnicutt EJ, Richardson GS, Nathanson JA. Atrial natriuretic factor and salt wasting after aneurysmal subarachnoid hemorrhage. Stroke. 1991;22:1519–24.
258. Wijdicks EFM, Schievink WI, Burnett Jr JC. Natriuretic peptide system and endothelin in aneurysmal subarachnoid hemorrhage. J Neurosurg. 1997;87:275–80.
259. Wijdicks EFM, Vermeulen M, ten Haaf JA, Hijdra A, Bakker WH, van Gijn J. Volume depletion and natriuresis in patients with a ruptured intracranial aneurysm. Ann Neurol. 1985;18:211–6.

260. Wilson SAK. On decerebrate rigidity in Man and the occurrence of "tonic fits". Proc R Soc Med. 1920;13:89–92.
261. Woodhall B, Devine Jr JW, Hart D. Homolateral dilatation of the pupil, homolateral paresis and bilateral muscular rigidity in the diagnosis of extradural hemorrhage. Surg Gynecol Obstet. 1941; 72:391–8.
262. Yaggi H, Mohsenin V. Obstructive sleep apnea and stroke. Lancet Neurol. 2004;3:333–42.
263. Yeomans ND. The ulcer sleuths: the search for the cause of peptic ulcers. J Gastroenterol Hepatol. 2011;26 Suppl 1:35–41.
264. Zafonte RD, Mann NR. Cerebral salt wasting syndrome in brain injury patients: a potential cause of hyponatremia. Arch Phys Med Rehabil. 1997;78:540–2.
265. Zaroff JG, Rordorf GA, Newell JB, et al. Cardiac outcome in patients with subarachnoid hemorrhage and electrocardiographic abnormalities. Neurosurgery. 1999;44:34–9.

First Descriptions of Clinical Syndromes

4

E.F.M. Wijdicks, *Famous First Papers for the Neurointensivist*,
DOI 10.1007/978-1-4614-3182-4_4,

Short Historical Note 19

MINIMALLY CONSCIOUS STATE

The Title of the Paper

Giacino JI, Ashwal S, Childs N, et al. The minimally conscious state: definition and diagnostic criteria. Neurology. 2002;58:349–53.

The Paper and the Times

It is expected that most comatose patients awaken even after a major acute injury. In the early weeks, the responsiveness and awareness varies. In some patients, there appears none, in others there is merely a hint. Following initial recovery in responsiveness, these patients may stay in the intensive care unit for treatment of systemic complications, but even if these intercurrent illnesses have come under control, a marked disability may remain.

Severe neurologic injury has been mostly dichotomized as "severe disability or persistent vegetative state." However, rehabilitation physicians recognized that patients in a supposedly persistent vegetative state (PVS) were sometimes more awake, albeit minimally so. These patients most typically showed inconsistent responsiveness, and therefore, an attempt was made to further define this condition, to name it *minimally conscious state* (MCS) and to set it apart from PVS. Estimates were brought forward that claimed MCS would be ten times more common than PVS. However, it did not appear obvious to neurologists that different states of prolonged consciousness could exist, different outcomes could be expected, and that there even could be different therapeutic approaches [21].

The Details of the Paper

In 2002, the Aspen Consensus Conference Work Group suggested a condition of severe disability with minimal awareness. Nine meetings were held with delegates in bioethics, neurology, neuropsychology, neurosurgery, physiatry, nursing, and allied health (Fig. 4.1). When patients did not fulfill the criteria of a PVS, they suggested using the term *minimally conscious state* (MCS). However, the definition (or boundaries) of this disabled state was neither based on prospective data nor was there much known about the chances of improvement. The working group emphasized that the distinction of MCS from PVS was mostly a partial presence of awareness. In the working group's opinion, this characteristic had medicolegal implications and questions about the use of resources, but there was no further explanation about the consequences of such a distinction.

Although patients in an MCS are aware, to recognize and demonstrate awareness is difficult if the patient does not follow a command. A simple motor task does not imply full awareness, and obviously, a gesture or verbalization is a more useful sign. To the physician observing these patients behaviors should be purposeful, although patients' responses could be slow. In all patients, the level of awareness was markedly diminished.

A definition of MCS was proposed: "The minimally conscious state is the condition of severely altered consciousness in which minimal but definite behavioral evidence of self or environmental awareness is demonstrated." Diagnostic criteria were proposed: "the following simple commands, gestural or verbal yes and no responses, intelligible verbalization, purposeful behavior including movement or effective behaviors that occur in contingent relation to relevant environmental stimuli and are due to reflexive activity." The working group also suggested future directions for research to study the incidence and prevalence of MCS, natural history, and recovery course but also interrater and intrarater reliability of the diagnostic criteria.

Criteria for emergence from MCS also were proposed and included the appearance of interactive communication and functional use of two objects.

The working group acknowledged that the incidence and prevalence, the ability to be diagnosed accurately, the course of recovery, and potential for treatment remained largely unknown.

AMERICAN ACADEMY OF NEUROLOGY

Special Article

CME

The minimally conscious state

Definition and diagnostic criteria

J.T. Giacino, PhD; S. Ashwal, MD; N. Childs, MD; R. Cranford, MD; B. Jennett, MD; D.I. Katz, MD; J.P. Kelly, MD; J.H. Rosenberg, MD; J. Whyte, MD, PhD; R.D. Zafonte, DO; and N.D. Zasler, MD

Abstract—*Objective:* To establish consensus recommendations among health care specialties for defining and establishing diagnostic criteria for the minimally conscious state (MCS). *Background:* There is a subgroup of patients with severe alteration in consciousness who do not meet diagnostic criteria for coma or the vegetative state (VS). These patients demonstrate inconsistent but discernible evidence of consciousness. It is important to distinguish patients in MCS from those in coma and VS because preliminary findings suggest that there are meaningful differences in outcome. *Methods:* An evidence-based literature review of disorders of consciousness was completed to define MCS, develop diagnostic criteria for entry into MCS, and identify markers for emergence to higher levels of cognitive function. *Results:* There were insufficient data to establish evidence-based guidelines for diagnosis, prognosis, and management of MCS. Therefore, a consensus-based case definition with behaviorally referenced diagnostic criteria was formulated to facilitate future empirical investigation. *Conclusions:* MCS is characterized by inconsistent but clearly discernible behavioral evidence of consciousness and can be distinguished from coma and VS by documenting the presence of specific behavioral features not found in either of these conditions. Patients may evolve to MCS from coma or VS after acute brain injury. MCS may also result from degenerative or congenital nervous system disorders. This condition is often transient but may also exist as a permanent outcome. Defining MCS should promote further research on its epidemiology, neuropathology, natural history, and management.

NEUROLOGY 2002;58:349–353

Precise estimates of the incidence and prevalence of severe disorders of consciousness are unavailable. In the United States, the number of individuals who sustain severe traumatic brain injury (i.e., brain injury caused by externally inflicted trauma[1]) with prolonged loss of consciousness each year is estimated to be between 56 and 170 per one million.[2,3] The economic impact of the problem is enormous. Projected average per person lifetime costs of care alone for severe traumatic brain injury range from $600,000 to $1,875,000.[4] A single case described by Paris[5] reported in-hospital lifetime costs of $6,104,590. In the last 5 years, there have been some attempts to clarify and define diagnostic, prognostic, and treatment issues concerning patients with severe disturbances of consciousness.[6-10] Disorders of consciousness include coma and the vegetative state (VS). Patients in coma have complete failure of the arousal system with no spontaneous eye opening and are unable to be awakened by application of vigorous sensory stimulation.[11] VS is characterized by the complete absence of behavioral evidence for self or environmental awareness. There is preserved capacity for spontaneous or stimulus-induced arousal, evidenced by sleep–wake cycles.[12] The locked-in syndrome, characterized by anarthria and quadriplegia with general preservation of cognition, must be distinguished from disorders of consciousness.[11] The table outlines the clinical features of disorders of consciousness and the locked-in syndrome.

Some patients with severe alteration in consciousness have neurologic findings that do not meet criteria for VS. These patients demonstrate discernible

Fig. 4.1 The title page

The Message and Acceptance

The American Academy of Neurology endorsed the document that was proposed by the Aspen Working Group.

Now looking back, the term *minimally conscious state* is most useful for patients with certain neurologic characteristics, but it likely is a mixed bag of neurologic conditions [37, 197, 198]. The transition to a better than minimal conscious state also is poorly defined, and using these aforementioned criteria may, on the surface, categorize quite a large proportion of patients with severe brain injury in this state. Those who care for patients in neurointensive care and trauma units may even question who is not in a MCS.

Moreover, a recent study found the current criteria of giving accurate answers to simple yes and no questions problematic in patients with traumatic brain injury and suggested the MCS criteria could result in misclassifying patients with cognitive disabilities [120].

Perception of pain in MCS- and perhaps suffering from it- has been very difficult to assess. One study applied a noxious stimulus (nerve conduction stimulus) to the median nerve and found activation of the primary sensory cortex, thalamus, frontoparietal and anterior cingulate cortex in MCS similarly as in controls, but much less so in PVS [31]. These findings, however, do not resolve the issue because it remains unclear how to reliably assess pain perception.

In the United States, MCS became accepted after the case of Terri Schiavo. Attorneys for the Schiavo family suggested Terri could be in a MCS. The publicity surrounding this case brought this category of abnormal consciousness into the mainstream and—incorrectly—suggested that an easy distinction between MCS and PVS was feasible clinically. Moreover, several years later, functional magnetic resonance imaging scan studies suggested that neurologic examination may not be sufficient and that these tests could actually identify patients in an MCS previously diagnosed as being in a PVS [108, 116, 166, 190]. Furthermore, studies suggested that MCS could result in further improvement and that PVS could potentially improve into an MCS. Most patients emerge from MCS in 3 months, and improvement may occur later, but more than 60% of the patients will remain severely disabled and fully dependent on others.

It is thus likely that MCS is a transitional condition leading to a severely handicapped state that requires full nursing care to maintain body integrity. Families cannot expect any participation in decision making. The emotional state, if any, may be bland and not responsive to medication. Attempts to change this deplorable situation with deep brain stimulation have resulted in some improvement in responsiveness, but whether this intervention will show promise is unclear [164, 165]. A recent study however suggested that amantadine could speed up recovery in some patients [68]

Short Historical Note 20

PERSISTENT VEGETATIVE STATE

The Title of the Paper

Jennet B, Plum F. Persistent vegetative state after brain damage: a syndrome in search of a name. Lancet. 1972;1:734–7.

The Paper and the Times

Severely injured patients with no evidence of awareness of their surroundings and no prospects for improvement have been known for centuries. When neurology matured as a specialty, there was not only an incentive to better diagnose these states, but also to mark the dismal nature of the condition.

Over the years, there have been many attempts to find a fitting and workable term. Dejerine possibly coined the term *coma vigil* to distinguish it from other types of coma. The more severe types of coma were mostly called *coma carus* and were defined as a patient who can hardly be aroused, would only open the eyes after a strong stimulus, and could barely move. In *coma vigil*, none of that would exist, but the patient's eyes were spontaneously open [56]. (*Coma dépassé* would become the next stage; see historical note 21). Jouvet introduced the term *la stupeur hypertonique post-comateuse*, but the term lacked sufficient details and was untranslatable. Other terms used by French neurologists were *vie vegetative* or *coma prolongé*. Kretschmer named it *Das apallische syndrom*. The term indicated an abnormality of a lesion of the pallium also known as the mantle of the gray matter forming the cortex. In 1969, in the United States, Adams and Jequier already described these patients as being in "a most primitive vegetative state" [6].

Since its original description, the term persistent vegetative state (PVS) has remained unchallenged [191]. Short of a better alternative, PVS has resonated well for physicians. Patient's families may occasionally say "he never wanted to be kept as a vegetable" (often referring to a less severe disability), or some may use the Terri Schiavo case as an example "she never wanted to be like the Schiavo case [10]."

The Details of the Paper

Bryan Jennett—having seen a significant number of patients after traumatic brain injury—approached Fred Plum to write this paper together (Fig. 4.2). In their 1972 communication, Jennett and Plum coined the term *persistent vegetative state*. In their 1972 *Lancet* communication, they wrote:

> The word vegetative itself is not obscure: vegetate is defined in the Oxford English Dictionary as "to live a merely physical life, devoid of intellectual activity or social intercourse," and vegetative is used to describe "an organic body capable of growth and development but devoid of sensation and thought."

Jennett used the term *vegetative* to emphasize the vegetative component of the nervous system. Plum noted that he could have called it "persistent autonomic state," but felt that it was less flexible.

The major focus of this paper was to call attention of a group of patients with undeniable clinical characteristics, but Jennett and Plum understood that transitional cases could exist. "Although we would not deny that a continuum must exist between this vegetative state and some of the others described, it seems wise to make an absolute distinction between patients who do make a consistently understandable response to those around them, by word or gesture, and those who never do."

Jennett and Plum were also quick to point out:

> New methods of treatment may, by prolonging the lives of patients with conditions which were formerly fatal, result in situations never previously encountered. And new situations call for new names if they are to be accurately understood and discussed. … There is a group of patients who never show evidence of a working mind. This concept may be criticized on the grounds that observation of behavior is insufficient evidence on which to base a judgment of mental activity; it is our view that there is no reliable alternative available to the doctor at the bedside, which is where decisions have to be made.

Jennett and Plum felt that hope for clinical recovery was unrealistic. In order to increase confidence in the diagnosis, they called for more clinical studies and questioned how long PVS should persist before it can be declared permanent. This would have to be determined by prospective studies.

Points of View

PERSISTENT VEGETATIVE STATE AFTER BRAIN DAMAGE

A Syndrome in Search of a Name

BRYAN JENNETT

Institute of Neurological Sciences, Glasgow GS1 4TF

FRED PLUM

New York Hospital—Cornell Medical Center, New York City, N.Y., U.S.A.

Summary Patients with severe brain damage due to trauma or ischæmia may now survive indefinitely. Some never regain recognisable mental function, but recover from sleep-like coma in that they have periods of wakefulness when their eyes are open and move; their responsiveness is limited to primitive postural and reflex movements of the limbs, and they never speak. Such patients are best described as in a persistent vegetative state, which should be clearly distinguished from other conditions associated with prolonged unresponsiveness. What is common to these patients is the absence of function in the cerebral cortex as judged behaviourally; the lesion may be in the cortex itself, in subcortical structures of the hemisphere, or in the brain-stem, or in all of these sites. But the exact site and nature of the lesion is unknown to the bedside clinician, and the name for the syndrome should not imply more than is known.

Fig. 4.2 Title page

The Message and Acceptance

The message by Jennett and Plum was very clear—some patients are permanently unconscious, and they should be recognized as a separate category [88]. The neuropathologic correlate is often a severe diffuse cortical injury with atrophy, but there may be more pronounced abnormalities in the thalami [4].

The clinical condition was further scrutinized by a Multi-Society Task Force (see historical note 57). Although a presumptive diagnosis could be made earlier, it was suggested that a diagnostic neurologic examination for the purpose of establishing a definitive diagnosis of a PVS should be postponed until at least 1 month has passed.

A basic neurologic examination may not capture the salient features of PVS. Careful examination of the eye movements has a high priority. Eyes may open wide when patient is touched, but visual pursuit—smoothly following an object—is absent or at the very least momentary and not reproducible. Visual fixation is absent, although it can appear later and mostly at random without other signs of improvement. A visual orienting reflex may occur with head turning when family members or nursing staff move in the room. Large objects or persons suddenly closely approaching the patient may result in the patient briefly turning the eyes and suggest target focusing, but the response extinguishes quickly. The task force recognized that one should not make a diagnosis of PVS when there is any degree of sustained visual pursuit or reproducible visual fixation.

In a later paper, Jennett summarized the current state of the terminology [89]:

> What attracts attention and curiosity is the dissociation between arousal and awareness—the combination of periods of wakeful eye opening with lack of any evidence of a working mind either receiving or projecting information. The advantage of the term "vegetative state" is that it simply describes observed behavior, without implying specific structural pathology.

Misdiagnosis of PVS has been reported [9, 118]. The reliability of the diagnosis of a PVS has been surveyed in the United Kingdom and in the United States, and traces of awareness were found in a considerable proportion of patients deemed to be in a PVS. Misdiagnosis was more likely in patients identified as being in a PVS within 3 months of injury and after trauma. Conversely, patients who reside in long-term care facilities may not have been diagnosed as being in a vegetative state. Indistinct terms (e.g., severe brain injury, or even comatose) may be used, and far more importantly, families may not have been informed about the permanent nature of the brain injury. The reasons are unclear, but most likely pertain to insufficient expert assessment of these patients and much less likely recovery when the patients—for some legal reason—are extensively reexamined. It also remains to be seen whether some subgroups of patients exist that may be in a condition in between PVS and MCS (MCS plus or PVS minus.)

For most expert neurologists, the diagnosis of PVS is quite simple and straightforward, recognizing that multiple examinations over time would be most accurate. For non-neurologists, the diagnosis can be challenging and not infrequently nursing staff or families may notice more. Ignoring their call is likely a major factor in misdiagnosis.

A European task force on disorders of consciousness suggested to rename the condition "unresponsive wakefulness syndrome." The reason was the alleged "negative connotation" and "pejorative undertone"; a concern so often put forward by pro-life groups. The working group also felt that once using the term *PVS*, the signs of recovery of consciousness would be missed. Whether changing the term to unresponsive wakefulness syndrome would prevent that from happening is unknown and unlikely [100].

Sadly, there is still a misunderstanding among some physicians and health care workers about the meaning of the terms *brain death* and *vegetative state*. In fact, most catastrophic injury spares the brainstem and does not lead to PVS or brain death. Both conditions represent the extremes of neurologic injury.

Short Historical Note 21

BRAIN DEATH

The Title of the Paper

Mollaret P, Goulon M. Le Coma Dépassé (memoire preliminaire). Rev Neurol. 1959;101:3–15.

The Paper and the Times

Death of the brain—meaning death of the person—was quite a departure from the traditional clinical diagnosis of death that required irreversible absent breathing and circulatory arrest. After a catastrophic neurologic injury, patients would follow a common pathway, become comatose, and develop respiratory failure leading to insufficient breathing, apnea, and circulatory arrest. The mechanical ventilator would change that course. Now, patients were placed on a ventilator and the brain injury could progress to involve the disappearance of all brainstem reflexes. Even before criteria were published, most physicians felt that these patients were essentially dead.

These clinical observations became more pertinent when electroencephalographers found that the electroencephalogram (EEG) showed no activity and neuropathologists found complete necrosis of the brain.

Although most initial observations pertained to EEG findings, Lofstedt and von Reis reported in 1956 six mechanically ventilated patients with absent reflexes, apnea, hypotension, hypothermia, and polyuria. Cerebral blood flow, determined by angiography, was absent [107]. Cerebral necrosis was present at autopsy in all cases.

In 1959, Wertheimer, Jouvet, and Descotes were among the first to propose criteria for this new clinical state [193]. This manuscript largely focused, as many before, on the significance of an isoelectric EEG but also documented shutting off the ventilator to stimulate the respiratory centers with increasing respiratory acidosis. Absent medulla oblongata function was further confirmed with no change in pulse rate with carotid compression, ocular pressure, and IV injection of atropine and amphetamine.

Both these papers, although introducing new findings lacked neurologic details that would come with the work by Mollaret and Goulon (Fig. 4.3). Almost 10 years would pass until the issue was comprehensively dealt with by a committee of physicians and other stakeholder specialties from Harvard Medical School.

The Details of the Paper

The paper involves 23 cases at Claude Bernard Hospital in Paris that were called *Coma dépassé*. The authors described in sufficient detail absent brainstem reflexes, apnea, and also polyuria and difficulty maintaining blood pressure with vasopressors. A flat EEG also was noted by the authors. Oxygen desaturation and respiratory metabolic acidosis were commonly observed, and intramuscular injection of vasopressor was needed to maintain a systemic hemodynamic stability. *Coma dépassé* was said to be characterized by immobility of the eyeballs in a neutral position, mydriasis, absent light reflex, absent blinking with stimuli, absence of swallowing reflexes, drooping of the jaw, absence of motor responses to any stimuli, muscle hypotonia, tendon areflexia, equivocal plantar reflexes, absence of spontaneous respiration after discontinuation of ventilation, immediate cardiovascular collapse as soon as vasopressors are stopped, and a disturbance of thermoregulation with core temperature, depending on the environmental temperature. The authors compared this clinical state with other types of coma and pointed out differences (Fig. 4.4).

Mollaret and Goulon found cases in which mechanical ventilation was controlled in the first days, only to deteriorate later, and they documented oxygen desaturation, acute hypercapnia, and combined respiratory and metabolic acidosis. Polyuria was present in most cases, and intramuscular injection of *d'hormone post-hypophysaire* resulted in reduced diuresis and concentration of urine. Hyperglycemia and glycosuria were observed, but there was a normal response to insulin. The heart rate slowed to 40–60 beats/min and was not changed by pressure on the eyeballs, carotid sinus, or by IV injection of atropine. This condition ended ultimately with cardiac arrest.

Fig. 4.3 Title page

REVUE NEUROLOGIQUE

MÉMOIRES ORIGINAUX

LE COMA DÉPASSÉ
(MÉMOIRE PRÉLIMINAIRE)

PAR MM.

P. MOLLARET et M. GOULON

Après quatre années de réflexion, nous croyons venu le moment d'ajouter un chapitre nouveau au domaine traditionnel des comas.

Précisons de suite que ce problème du coma dépassé a été mis, l'année dernière, au programme de la prochaine Journée de Réanimation de l'Hôpital Claude-Bernard du 7 octobre 1959, en vue d'une mise au point intégrale.

La présente communication, qui n'a ainsi qu'une valeur préliminaire, peut être offerte, peut-être, en hommage à la XXIIIe Réunion Neurologique Internationale, qui a accepté de tenir une de ses séances dans le Centre de Réanimation où fut élaboré ce travail. Précisons également que le coma dépassé a déjà conquis droit de cité dans l'important volume qui vient de paraître de H. Fischgold et P. Mathis (*Obnubilations, comas et stupeurs*, Masson édit., Paris, 1959, p. 5 et pp. 51-52) ; nous remercions ces auteurs d'être venus se faire présenter les premiers malades et d'avoir donné place à quelques-uns de nos documents.

DÉFINITIONS.

Selon les traités classiques, le coma est un état caractérisé ***par la perte des fonctions de la vie de relation*** (conscience, motilité, sensibilité et réflexes), ***avec conservation des fonctions de la vie végétative*** (avant tout respiration, circulation et thermorégulation).

Guy Tardieu, dans sa thèse de 1942, qui fit date à l'époque, a repris cette définition mais en ajoutant qu'elle est, à plusieurs égards, inexacte. D'une part, dans nombre de comas, il y a, non abolition complète, mais

REVUE NEUROLOGIQUE, T. 101, N° 1, 1959.

P. MOLLARET ET M. GOULON

TABLEAU I.

		Degrés du coma	C. vigile	C. type	C. carus	C. dépassé
Fonctions de relation		Hypersomnie	++	+++	++++	++++
		Réveil provoqué	possible	0	0	0
		Conscience	diminuée	0	0	0
		Confusion mentale	possible	0	0	0
		Contrôle des besoins élément.	possible ±	0	0	0
		Hypertonie de décérébration	0	Rare	moins rare	0 (ou transitoire) au début
		Réflexes mésencéphal.	+	0 ou ±	0	0
	Déglutition	Premier temps	+	0	0	0
		Dernier temps	+	±	0	0
Fonctions végétatives		Respiration	conservée	conservée	perturbée	abolie
		Circulation	conservée	conservée	perturbée	collapsus progressif
		Régulation thermique	conservée	conservée	perturbée	perturbée

Fig. 4.4 Comparison with other types of coma (most notable difference with coma carus [deep coma]) is *respiration* pertubeé (abnormal breathing) to *respiration abolie* (absent breathing) and *circulation collapsus progressif* (progressive circulatory collapse)

The Message and Acceptance

There has been some historical discussion as to whether neurologists Mollaret and Goulon or neurosurgeon Wertheimer and neurologist Jouvet were the first to describe brain death. Both papers—published the same year and even months in between—have important comparable attributes. A strong argument can be made that Mollaret and Goulon had a more detailed paper, larger series of patients, significant more detail on how the patient's absence of brain function impacted on systemic instability, and further characterization of laboratory abnormalities.

Jouvet and Wertheimer were set on defining brain death by electrophysiologic criteria. They described patients as "heart-lung preparations." The authors felt objective criteria were needed and inserted fine bipolar electrodes into the medial thalamic structures, applied strong electrical currents, and found no motor response.

After these observations, very few papers were published between 1959 and 1968. Studies largely concentrated on isoelectric EEGs and findings of absent intracranial flow. In the United States, Schwab is credited for providing a more detailed description of an isoelectric EEG in brain death and merging the EEG into diagnostic criteria [168]. These criteria would allow the physician to indicate that the patient was dead:

Absence of spontaneous respiration for 30 min
No tendon reflexes of any type
No pupillary reflexes
Absence of oculocardiac reflex (eyeball pressure slowing heart rate)
Thirty minutes of isoelectric EEG

These early observations in 1963 were a prelude to a more comprehensive definition of brain death. This focused effort would appear in 1968. In Boston, the Harvard Medical School Ad Hoc Committee to Examine the Definition of Brain Death [1] set out to "define irreversible coma as a new criterion for death" [1, 196]. The criteria of brain death were based on the collective experience of the committee members. The Harvard criteria were published in the *Journal of the American Medical Association* (*JAMA*) on August 5, 1968 (Fig. 4.5). The document, a collection of brief statements included a definition of brain death, a legal commentary, and an explanation of an address by his holiness Pope Pius XII.

In the next development, which turned out to be crucial in the way brain death was diagnosed, Mohandas and Chou published the Minnesota Code of Brain Death [114], also known as the Minnesota criteria. Major changes from the Harvard criteria included definition of time of apnea (4 min of disconnection), exclusion of metabolic derangements, and shorter observation time of 12 h, but the paper did not present validating data. Mohandas and Chou should be credited for first introducing into the brain death literature the information that damage of the brainstem was a critical component of severe brain damage.

The centrality of the brainstem had been recognized by many. During this time, a confusing discussion appeared with new terminology. Brain death was now described by some bioethicists as whole brain death (hemispheres and brainstem irreversibly damaged) but also as higher brain death (hemispheres irreversibly damaged), brainstem death (brainstem irreversibly damaged), and even a super locked-in syndrome (brainstem irreversibly damaged but hemispheres functioning), dividing the death of the brain into segments. This discussion largely was helpful in distinguishing persistent vegetative state (higher brain death) from brain death (whole brain death), but such a categorization would ignore the typical course of massive hemispheric damage that would eventually, in a rostrocaudal way, damage the brainstem.

These discussions, culminated in a report of the *Medical Consultants on the Diagnosis of Death to the President' Commission on Ethical Issues in Medicine and Biomedical and Behavioral Research* and were published in 1981 [8]. The report led to the Uniform Determination of Death Act. The American Academy of Neurology published its guidelines in 1995 and 2010 and no other society guidelines have been published since [203].

The British neurologists understood as one of the first that the "brainstem death is the infratentorial repercussion of supratentorial events [51]." In a series of papers, Pallis described the diagnosis of brainstem death, the pitfalls and preconditions

A Definition of Irreversible Coma

Report of the Ad Hoc Committee of the Harvard Medical School to Examine the Definition of Brain Death

Our primary purpose is to define irreversible coma as a new criterion for death. There are two reasons why there is need for a definition: (1) Improvements in resuscitative and supportive measures have led to increased efforts to save those who are desperately injured. Sometimes these efforts have only partial success so that the result is an individual whose heart continues to beat but whose brain is irreversibly damaged. The burden is great on patients who suffer permanent loss of intellect, on their families, on the hospitals, and on those in need of hospital beds already occupied by these comatose patients. (2) Obsolete criteria for the definition of death can lead to controversy in obtaining organs for transplantation.

Irreversible coma has many causes, but *we are concerned here only with those comatose individuals who have no discernible central nervous system activity.* If the characteristics can be defined in satisfactory terms, translatable into action–and we believe this is possible–then several problems will either disappear or will become more readily soluble.

More than medical problems are present. There are moral, ethical, religious, and legal issues. Adequate definition here will prepare the way for better insight into all of these matters as well as for better law than is currently applicable.

The Ad Hoc Committee includes Henry K. Beecher, MD, *chairman;* Raymond D. Adams, MD; A. Clifford Barger, MD; William J. Curran, LLM, SMHyg; Derek Denny-Brown, MD; Dana L. Farnsworth, MD; Jordi Folch-Pi, MD; Everett I. Mendelsohn, PhD; John P. Merrill, MD; Joseph Murray, MD; Ralph Potter, ThD; Robert Schwab, MD; and William Sweet, MD.

Reprint requests to Massachusetts General Hospital, Boston 02114 (Dr. Henry K. Beecher).

Characteristics of Irreversible Coma

An organ, brain or other, that no longer functions and has no possibility of functioning again is for all practical purposes dead. Our first problem is to determine the characteristics of a *permanently* nonfunctioning brain.

A patient in this state appears to be in deep coma. The condition can be satisfactorily diagnosed by points 1, 2, and 3 to follow. The electroencephalogram (point 4) provides confirmatory data, and when available it should be utilized. In situations where for one reason or another electroencephalographic montioring is not available, the absence of cerebral function has to be determined by purely clinical signs, to be described, or by absence of circulation as judged by standstill of blood in the retinal vessels, or by absence of cardiac activity.

1. *Unreceptivity and Unresponsitivity.*–There is a total unawareness to externally applied stimuli and inner need and complete unresponsiveness–our definition of irreversible coma. Even the most intensely painful stimuli evoke no vocal or other response, not even a groan, withdrawal of a limb, or quickening of respiration.

2. *No Movements or Breathing.*–Observations covering a period of at least one hour by physicians is adequate to satisfy the criteria of no spontaneous muscular movements or spontaneous respiration or response to stimuli such as pain, touch, sound, or light. After the patient is on a mechanical respirator, the total absence of spontaneous breathing may be established by turning off the respirator for three minutes and observing whether there is any effort on the part of the subject to breathe

Fig. 4.5 Title page

eventually bundled in the ABC of brainstem death [132–134] (Fig. 4.6).

These preconditions were essential in the approach to the patient. "Testing for brainstem death should not be undertaken unless the cause of coma has been established beyond all doubt." Pallis clearly emphasized the importance of an apnea test and using blood gas determination. Pallis warned against apnea testing by only looking at overriding the ventilator for 15 min. "The test for apnea without ensuring and documenting an appropriate rise in $PaCO_2$ has been likened to testing the pupils without a battery in the torch."

Cardiac arrest is inevitable when all brainstem functions are lost. Pallis noted in 1990:

> To date not a single case seems to have been recorded—in a reputable and widely accessible journal- of a patient with well documented structural brain damage (from trauma or intracranial hemorrhage, for instance) who recovered brainstem function after fulfilling properly applied clinical criteria of brain stem death [134].

ABC of Brain Stem Death CHRISTOPHER PALLIS

FROM BRAIN DEATH TO BRAIN STEM DEATH

Historical background

Harvard criteria

1 Unreceptivity and unresponsivity

2 No movements (observe for 1h)

3 Apnoea (3min off respirator)

4 Absence of elicitable reflexes

5 Isoelectric EEG "of great confirmatory value" (at 5μV/mm)

All of the above tests shall be repeated at least 24 hours later with no change

The first insight

"What we are attempting to define and establish beyond reasonable doubt is the state of irreversible damage to the brain stem. It is the point of no return."

Mohandas and Chou[4]

Brain death was first described clinically in 1959 when two French physicians[1] identified a condition they called "coma dépassé"—literally, a state beyond coma. Twenty of their 23 patients were suffering from primary intracranial disorders and the other three from the cerebral sequelae of cardiorespiratory arrest. All the classic features of brain death are found in this early report. Articles published in the early 1960s already suggested that the cerebral circulation was "blocked" by raised intracranial pressure in most of these cases.

The report of the Ad Hoc Committee of the Harvard Medical School in 1968[2] brought awareness of brain death to a much wider audience. The Harvard criteria demanded that the patient should be unreceptive and unresponsive, the most intensely painful stimuli evoking "no vocal or other response, not even a groan, withdrawal of a limb or quickening of respiration." There had to be no movements during observation for one hour. Apnoea was to be confirmed by three minutes off the respirator (the centrality of apnoea, properly defined and tested for, had already been appreciated). The Harvard criteria also required that there should be "no reflexes," the emphasis being on brain stem reflexes. A flat or isoelectric electroencephalogram at high gain was of "great confirmatory value." All the tests were to be repeated at least 24 hours later, with no change in the findings.

The report unambiguously proposed that this clinical state should be accepted as death; recognised the moral, ethical, religious, and legal implications; and boldly saw itself as preparing the way "for better insight into all these matters as well as for better law than is currently applicable." A year later Beecher, the chairman of the Harvard committee, stated that this body was "unanimous in its belief that an electroencephalogram was not essential to a diagnosis of irreversible coma," although it could provide "valuable supporting data."[3]

Within three years of this radical yet humane proposal two neurosurgeons from Minneapolis made the challenging suggestion that "in patients with known but irreparable intracranial lesions" irreversible damage to the brain stem was the "point of no return." The diagnosis "could be based on clinical judgment."[4]

The Minnesota workers introduced the notion of aetiological preconditions. (Twenty of their 25 patients had sustained massive craniocerebral trauma and the others were suffering from other primary intracranial disorders.) They emphasised the importance of apnoea to the determination of brain death; in fact, they insisted on four minutes of disconnection from the respirator. They demanded absent brain stem reflexes, stated that the findings should not change for at least 12 hours, and emphasised that the electroencephalogram was not mandatory for the diagnosis. Their recommendations later became known as the Minnesota criteria and were to influence thinking and practice in the UK considerably. I am emphasising this because it has been suggested that physicians in the UK have been overcritical of much American work on this subject.

Fig. 4.6 Pallis' opening paper arguing brainstem death in a series of articles published in *BMJ* in 1982

Short Historical Note 22

LOCKED-IN SYNDROME

The Title of the Paper

Nordgren RE, Markesbery WR, Fukuda K, Reeves AG. Seven cases of cerebromedullospinal disconnection: the "locked-in" syndrome. Neurology. 1971;21:1140–8.

The Paper and the Times

One of the most existential fears one could have is being trapped in one's own body and being misdiagnosed as comatose. In 1844, Alexandre Dumas described such a state in the fictional character of Monsieur Noirtier, who was in this condition for more than 6 years and was described as a "corpse with living eyes." Later descriptions of a locked-in syndrome in a novel included one by Emile Zolá in *Therese Raquin*, in which Madame Raquin had a stroke. The features of the syndrome were translated by Pearce as "her tongue turned to stone," "she was struck dumb and motionless," "she only had the language of her eyes," and "she could communicate quite easily with an imprisoned mind buried alive in a dead body" [137].

The medical literature, however, lacked a clinicopathologic correlation and a detailed description of the eye movement abnormalities. Being paralyzed and unable to communicate while wide awake was perhaps best known from using neuromuscular drugs during anesthesia. Decamethonium, gallamine, and suxamethonium were discovered in the early 1950s. Neurologic causes for being "locked-in" were often intoxications. For example, Davis et al. described a case resembling locked-in syndrome caused by diazepam toxicity, which caused "prolonged semi-coma followed by transient muteness and tetraplegia in a patient with tetanus [53]." Most noteworthy was buckthorn neuropathy with a rapid paralysis and bulbar involvement. A brainstem location for locked-in-like syndrome had been noted by Adams and Victor in central pontine myelinolysis.

The term *locked-in* syndrome was based on a single case described in detail in the first edition of Plum and Posner's monograph on stupor and coma (Fig. 4.7). The 44-year-old man described had a basilar artery thrombosis. He was examined 1 month after the ictus. He was awake and appropriately moved his eyes up and down on commands and to indicate yes or no. There was no "lateral motion of the eyes either on command or on passive head turning." In addition, "there was no voluntary movement in structures innervated by cranial nerves IX–XII." The electroencephalogram (EEG) was normal. The patient developed some motion in the ankle, but died from pneumonia. Autopsy confirmed the diagnosis with severe atherosclerosis of the basilar artery, a cystic infarct in the upper two-thirds of the base of the pons and an infarction of the cerebellar peduncle. Autopsy also revealed that the reticular formation was not involved. One of the first mentions after this case report was by Chase et al. [48] and most notably by Nordgren, who summarizes the literature adding four cases (Fig. 4.8).

The Details of the Paper

Nordgren and associates saw an extraordinary number of cases in a short time period. Three cases were due to basilar artery thrombosis, and one was a hemorrhage into the fourth ventricle. A careful clinicopathologic correlation was described with illustrations showing the extent of involvement in some cases. The authors considered it a variant of akinetic mutism, but were quick to point out the major differences in neurologic examination and site of the lesion. Consciousness was preserved, but patients had decerebrate posturing after a noxious stimulus was applied.

In one case with bilateral involvement of the pontine tegmentum, the patient remained alert, suggesting that the reticular formation rostral to the pons was preserved. Further extension into the rostral tegmental levels resulted in loss of consciousness, and extension into the medulla oblongata resulted in fatality.

Most patients had an ataxic breathing defined as "unpatterned in amplitude, rhythm and rate." Apneustic breathing with deep inspiratory holding—previously associated with pontine tegmentum lesions—was not found. Others had deep and rapid respirations as seen in central neurogenic hyperventilation.

Comment: Like M. Noirtier de Villefort in Dumas' *The Count of Monte Cristo*, this patient was awake but had lost all power to communicate except with his eyes—"a corpse with living eyes." Although both akinetic and mute, he did not suffer from the syndrome of akinetic mutism in which patients are unconscious and make no appropriate responses.[41, 60] Great care must be exercised in distinguishing "a mind . . . encumbered by a body over which it has lost the power of compelling obedience" from typical akinetic mutism, since the former usually results from a low or midpontine lesion, as with this patient, and the latter, from midbrain and diencephalic lesions. The implications for humane patient care are profound. This constellation of alert wakefulness accompanied by mute tetraplegia of brainstem origin we have termed "the locked-in syndrome" to distinguish it from akinetic mutism, which is properly a form of coma.

Fig. 4.7 First mention of a locked-in syndrome in Plum and Posner's monograph on the diagnosis of stupor and coma

Seven cases of cerebromedullospinal disconnection: The "locked-in" syndrome

R. E. Nordgren, M.D., W. R. Markesbery, M.D.,
K. Fukuda, M.D., and A. G. Reeves, M.D.

THE TERM "AKINETIC MUTISM" was coined by Cairns et al.[1] in 1941 to describe a patient with an epidermoid cyst of the third ventricle. In the original description, the patient did not speak or move but followed the observer with her eyes. "Usually there are no movements of a voluntary character" though the patient could be made to carry out simple commands and would withdraw from painful stimuli. In contradistinction, Plum and Posner[2] use the term "locked-in" syndrome to describe a patient who, with bilateral basis pontis infarction, had no motion at all other than vertical eye movements. This patient was alert and communicated intelligently by using his eyes, differing from the classic akinetic mute who has the ability to move his extremities but usually does not do so.

The purpose of this paper is to present seven patients who, at some time during their illness, were alert and totally paralyzed save for mesencephalic-controlled eye and lid movements, their only means of communication. Seven patients with similar difficulties are abstracted from the literature (see table). All cases are considered to have had bilateral lesions in the pons as determined by clinical evaluation, verified in most cases by postmortem examination.

CASE REPORTS

Case 1. A 69-year-old white man with hypertension and electrocardiographic evidence of ischemic cardiac disease was admitted to Strong Memorial Hospital following loss of responsiveness. One day prior to admission he had suffered a short episode of vertigo, vomiting, and double vision. One year previously he had a vertiginous spell with loss of consciousness and since that time had been treated for occasional transient episodes of vertigo with an antihistaminic preparation.

Blood pressure on admission was 180/110 mm. Hg, pulse was 100 per minute and regular, and temperature was 37.5° C. Respirations were 14 per minute, regular in rhythm, and normal in depth. The patient could not modify his respiratory pattern in any way. He was alert and responded appropriately to "yes-no" questioning by elevating or depressing his eyes. No other means of communication was available. Visual fields were full to confrontation and hearing was intact bilaterally. The pupils were 1 to 2 mm. in size, constricted to light and accommodation, and dilated on cervical pinch. Eye opening was accomplished facilely, and vertical upward and downward versions were conjugate and full. Voluntary convergence was present. There was no response to vertical or horizontal oculocephalic maneuvers. Both unilateral and bilateral simultaneous hot and cold caloric irrigation produced no ocular deviations. A corneal response was present on the right and absent on the left, and the patient signaled perception on the right. The left face was totally paralyzed and the right was paretic. No gag response was elicited; however, a cough was elicited during nasotracheal stimulation. No head rotation or shoulder or tongue movement was possible. The patient was quadriplegic and had some increase of muscular tone of a spastic nature, variably brisk deep tendon reflexes, and consistently extensor plantar responses bilaterally. Right extremity decerebrate posturing and left extremity decorticate posturing were elicited simultaneously during ice-water irrigation of the auditory canals. The patient survived for five months with only minimal change in his neurological picture. Five degrees of voluntary right conjugate horizontal gaze were regained after one month in the hospital. Minimal percep-

From the Departments of Neurology and Pathology and The Waasdorp Laboratories for Stroke Research, University of Rochester Medical Center, Rochester, N.Y.

This study was supported in part by USPHS training grant No. NS 5084.

Submitted for publication Feb. 18, 1971; accepted March 5, 1971.

Dr. Reeves' address is Division of Neurology, Dartmouth-Hitchcock Medical Center, Hanover, N. H. 03755.

Fig. 4.8 Title page

The authors warned, "many presumed comatose patients could well be in this alert but helpless state. Unless commanded to elevate or depress their eyes, alertness would go unrecognized and they remain truly locked in."

The authors also elaborated on some of the ethical issues associated with being in a locked-in syndrome:

> While most patients with the lesions described herein will extend their infarction or hemorrhage and not survive, Case 1 of this series raises moral and ethical considerations that can be distressing for the personnel and family involved. He survived with a minimum of support for many months in an alert but completely helpless state. He was indeed completely locked in, except for his eye movements, and appeared to have no intellectual deterioration in spite of his profound motor deficit. It is worth emphasizing that considerable effort should be made to enrich the environment of these unfortunate individuals by whatever means are available to the auditory and visual spheres.

The Message and Acceptance

The term *locked-in syndrome* was introduced by Plum and Posner in 1966 but other terms, such as *pontopseudocoma*, *ventral pontine syndrome*, *deefferented state*, *pontine disconnection syndrome*, and *Montecristo syndrome* continue to surface. One of the first citations of locked-in syndrome was made 2 years later by Shafey et al. who called it *the ventral pontine syndrome* [171]. In 1974, Hawkes et al. confirmed a normal EEG in a patient with locked-in syndrome. His seven patients showed an α- or τ-rhythm that reacted to noise, painful, or photic stimuli [75, 76].

The term has been overused. It has been confused with persistent vegetative state and minimally conscious state. The crucial distinction of the presence of a disconnect between horizontal and vertical eye movements in an alert patient with a paralysis of all motor function below the mesencephalon should be appreciated. Locked-in syndrome may not be recognized in patients who appear motionless.

The pathologic lesion in locked-in syndrome interrupts the corticobulbar and corticospinal tracts, but the tegmentum of the pons and midbrain, which harbors the reticular formation, is preserved, and thus, consciousness is fully retained. In patients with a basilar artery occlusion, extension of the infarct into the tegmentum and involvement of the thalamus, however, may further decrease the level of consciousness.

Voluntary eye movements in the vertical plane and blinking remain because the oculomotor and trochlear nuclei and the center for vertical gaze remain intact. A significant skew deviation may occur along with ocular bobbing.

The most recent dramatic and sad description of locked-in syndrome is that by Jean-Dominique Bauby, editor in chief of the Parisian magazine *Elle*, who had a devastating stroke in the brainstem. His book is titled, *The Diving Bell and the Butterfly*, referring to the heavy corporeal trap—the "Diving Bell"—and his imagination wandering off in space or time—the lightness of a "Butterfly." Bauby often strove to savor the pleasures that were left to him, such as smells and vision. With a feat of great willpower and a devoted speech therapist, he blinked at the letter he wanted to produce a 137-page book describing his ordeal before he died [14]. The book provides useful insight into the terror of this condition.

In most patients, the locked-in state remains unchanged, but incomplete states have a much higher proclivity of major improvement. In complete states, some improvement may occur, such as movement of fingers that allows better signaling. However, recovery from locked-in syndrome has been reported in patients with herpes simplex encephalitis, after a bout of basilar artery migraine, multiple sclerosis, and following uncal herniation from a lobar hematoma [24, 26, 36, 177, 200]. In most of these cases, improvement occurred within days to weeks after presentation. Late recovery has not been reported, but patients may remain cognitively intact for years [43, 125, 126, 180]. A large proportion of patients die from pulmonary complications, but some patients have survived for many years, including one patient who survived for up to 27 years [72, 135].

Short Historical Note 23

ANOXIC ENCEPHALOPATHY AFTER CARDIOPULMONARY RESUSCITATION

The Title of the Paper

Howkins J, McLaughlin CR, Daniel T. Neuronal damage from temporary cardiac arrest. Lancet. 1946; 1:488–92.
Bell JA, Hodgson HJF. Coma after cardiac arrest. Brain. 1974;97:361–72.

The Paper and the Times

Resuscitation after cardiac standstill likely started in the operating room and in extreme circumstances. Intraoperative massage after cardiac arrest had been used for many decades. How it would affect the brain and how it would present itself was less well known. Very few neurologists concerned themselves with postsurgical disasters and descriptions were done by non-neurologist clinicians. Most initial observations came from surgeons who experienced intraoperative cardiac arrest during surgery and were left with a patient who never awakened. Perhaps one of the first cases describing clinically injured brain after successful resuscitation is by Mollison, an ear, nose, and throat surgeon from Guy's Hospital in England in 1917 [115]:

> A 6-year-old boy developed shock was flaccid, stopped breathing with absent corneal and pupil reflexes. After abdominal opening the right hand was inserted between the liver and diaphragm and the left hand on the chest wall and fingers of the right hand behind the heart. Pressure was exerted at about the rate of ninety times a minute. … Some respiration movement began attributed to blood driven to the medulla and stimulating the respiratory center but no heart contractions occurred. One cc of pitruitin was injected into the heart resulting in "strong heart beating. … For seven days the boy was more or less unconscious…for ten days there was rigidity of the limbs or choreic movements. At one time both feet and hands were held in the position of tetany. … For thirty-six hours the screaming was almost continuous … [and] has symptoms of severe cerebral irritation, no doubt due to the damage done to the brain during cessation of the circulation. … He made eventually a perfect recovery.

With the introduction of cardiopulmonary resuscitation (CPR), cerebral damage became recognized by clinicians and first by Negovsky who named it *postresuscitation disease* [121]. Some of the early explanations included cerebral reoxygenation injury or postischemic vasospasm leading to a necrotic process.

The devastating consequences to the brain became gradually known through careful examinations. When the more severe cases came to autopsy, neuropathologists would notice congestion of the gray matter and poor demarcation of the gray/white matter areas. Under the microscope, necrotic zones were seen in the cortical laminae, with bands of cellular vacuolization [7, 103, 117, 167]. Some of the attention was directed to the different vulnerability of gray and white matter, and it became clear that the cerebral and cerebellar cortices were more affected from ischemia than the basal ganglia—with the reverse in hypoxemia. Animal experiments also showed that white matter was more resistant to anoxic–ischemic injury than gray matter [103].

Overtime—only after carefully examining patients in persistent coma—the clinical descriptions and methods of prognostication became more sophisticated, but had to wait until the 1980s.

The Details of the Paper

Howkins paper on neuronal damage from cardiac arrest can be considered one of the first comprehensive papers on the evaluation of a patient who had successful cardiac massage (Fig. 4.9). The report is before CPR became common place. The patient is a 32-year-old woman who—after surgery was almost completed—had a sudden cardiac failure and transdiaphragmatic cardiac massage was started and lasted 7 min. She also received intracardiac adrenaline. Six hours later, her neurologic examination showed absent corneal reflexes, increased knee jerk, clonus, extensor plantar responses, and significant decerebrate rigidity. Lumbar puncture was performed and showed normal pressure. She remained comatose. The case report describes a rather complete neurologic examination with examination of the cranial nerves, motor function, tone, and reflex pattern. The EEG report showed very low voltage waves. Additionally, at autopsy, many of the anterior

NEURONAL DAMAGE FROM TEMPORARY CARDIAC ARREST

JOHN HOWKINS, M.D., M.S. Lond., F.R.C.S.
C. R. McLAUGHLIN, M.B. Camb., F.R.C.S.E.
LATE WING-COMMANDERS R.A.F.V.R., I/C A SURGICAL DIVISION

PETER DANIEL, M.A., M.B. Camb.
NUFFIELD GRADUATE ASSISTANT IN PATHOLOGY, RADCLIFFE INFIRMARY, OXFORD

EXAMPLES of successful cardiac massage where the heart has stopped beating at operation are now numerous, but permanent success without cerebral damage is governed by the duration of cardiac arrest, the critical limit of which is at most 5 minutes. If this critical period has been exceeded and the heart has started again as a result of resuscitation, neuronal damage is likely to be proportionate to the duration of anoxia. The extent of this damage can only be fully assessed in those infrequent cases where "life" lasts for several days or weeks after the cardiac disaster. A case of this kind is reported here, in which there were opportunities for full neurological, electroencephalographic, and histological investigations.

The published work on this subject is limited. Tureen (1936, 1938) studied the functional and histological effects of complete experimental vascular occlusion of the spinal cord of animals by clamping the thoracic aorta. He checked the efficiency of the occlusion by a method of intravital staining. Complete occlusion for 15 min. was compatible with complete physiological and histological recovery of the anterior horn cells. Motor and sensory function recovered within 24 hours. Histological changes were present at 7 hours and maximal between 7 and 72 hours. Histological normality was reached in 6 days. The nerve-cell changes consisted of chromatolysis, nuclear changes, neuronophagia, and satellitosis. The interstitial reaction was apparently an inflammatory one, with capillary dilatation and proliferation, and lagged behind the demonstrable appearance of nerve-cell damage. It was therefore the anoxia that damaged the nerve-cells, not the interstitial reaction. Complete functional recovery was possible in spite of chromatolysis. The spinal cord was therefore less sensitive than the brain to anoxia. Motor power did not appear in any animal with an occlusion period of 20 min.; the critical period for the anterior horn cells appeared to be 15 min. Greenfield (1938) reviewed the experimental work on ischæmia and anoxæmia of the neurone and found that all experimenters had noted considerable differences in the resistance of different nerve-cells to ischæmia.

Fig. 4.9 Title page

horn cells were shrunken and stained darkly on the lumbar cord. The midbrain showed little abnormality, and the medulla oblongata and pons also were largely spared with a few shrunken cells. The Purkinje cells in the cerebellum were reduced in number with many empty baskets. The basal ganglia showed extensive and severe changes, particularly in the caudate nucleus and putamen. Great loss of pyramidal cells was also found in the cornu ammonis.

Another work that has been often cited and was one of the largest series of coma after cardiac arrest is by Bell and Hodgson [17] (Fig. 4.10). This series shows the outcome of patients studied in the Saint Thomas Hospital: 284 patients resuscitated from cardiac arrest with 133 patients comatose. For the first time, this paper analyzes the poor prognosis of coma after cardiac arrest with only 19% of comatose patients living to be discharged from the hospital compared with 54% of noncomatose patients.

The Message and Acceptance

These reports introduce the neurology of prolonged coma after cardiac arrest and in some the evolution of a persistent vegetative state. The authors made the observation that cortical neurons die after 5 min of complete arrest.

These observations became even more important when the clinical landscape changed with the introduction of CPR standards set by the American Heart Association in 1966 [45]. Clinicians now noted that despite successful intervention, the brain still could have irreparable damage.

A major change came when Peter Safar from the University of Pittsburgh introduced "brain-oriented intensive care for coma" also known as "cerebral resuscitation [158–160]." An ambitious plan was created that included corticosteroids, temperature control, osmotic agents, and the use of barbiturates. Unfortunately, clinical trials with possible neuroprotective drugs were unsuccessful, and none of the interventions proved to be successful. A breakthrough came with the observation that early induced hypothermia to 33°C could improve mortality and morbidity [81].

As recently as 1970, there was little known on prognostication of neurologic injury after cardiac arrest. By that time, absent brainstem reflexes were clearly identified as indicative of poor outcome, and over the years, a more detailed definition of brain death emerged. However, most patients after cardiac arrest did not lose all brainstem reflexes but remained comatose with normal pupil, corneal, and oculocephalic reflexes.

How the neurologic examination could predict outcome remained elusive, and the leading neurology textbooks did not address the topic. The general impression was that duration of anoxia to the brain, duration of coma, and EEG were indicators of poor outcome [47, 172]. Studies correlating EEG with clinical findings often found in retrospect that coma lasting less than 2 days resulted in good outcome. A major study from Royal Adelaide Hospital in New Zealand reported by neurologist John Willoughby, who examined all 48 cases personally in detail, found that patients who did not respond purposefully 1 h after cardiac arrest had a 56% mortality and high likelihood of "intellectual impairment [205]". A prospective series focused on prognosticating morbidity, and mortality was published by Levy and associates (see Historical Note 53 [105]).

Brain (1974) **97**, 361–372

COMA AFTER CARDIAC ARREST

BY

J. A. BELL AND H. J. F. HODGSON

(*From the Intensive Care Unit, St. Thomas' Hospital, London, S.E.1*)

In the years since Kouwenhoven, Jude and Knickerbocker (1960) described the technique of external cardiac massage there have been many published series and sporadic reports of the results of cardiac resuscitation. Claims for successful resuscitation with discharge from hospital with an intact nervous system range from 5 per cent (Baringer *et al.*, 1961) to 44 per cent (Lawrie *et al.*, 1967) of cardiac arrests.

Early fears that cardiopulmonary resuscitation would produce a large number of permanently brain-damaged patients have not proved justified. In one series, of 65 patients discharged from hospital after resuscitation from ventricular fibrillation, and all previously employed, only one was prevented from returning to work by cerebral damage (McNamee *et al.*, 1970). Other series giving figures for the incidence of permanent neurological sequelæ all show a low incidence. Recently 6 patients surviving with permanent brain damage after cardiac arrest have been described (Norris and Chandrasekar, 1971), but the size of the population from which the 6 are drawn is not stated.

Most authors are agreed that short-term survivors who are resuscitated, yet die before leaving hospital, outnumber those who are eventually discharged from hospital. In Kaplan and Knott's (1964) series of 100 patients, out of 29 short-term survivors only 6 were discharged. In a larger series, Johnson *et al.* (1967) showed that 31·7 per cent lived for more than twenty-four hours yet only 14·9 per cent were discharged. Many of the short-term survivors after cardiac arrest have severe anoxic brain damage, and it is surprising that the commonest neurological problem after cardiac arrest, coma, has received little attention.

With the advent of more intensive care units and the concentration of available techniques, the management of patients after cardiac arrest has become almost a routine matter, yet there are no detailed analyses of either the prevalence or the prognosis of coma in these patients. It is the purpose of the present paper to analyse these factors in 284 patients resuscitated from cardiac arrest seen in a general purpose intensive care unit over six years of operation.

Fig. 4.10 Title Page

Short Historical Note 24

PERIMESENCEPHALIC HEMORRHAGE

The Title of the Paper

van Gijn J, van Dongen KJ, Vermeulen M, Hijdra A. Perimesencephalic hemorrhage: a nonaneurysmal and benign form of subarachnoid hemorrhage. Neurology. 1985;35:493–7.

The Paper and the Times

Aneurysmal subarachnoid hemorrhage in the early 1980s had been well characterized clinically, not only its initial presentation but also its complications. In this time period, most patients with aneurysmal subarachnoid hemorrhage (SAH) were operated on usually after the period of cerebral vasospasm had subsided and often at the end of the second week from presentation.

Most patients with an aneurysmal SAH had a cerebral angiogram except those presenting in a very poor condition or the very old, When the first cerebral angiogram showed no aneurysm, a second and even a third cerebral angiogram was performed to reliably exclude a ruptured aneurysm. The yield of these repeated studies was initially relatively high with up to 20% of cases showing an aneurysm on the second cerebral angiogram. For neurosurgeons, some concern remained even when patients had negative cerebral angiograms. Repeatedly, studies appeared that emphasized a much better outcome when no aneurysm could be demonstrated. The assumption was that the aneurysm had destroyed itself during rupture and the artery had healed naturally. Rebleed rates in these patients were very low.

After a retrospective review of all computed tomography (CT) scans of patients with such a negative angiogram—conducted in Rotterdam, Erasmus University Hospital (Dijkzigt)—a pattern became apparent that had not been noted before. Patients with a normal cerebral angiogram but demonstrable SAH on CT scan had blood mainly or only in the cisterns around the midbrain [185]. This prompted the term *perimesencephalic subarachnoid hemorrhage*.

This finding led to a fundamentally new insight in the evaluation of a patient with a SAH and had great consequences for treatment and follow-up of the patients.

The Details of the Paper

The initial paper involved 28 patients with SAH and a normal cerebral angiogram. In 13 patients, blood was largely located in front of the brainstem, ambient cistern, and quadrigeminal cistern. This pattern was different from an aneurysmal pattern where blood was distributed throughout the cisterns and fissures (Fig. 4.12). When the clinical features of nonaneurysmal perimesencephalic hemorrhages were compared with patients who did have more aneurysmal patterns, striking differences were noted. Headache was more gradual in the perimesencephalic hemorrhage group, and outcome was invariably good with no rebleeding or cerebral infarction, although acute hydrocephalus was found with one patient requiring a ventriculostomy. The authors speculated that this type of hemorrhage was not an arterial hemorrhage, but more likely venous. This was also considered plausible because several patients had a sudden head turn at the onset of headache, or headache started after the patient overreached—all tentatively suggesting friction of a cerebellar vein against the tentorial margin.

The Message and Acceptance

A major study followed that further refined the disorder in a larger series of patients [146–149]. According to van Gijn, acceptance of this variant started with the publication of a larger paper in *The Lancet*, and citations increased exponentially over the years [147, 184].

The main premise has remained unchallenged. Patients invariably presented in a good clinical condition and were rarely very much affected by it. Once a cerebral angiogram had excluded a posterior circulation aneurysm, rebleeding did not occur, cerebral vasospasm did not lead to cerebral infarction, and the outcome was exceptionally good.

Later, magnetic resonance imaging found that the hemorrhage was not so much in the

Article abstract—We studied 28 patients with subarachnoid hemorrhage and normal angiograms. On early CT (within 5 days) in 13 cases, blood was seen mainly or only in the cisterns around the midbrain. This pattern of hemorrhage was found in only 1 of 92 patients with a ruptured aneurysm. None of the unexplained perimesencephalic hemorrhages was associated with intracerebral hematoma or intraventricular hemorrhage. The clinical features also differed from those of aneurysmal hemorrhage; loss of consciousness was rare, and after 3 months, all 13 patients had returned to normal life. The cause of this benign disorder remains elusive, but a venous or capillary source seems likely.

NEUROLOGY 1985;35:493-497

Perimesencephalic hemorrhage: A nonaneurysmal and benign form of subarachnoid hemorrhage

J. van Gijn, K.J. van Dongen, M. Vermeulen, and A. Hijdra

A recurring enigma is the patient with all the evidence of a spontaneous hemorrhage in the cerebral subarachnoid space, but without an aneurysm or other source of bleeding on four-vessel angiography. A favorable outcome is the rule,[1-4] in marked contrast to the devastating natural history of patients with a demonstrable aneurysm.[5] "Occult aneurysms" have often been invoked to explain these hemorrhages,[6] even in the era of selective angiography.[7] Failure of an aneurysm to fill with contrast medium has been attributed to local thrombosis[8] or to arterial spasm.[9] However, we have found by early CT that patients with negative angiograms rarely show extravasated blood in the basal cisterns and fissures, whereas this is the rule with ruptured aneurysms.[10] Here, we report a larger and prospective study in which patients without aneurysms did show basal hemorrhages, but of a distinct kind: mainly or only in the perimesencephalic cisterns.

Subjects and methods. From July 1, 1979, to May 1, 1983, we prospectively studied 226 patients with subarachnoid hemorrhage who were admitted and investigated by CT within 5 days of the first symptoms. One hundred and twenty patients underwent angiography; they form the basis of this study. Angiography was carried out only in view of surgical treatment, and at the time of investigation, these 120 patients showed no alteration of consciousness or ischemic cerebral deficits. All patients were under 65 years old. The criteria for the diagnosis of subarachnoid hemorrhage were (1) spontaneous onset of headache or unconsciousness without associated head trauma, and (2) presence of blood in the CSF proven by CT or, if this was negative, by spectrophotometric analysis of lumbar CSF,[11] in combination with previous neck stiffness. We excluded patients with primary intraparenchymal hemorrhage or arteriovenous malformations.

Results. *Perimesencephalic hemorrhages in patients without aneurysms.* Of the 120 patients who had four-vessel angiograms, 92 proved to have one or more aneurysms. In the remaining 28 patients (23%), no source of hemorrhage was found; in 11 of them, especially those with some narrow arterial segments, the angiographic study was repeated once or twice with the same result. The first CT showed evidence of extravasated blood in basal cisterns or fissures in 86 of the 92 patients with an aneurysm (93%), and in 20 of the 28 patients with a negative angiogram (table 1).

In 13 of the 20 patients with negative angiography and with subarachnoid blood at the base of the brain, the main site of hemorrhage was one of the cisterns around the midbrain (figure 1). Nine of these 13 patients also showed blood in other basal cisterns, but much less. This pattern of hemorrhage would be unusual for aneurysms (figure 2).

To quantify this distinction, we graded the density of extravasated blood in each separate cistern from 0 to 3, for patients with or without aneurysms. Patients with aneurysms that had bled in the perimesencephalic cisterns showed more, or at least an equal amount of, blood in the anterior and lateral cisterns (chiasmatic cistern, frontal inter-

Fig. 4.11 Title page

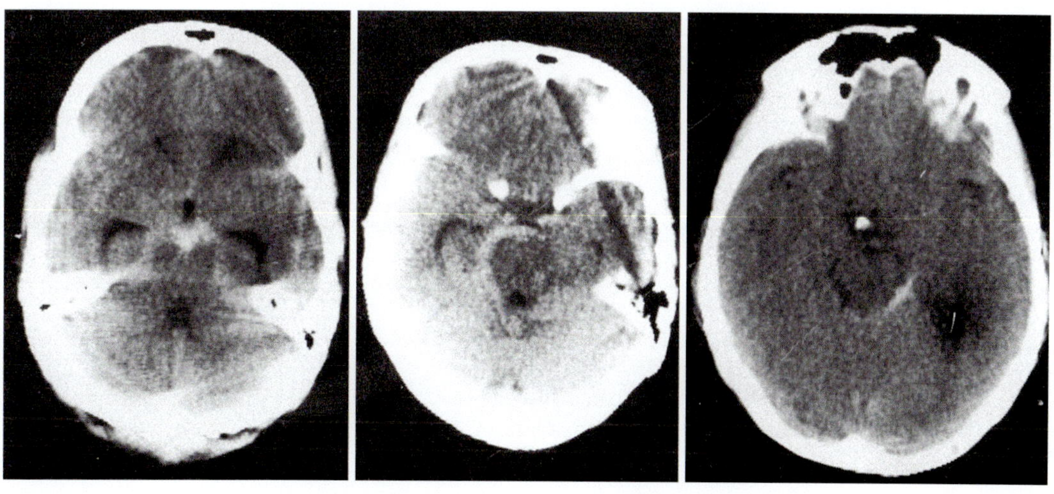

Fig. 4.12 Computed tomography scans showing perimesencephalic hemorrhage patterns

perimesencephalic region, but largely in front of the entire brainstem [163]. Over the years, multiple observations have claimed to have found the cause of a nonaneurysmal perimesencephalic hemorrhage.

Candidate vessels for rupture into the prepontine and interpeduncular cistern are the basilar artery, anterior pontomesencephalic vein, superior cerebellar artery, and any of the perforating arteries in the vicinity [80, 201, 202]. Intramural dissections may have been the culprit. Arguments for this explanation included: (1) small hemorrhage would fit with a dissection, (2) common wall irregularity, often misinterpreted as early vasospasm, and (3) presence of infarcts in the pons in some cases [163].

More recently, a three-dimensional cerebral angiogram in a patient showed that small basilar artery outpouches may appear and then disappear. Thrombosis and recanalization may explain the radiologic findings of reappearance of a small aneurysm after follow-up angiogram [194].

Other studies have repeatedly shown abnormal venous patterns in patients with perimesencephalic nonaneurysmal hemorrhage, but in patients examined, venous structures in the interpeduncular or prepontine cisterns are without any abnormalities except for an occasional engorged anterior pontomesencephalic vein. No patient with a nonaneurysmal perimesencephalic hemorrhage has come to autopsy soon after the initial hemorrhage.

The discovery of a separate entity in a population of patients with "angiographic-negative subarachnoid hemorrhage" meant that neurologists and neurosurgeons now had to specifically distinguish between three CT patterns: "perimesencephalic," "aneurysmal," and "nonaneurysmal–nonperimesencephalic." Each of these CT scan patterns could indicate a certain vascular lesion on cerebral angiogram or could indicate there was none. Outcome would be much different. The CT pattern has now been recognized in most medical centers throughout the world.

Short Historical Note 25

BASILAR ARTERY OCCLUSION

The Title of the Paper

Kubik CS, Adams RD. Occlusion of the basilar artery: a clinical and pathological study. Brain. 1946;69: 73–121.

Caplan LR. "Top of the basilar" syndrome. Neurology. 1980;30:72–9.

The Paper and the Times

Ronnov-Jensen claims the very first description of a basilar artery occlusion may have been in Dumas' *Three Musketeers* where he describes symptoms that could have been a traumatic vertebral dissection [154]. Pathologists were aware of an acute embolus to basilar artery as early as 1900s. The first description is most likely by the Scottish physician John Abercrombie in his book, *Pathological and Practical Researches on Disease of the Brain and the Spinal Cord.* This observation was recently summarized in a historical article [96]. The paper describes an 18-year-old man who had a left hemiplegia followed 1 month later by loss of speech and dysphagia, and at autopsy a blocked basilar artery filled by "a firm white matter without any appearance of blood." The diagnosis was considered "plugging of the basilar."

Other incidental cases have been described by several physicians, and the contributions of French neurologists—Charles Foix in particular—have been recognized, leading to multiple eponyms associated with brainstem syndromes [41, 64, 65, 169]. Foix gained an eponyrm after describing a vascular syndrome in the brainstem involving the red nucleus, but he became better known by the Foix-Alajounine syndrome of the spinal cord.

According to Raymond Adams, the most completely examined case of basilar artery thrombosis was in 1932 by Pines and Gilinsky and showed a serial section of the brainstem and clear delineation of the infarctions [141]. At the time, the diagnosis or warning signs were seldom made while the patient was still alive, and autopsy often revealed surprising findings [86]. Denny-Brown may have introduced the term *vertebrobasilar insufficiency*, which gradually has been replaced by the term *vertebrobasilar transient ischemic attacks* [57].

The Details of the Paper

Kubik and Adams' paper summarizes 18 carefully examined cases with autopsy (Fig. 4.13). The paper summarized multiple areas of occlusion with concomitant clinical features. The paper by Kubik and Adams was important because it documented for the first time that the clinical syndrome of progressive brainstem dysfunction could be associated with thrombosis of the basilar artery. The mortality was as high as 90%. The paper described single cases that presented with progressive clinical signs that included tinnitus and vertigo followed by swallowing difficulties and pupillary abnormalities and gradually lapsing into coma:

> The onset is abrupt, frequently with loss of consciousness and with signs indicating a lesion in the mid-brain and/or pons. In the majority of cases there was evidence of bilateral involvement. Outstanding features are various combinations of (1) pupillary disturbances: (2) ocular palsies and other cranial nerve palsies; (3) dysarthria: (4) bilateral extensor plantar reflexes; (5) hemiplegia, quadriplegia: (6) commonly a marked remission of symptoms which is usually temporary but may occasionally end in recovery.

The paper focused on a clinical pathologic correlation. Many patients had thrombi formed on severe atherosclerotic vertebrobasilar arteries. Cardiac emboli were considered another possibility in 7 of 18 patients, but the embolus was rarely seen and probably had lysed.

In the past, cerebral vasospasm often was put forward as a cause of this syndrome, but Adams completely discounted that as a possibility. They concluded that the entity could be recognized and that patients could recover. "It should be possible in most cases of basilar artery occlusion to make a correct diagnosis. The disease is not always fatal. Histories are submitted of four patients who have recovered."

Another major work was by Louis Caplan, who suggested a clinical diagnosis of an embolus lodged at the top of the basilar artery (Fig. 4.14). These patients presented with a rostral brainstem infarction. The concept here was that an embolus that

BRAIN

VOL. 69, PART 2.

OCCLUSION OF THE BASILAR ARTERY—A CLINICAL AND PATHOLOGICAL STUDY.

BY CHARLES S. KUBIK[1] AND RAYMOND D. ADAMS[2].

AT the outset we wish to state that it is not intended to include in this article an account of all the diverse brain-stem syndromes which may follow occlusion of the branches of the basilar artery. These have been discussed in numerous publications and are well known to neurologists under such eponyms as the syndrome of Millard-Gubler, Foville, Weber, Benedict and others. Instead, it is our purpose to discuss the symptomatology and pathology of occlusion by thrombosis and embolism of the basilar artery itself. We believe that pertinent facts and observations have come into our possession which permit some clarification of a heretofore obscure clinical syndrome and also cast some light on the phenomenon of acute decerebration in man.

The report is based on the study of 18 cases, some of which were examined by us during life, and all of which were submitted to autopsy. The cases were gathered from the records of the Department of Pathology at the Massachusetts General Hospital and the Mallory Institute of Pathology at Boston City Hospital. In all we have found 13 cases among 4,200 consecutive autopsies at the Massachusetts General Hospital and 12 cases among the last 3,200 autopsies at the Boston City Hospital. Thus the average incidence was about 1 case in every 300 autopsies. Of these 25 cases, 7 were discarded because of inadequate clinical records.

HISTORICAL NOTES.

Whereas most of the vascular syndromes of the brain-stem have been the subject of a voluminous literature, basilar artery occlusion has

[1]From the Neuropathological Laboratory, Massachusetts General Hospital, and the Department of Neuropathology, Harvard Medical School.

[2]From the Neurological Unit, Boston City Hospital and the Department of Neurology, Harvard Medical School.

Fig. 4.13 Title page

could traverse a smaller vertebral artery would not necessarily occlude the basilar artery, except more distally where the basilar artery was tapered. Atherosclerosis of the vertebral basilar system was widespread in the reported patients.

The syndrome was characterized by visual field defects, disorders of vertical gaze, convergence, a skew deviation, and pupillary abnormalities mostly resulting in small and poorly reactive pupils. Behavior abnormalities that included hallucinosis were common, and visual field defects including visual perseverations and scintillations in an optic field were described. Many of the infarcts were bilateral and a cortical blindness or a Balint's syndrome was noted. Patients with thalamic lesions could not form new memories and could be permanent in patients with paramedian thalamic infarcts.

The Message and Acceptance

Initially smaller brainstem infarcts were described in which patients have a constellation of findings that could localize to a specific lesion in the pons, medulla, or even mesencephalon. In some patients, rapid infarction involving the pons, thalami, and the occipital lobes could be associated with occlusion of the basilar artery or the more distal portions. Both papers from Harvard Medical School clearly defined syndromes of acute occlusion of the basilar artery with rapid progression.

Raymond Adams studied 1,400 brains at the Mallory Institute of Pathology. According to his biographer Laureno, this detailed manuscript brought Raymond Adams international recognition [99]. The "top of the basilar" syndrome also has become a medical classic and has been recognized as a devastating stroke. One of Caplan's major achievements has been the establishment of the New England Medical Center posterior circulation registry that allowed more detailed study of patients over time or in Miller Fisher's words "stroke by stroke" [42, 189].

A basilar artery thrombus most permanently infarcts the pons and is associated with either prolonged coma or a locked-in syndrome, both with major clinical consequences. Early recognition of acute basilar artery embolus remains problematic and clinical signs often are not appreciated by non-neurologists.

Patients may present with difficulty clearing secretions from acute dysphagia and level of consciousness may fluctuate initially resulting in respiratory problems. Not uncommonly, the patient arrives intubated in the emergency department. Computed tomography (CT) scan often is initially normal, and a hyperdensity in the basilar artery representing clot also is often not recognized in an acute hectic setting [97]. CT angiogram is now the diagnostic test of choice, or the patient goes straight to a cerebral angiography. Early endovascular therapy in basilar artery occlusive disease has been a breakthrough intervention and there is a high likelihood of improving clinical signs with recanalization.

Article abstract—Infarction of rostral brainstem and cerebral hemispheral regions fed by the distal basilar artery causes a clinically recognizable syndrome characterized by visual, oculomotor, and behavioral abnormalities, often without significant motor dysfunction. Rostral brainstem infarction produces oculomotor and pupillary signs that are identical to those in thalamic hemorrhage. Somnolence, vivid hallucinations and dreamlike behavior may also accompany rostral brainstem infarction. Temporal and occipital infarctions are frequently accompanied by hemianopia with distinctive characteristics, fragments of the Balint syndrome, amnestic dysfunction, and agitated behavior. The "top of the basilar" syndrome is most often due to an embolus.

NEUROLOGY 30: 72-79, **January 1980**

"Top of the basilar" syndrome

Louis R. Caplan, M.D.

Occlusive vascular disease of the rostral basilar artery frequently causes infarction of midbrain, thalamus, and portions of the temporal and occipital lobes fed by posterior communicating and posterior cerebral arterial tributaries of the basilar artery. Clinical signs include an array of visual, oculomotor, and behavioral abnormalities, usually without prominent motor dysfunction, which may confuse those inexperienced with these findings. Segarra[1] used the term "the syndrome of the mesencephalic artery" to describe rostral paramedian brainstem infarction, and analyzed one type of behavioral manifestation ("somnolent mutism"). Others have described clinicopathologic aspects of isolated neuroophthalmologic[2-19] and behavioral[19-32] features. This report, based principally on experience from personally examined cases with autopsy, computerized tomography (CT), or angiographic verification, reviews the major clinical features. Aspects of the syndrome considered in detail elsewhere (e.g., memory loss[20,22,33,34] and alexia without agraphia[22]) are given only passing attention. The "top of the basilar" syndrome is a recognizable subdivision that can be distinguished from the large group of heterogeneous conditions usually lumped together under the term "vertebrobasilar ischemia" or "insufficiency."

Infarction of rostral brainstem and posterior hemispheres often coexists because of the common vascular supply. However, because either may occur in isolation, it is appropriate to consider brainstem and hemisphere manifestations separately.

rostral midbrain and posterior thalamus is indistinguishable from that in patients with thalamic hemorrhage.[35,36] The signs include:

Disorders of vertical gaze. Voluntary or reflex vertical gaze (tested by oculocephalic and caloric maneuvers and Bell phenomenon) is often abolished. One or both eyes may rest in a downward position. Isolated paralysis of upward or downward gaze occurs less frequently. In human patients with vertical gaze paralysis due to vascular disease, bilateral lesions are found in the midbrain tegmentum.[4,11,17] In monkeys and humans,[4,11] lesions of the pretectum, in the region of the posterior commissure, are necessary to produce paralysis of upward gaze. Isolated downward gaze palsy is rare, and may be associated with lesions medial and dorsal to the red nucleus;[8,9] lesions causing paralysis of downward gaze are more ventral and caudal in the midbrain tegmentum than those responsible for deficits of upward gaze.

Disorders of convergence. One or both eyes may rest in an inward position. Hyperconvergence or convergence spasm may be observed when the patient attempts conjugate lateral or vertical gaze. Convergence retraction nystagmus,[37] a rhythmic inward beating movement of the eyes, may be spontaneous, but is best elicited by having the patient fix on an optokinetic stimulus which is moving upward.

Fig. 4.14 Title page

Short Historical Note 26

DELAYED TRAUMATIC CEREBRAL HEMATOMA

The Title of the Paper

Baratham G, Dennyson WG. Delayed traumatic intracerebral hemorrhage. J Neurol Neurosurg Psychiatry. 1972;35:698–706.

The Paper and the Times

Nonpenetrating traumatic brain injury could produce rapid injury to brain tissue, resulting in diffuse swelling or hemorrhagic contusions. For many decades, it was known that a so-called lucid interval existed. Perfectly fine patients with no overt injury after a major accident were looked at with trepidation by neurosurgeons who knew they could get worse and dramatically quick. In the majority of cases, expanding subdural or epidural hematoma could be implicated [52].

In 1891, Bollinger described for the first time delayed intracerebral hemorrhage (ICH) after trauma and named it *traumatische spät-apoplexie* [28]. However, neuropathology was poorly defined, and the term included different causes of traumatic brain injury. Bollinger pointed out that trauma could cause progressive cerebral infarction followed by hemorrhage. Others attributed it to "vasoparalysis" [63] or to compression of a surface collection causing hemorrhage.

The Details of the Paper

Experience from the Surgical Neurology University of Edinburgh revealed 21 patients (from 7,866 head injuries) with delayed hemorrhages (Fig. 4.15). All 21 patients had a trauma, transient period of recovery ("asymptomatic interval"), followed by secondary deterioration. The age ranged from 5 to 83 years. The interval was 90 min to 1 day. None had neurologic deficits in the asymptomatic interval. The hematoma location is shown in Fig. 4.16.

In 6 of 21 patients, there was rapid deterioration and coma before surgery. Ten of 21 patients had skull fractures. Most hematomas were in the frontal lobe. All patients required surgical treatment. The authors speculated the following:

> A combination of factors, therefore, operates in the production of the delayed variety of traumatic intracerebral hemorrhage. Focal trauma produce increased flow within and around traumatized brain. Hypoxia, carbon dioxide retention, and any cause for elevation of venous pressure will increase this tendency, thus producing ideal conditions for the gradual development of an intracerebral hematoma.

The Message and Acceptance

Years later, after the use of computed tomography (CT) scan became more widespread, delayed traumatic cerebral hematoma was more easily recognized [79, 122, 124, 174]. In Soloniuk's study, ICH was immediate (<3 h) in 20% within 3–6 h in 6% delayed (6–24 h) in 29% and much delayed (>24 h) in 46%. None of the patients had intracerebral hematoma on initial CT scan. Mortality despite surgery was 50% [173].

Another study found better outcomes, but only if patients had not deteriorated to coma. It is unclear if hypercapnia or hypoxemia played a role, but coagulopathy or prior antiplatelet agents often could be implicated.

Reilly and coworkers from the Institute of Neurologic Sciences in Southern General Hospital in Glasgow coined the term *patients who talked and died*. In a series of 66 patients, 70% died from parenchymal contusions. A "lucid interval" without any neurologic signs (and not even acute confusion) was found in 39% [144]. Later studies showed multifocal patterns in patients who died from traumatic brain injury, many with additional ischemic injury [6].

This asymptomatic lucid interval is a most interesting phenomenon. The lucid interval may be not so lucid if the patient is examined well cognitively and if physicians in overcrowded emergency departments have not taken the time

Fig. 4.15 The title page

Delayed traumatic intracerebral haemorrhage

GOPAL BARATHAM AND WILLIAM G. DENNYSON

From the Department of Surgical Neurology, University of Edinburgh

SUMMARY Twenty-one out of 7,866 head injuries were complicated by the development of delayed intracerebral haematomata. The age distribution of patients with this condition closely resembled that of patients with subdural haematomata and differed sharply from patients with extradural haemorrhage. This finding, combined with the fact that the two conditions often coexisted, suggests the possibility of similar aetiological factors operating in their production. The injury producing the lesion was often minor and the larger haematomata appeared to be associated with longer 'asymptomatic' intervals. The neurological deterioration was in most instances clearly the result of an increase in intracranial pressure. When possible, angiography followed by definitive craniotomy was the most satisfactory method of management and multiple burr holes even when combined with needling of the hemisphere yielded unsatisfactory results. The distribution of lesions tended to confirm their traumatic origin. On no occasion was there a vascular abnormality to account for the haemorrhage and, despite the fact that the ages of most patients were in the seventh and eighth decades, the incidence of degenerative vascular disease was small. Contusional injury causes a local failure of the mechanisms that regulate cerebral blood flow. Hypoxia, hypercapnia, and venous congestion produce cerebral hyperaemia which encourages gradual haematoma formation particularly at the sites of injury. This explains not only the situation of the lesions but also the latency between the trauma and their development.

The prognosis in severe head injuries with extensive cerebral contusions, cerebral lacerations, generalized neuronal disruption, or primary lesions of the brain-stem is notoriously bad. Such cases are recognizable by the unrelenting coma which exists from the moment of injury. Therapeutic attention has therefore been directed towards those patients who develop intracranial space-occupying lesions some time after the initial head injury. These tend to be recovering from the coma due to the concussional injury (even if the classical lucid interval is not always present) and to deteriorate secondarily because of a rise in intracranial pressure. The lesion which most commonly produces this picture is haemorrhage into the extradural or subdural space. The majority of patients with a traumatic intracerebral haemorrhage, usually resulting from severe cerebral lacerations, are profoundly unconscious from the time of injury. In a small minority, however, the intracerebral haemorrhage appears to occur some time after the impact. The trend in these patients is one of recovery, complete or partial, from the concussional injury, followed by a deterioration in the level of consciousness or the development of neurological deficits which were initially absent; such patients are clinically indistinguishable from those with extradural and subdural haematomata. Though the incidence of such cases is small, our interest in them is occasioned by the fact that they are potentially treatable by removal of the compressing haematoma though, because of destruction of cerebral tissue, treatment is less likely to be as effective as in those situations where the compressive lesions are entirely extracerebral.

Bollinger (1891) originally described the condition of delayed intracerebral haemorrhage associated with trauma, and proposed the term 'traumatische Spät-Apoplexie'. The original description and that of subsequent workers (Michel, 1896; Bailey, 1904; Symonds, 1940; Grant and Asutin, 1950; McLaurin and McBride,

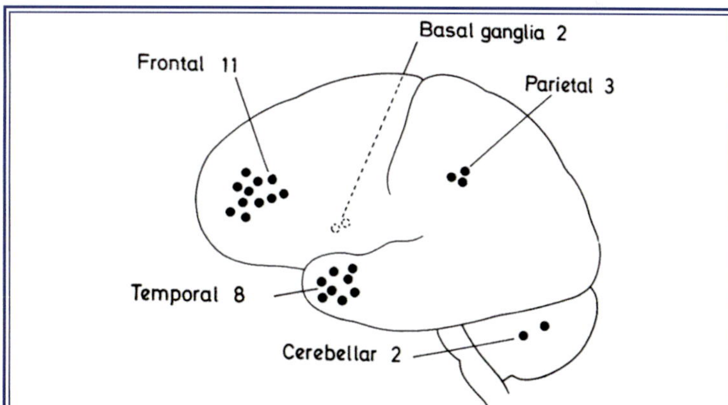

FIG. 2. *Distribution of haematomata. Five occurred at multiple sites.*

Fig. 4.16 Location of delayed cerebral hematomas

to comprehensively assess cognition and reaction speed. This lucid interval may not have a satisfactory pathophysiologic explanation, and most likely patients have a mild deficit, which will become much worse. Patients may be unconscious from the initial injury, then recover and be quite alert and rational; however, after 24–48 h, they deteriorate rapidly from frontotemporal hematomas (coup and contrecoup) [85, 91, 94].

The delayed traumatic cerebral hematomas occur more often in elderly patients in the 80's age group. Many of these patients experience a deterioration from enlargement of a hemorrhagic contusion. A bifrontal hematoma or temporal lobe hematoma increases the chance of herniation and marked deterioration. These patients, who "talk and deteriorate," – a more optimistic designation – need emergency neurosurgical evacuation at the first signs of deterioration [208]. If the temporal lobe is damaged, a lobectomy is done in the inferior segment of the damaged temporal lobe, and any other severely damaged brain tissue is resected [150].

Short Historical Note 27

GUILLAIN-BARRÉ SYNDROME

The Title of the Paper

Guillain G, Barré J, Strohl A. Sur un syndrome de radiculo-néurite avec hyperalbuminose du liquide céphalo-rachidien sans réaction cellulaire. Remarques sur les caractères cliniques et graphiques des reflexes tendineux. Rev Neurol. 1916;40:1462–70.

The Paper and the Times

This neuroimmunologic disorder with rapid paralysis, now known as Guillain-Barré syndrome (GBS), was already familiar to William Osler, who called it an acute febrile polyneuritis in his famed 1892 textbook, *The Principles and Practice of Medicine*. Even earlier, in 1859, manifestations of this affliction had been described by Landry, who reported a 43-year-old man with progressive weakness starting in all four limbs and difficulty walking followed by worsening weakness involving the diaphragm, facial, laryngeal, and jaw muscles. The patient died within 1 week. Before the paralysis started, the patient complained about fevers and bouts of severe pain. In Landry's paper, the peripheral nerves were not examined during autopsy [98].

The first pathology and microscopic examination of the nerves in this entity was by Duménil in 1864, who found "a genuine atrophy of the medullary substance of the peripheral nerve tubes," particularly in areas where there was significant muscle weakness and wasting [61]. The entity was considered separate from acute poliomyelitis but was understood as a postinfectious or infectious disorder.

In 1916, George Guillain, Jean Barré, and André Strohl described what became known as the eponym Guillain-Barré syndrome [70, 71, 83]. Guillain and Barré considered Landry's patient different than their cases because of fatal outcome. Landry's disorder was conveniently named Landry's ascending paralysis [138].

The Details of the Paper

The paper described two infantry soldiers who were admitted with tingling and progressive weakness causing major difficulty with walking (Fig. 4.17). Tingling progressed to the upper limbs and lower part of the face. Guillain and Barré considered the possibilities of syphilis, food poisoning, and alcohol abuse in both patients.

On examination, they found that the muscles were tender to touch and pressure. There was a mild sensory loss of touch, temperature, and pinprick. Severe weakness of all four extremities was present, and they noted areflexia [157]. This was also confirmed by electrophysiologic studies performed by André Strohl, who found absent reflexes, but retained idiomuscular contractions. One patient improved strength after 2 months. The other patient improved in the first month before he was transferred to another institution and was lost to further follow-up. Guillain and Barré described what they called a unique phenomenon, *hyperalbuminose du liquide céphalorachidien sans réaction cellulaire* also known as cerebrospinal fluid (CSF) albuminocytologic dissociation. In one of the soldiers, the CSF protein was 2.5 g/L.

Data derived from the tracings of delayed reflexes and speed of the reflex response and muscular contraction indicated that the entire peripheral neuromuscular motor apparatus was involved (Fig. 4.18). Guillain particularly emphasized an increased CSF albumin content without cellular reaction and reiterated that this observation had not been previously published [61, 71].

Guillain summarized the clinical characteristics as motor difficulties, loss of deep tendon reflexes with preservation of the cutaneous reflexes, paresthesias with slight impairment of objective sensation, muscle tenderness, and slight alterations in nerve conduction and electromyographical patterns.

This process appeared to simultaneously involve nerve roots, peripheral nerves, and muscles. It was distinct from "simple" radiculopathies, "pure" polyneuropathies, and polymyositis [71, 157].

The Message and Acceptance

Several months later, a similar report was published by Pierre Marie and Charles Chatelin confirming the diagnosis [110]. The first mention of the eponym was by Baker who designated it

SUR UN SYNDROME DE RADICULO-NÉVRITE AVEC HYPERALBUMINOSE DU LIQUIDE CÉPHALO-RACHIDIEN SANS RÉACTION CELLULAIRE. REMARQUES SUR LES CARACTÈRES CLINIQUES ET GRAPHIQUES DES RÉFLEXES TENDINEUX,

par MM. GEORGES GUILLAIN, J.-A. BARRÉ et A. STROHL.

Nous attirons l'attention, dans la présente note, sur un syndrome clinique que nous avons observé chez deux malades, syndrome caractérisé par des troubles moteurs, l'abolition des réflexes tendineux avec conservation des réflexes cutanés, des paresthésies avec troubles légers de la sensibilité objective, des douleurs à la pression des masses musculaires, des modifications peu accentuées des réactions électriques des nerfs et des muscles, de l'hyperalbuminose très notable du liquide céphalo-rachidien avec absence de réaction cytologique (dissociation albumino-cytologique). Ce syndrome nous a paru dépendre d'une atteinte concomitante des racines rachidiennes, des nerfs et des muscles, vraisemblablement de nature infectieuse ou toxique. Il doit être différencié des radiculites simples, des polynévrites pures et des polymyosites. Des recherches expérimentales par la méthode graphique sur la vitesse des réflexes et leur temps perdu, sur les modalités, la contractilité musculaire, montrent la réalité de la participation, dans ce syndrome, de tout l'appareil moteur neuro-musculaire périphérique. Nous insistons particulièrement aussi sur l'hyperalbuminose du liquide céphalo-rachidien sans réaction cytologique, fait qui, à notre connaissance, n'a pas été mentionné dans des cas semblables.

Fig. 4.17 The title page

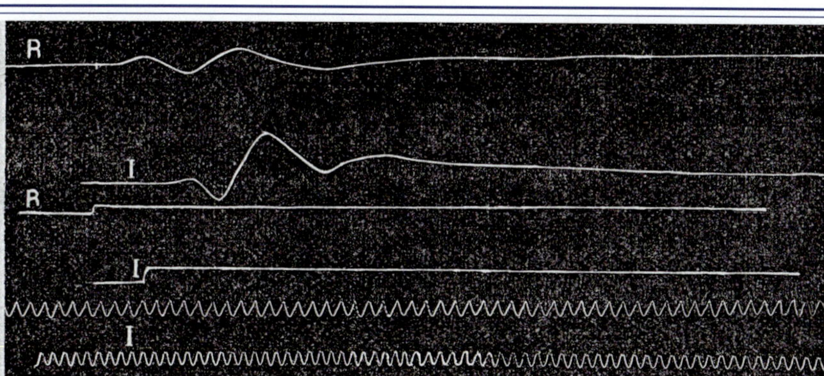

FIG. 1.

R, R, R, courbe myographique du quadriceps fémoral au cours du réflexe rotulien, avec le signal de Desprez indiquant le moment de la percussion et le temps en 1/100 de seconde.
I, I, I, les mêmes tracés pour la percussion directe du muscle quadriceps fémoral.
Enregistrement du 21 août 1916.
On remarque l'absence presque totale de contraction « réflexe » qui suit la percussion du tendon rotulien, alors qu'elle existe très nettement pour la percussion directe du muscle.

Fig. 4.18 Electrographic recording of areflexia. The knee reflex (reflex rotulien) is shown in *R* and direct quadriceps muscle percussion in *I*

Guillain-Barré disease [138]. Strohl was not included in the eponym for unknown reasons, but Guillain and Barré themselves quickly referenced to it as *nôtre syndrome* (our syndrome) several years later.

The original description was followed by a major clinical pathological paper of 50 fatal cases that called the disorder Landry–Guillain-Barré syndrome [77]. Neuropathologists Haymaker and Kernohan published on the findings in 50 fatal cases of GBS, curiously also in the military, but now employed during World War II and not during World War I as in Guillain and Barré's paper. They emphasized demyelinating edema of the nerve roots within the first 4 days as the most characteristic finding but also found lymphocytes and phagocytes after 1–2 weeks. The late appearance of inflammatory cells in patients made them refine the disorder as a polyradiculoneuropathy "and not primarily polyradiculoneuritis." Their clinical description of fatal cases is legendary. Additionally, they described variability in presentation, with some patients not presenting with sensory symptoms or an increased CSF protein. According to Pearce, Guillain was angered by the inclusion of Landry's name. He felt that Landry was an acute bulbar form and a separate condition and said the inclusion of his name confused the nomenclature, "Une confusion nosographique absolue" [71, 138].

The characterization of GBS over time involved mostly further neuropathologic characterization. A more detailed pathologic study appeared from Massachusetts General Hospital and found lymphocytic infiltration in peripheral nerves and spinal roots, which confirmed the disorder was inflammatory in nature [11].

Guillain wrote his last paper on this syndrome in 1953. In this paper, he acknowledged that there were bulbar forms and that autonomic involvement could occur. He also expressed uncertainty that a chronic forum would exist. One of his cases took 3 years to recover, but no relapses were noted [71].

A better pathologic understanding of the disorder emerged with further classification in subsets. Variants of GBS have been described by Miller Fisher and Ropper [155].

Further insights came with the development of an animal model. Waxman developed an experimental autoimmune neuritis in rabbits that were injected with peripheral nerve tissue with adjuvants [192]. Advances in immunologic understanding have included the discovery of antibodies, but they are likely nonspecific. The current understanding—as it was several decades ago—is that both an antibody and cell-mediated response exist. The treatment of GBS is based on the assumption that modulating this response with plasma exchange or immunoglobulin could reduce demyelination and speed up recovery.

GBS has now been subclassified into several forms. These are acute axonal forms that include acute motor–sensory axonal neuropathy, acute motor axonal neuropathy, and Miller Fisher syndrome. GBS has been associated with a preceding illness, mostly an upper respiratory infection or acute enterocolitis. Although respiratory illness suggests seasonal predominance, in northern China, a seasonal predominance was evident in the summer months among children and in young adults [111]. Some infections might result in an increase in cross-reactive antibodies to neural gangliosides, which could cause inflammatory neural damage. An association between pandemic influenza vaccines and GBS has remained controversial, with most studies finding no such association. More recently, one study found that during the 2009 influenza A (H1N1) pandemic the vaccines did not substantially increase the risk for GBS [58].

Next to immunotherapies, treatment of the disorder has been mostly supportive and only after the 1950s would include mechanical ventilation, initially negative pressure ventilation. Patients with severe oropharyngeal weakness and inability to clear secretions would still be at risk for pulmonary complications and succumb, but they could later be saved with the introduction of endotracheal intubation and positive pressure ventilation.

Short Historical Note 28

MYASTHENIC CRISIS

The Title of the Paper

Rowland LP, Hoefer PFA, Aranow H Jr, Merritt HH. Fatalities in myasthenia gravis: a review of 39 cases with 26 autopsies. Neurology. 1956;6:307–26.

The Paper and the Times

The name of this disorder was given by Jolly [16, 90] who called it *pseudoparalysis myasthenia* in 1895, and the disorder gradually entered the medical lexicon. However, 1935 was a landmark year after Mary Walker showed a dramatic response in a myasthenic patient to a subcutaneous injection of physostigmine or neostigmine [92]. A synthetic preparation of curare at the time was used by anesthesiologists to achieve muscle relaxation, and neostigmine was used as an antidote. Walker's reasoning at the time was that neostigmine could be used for the "curare-like" symptomatology of myasthenia gravis (MG).

Already in 1945, Viets, a world-renowned expert in MG, reported 60 cases from Massachusetts General Hospital, [186–188] and his experience was regularly updated in the literature by others.

Myasthenic crisis has been recognized as worsening disease with respiratory symptoms requiring mechanical ventilation. In many instances, there was also upper airway weakness with obstruction of the pharynx, repeated coughing, and particularly a significant acute neuromuscular respiratory failure with weakness of the diaphragm, intercostals, and abdominal muscles. Worsening MG often was described as attacks of dyspnea, rapid exhaustion of respiratory muscles, or asphyxia due to choking [93, 175].

MG could become particularly severe. Viets recommended:

> When the patient is more seriously ill than the average occurring in the ambulatory clinica, neostigmine is of necessity given in the form of neostigmine methylsulfate by subcutaneous or intramuscular injection. ... A respiratory embarrassment due to weakness of the diaphragm and chest muscles may be of rapid onset. It is well to have all patients prepared for this possibility.

The word crises was mentioned in several reviews, but it was not part of the commonly used Osserman classification (group 3 was defined as "acute severe myasthenia gravis developing over a period of weeks to months with severe bulbar involvement often needing tracheostomy and respirator") [129–131]. In the 1951 paper by Rider, a patient in myasthenia crisis was reportedly showing dyspnea, weakness, and much mucous and saliva, which resulted in the patient choking on increased secretions requiring 336 mg of intramuscular neostigmine over 24 h [145].

The Details of the Paper

Thirty-nine cases are reported during the 1930–1955 time period (Fig. 4.19). Sixteen patients had a major concurrent illness that could possibly contribute to fatality. These included thyreotoxicosis, seizures and myocarditis (2). Two patients died after thymectomy, one from cardiac arrest, and another associated with pneumothorax.

The paper divided patients into 13 patients not on a ventilator, but with acute myasthenic attacks starting abruptly with sudden obtundation, dyspnea, and cyanosis. Respiratory weakness with or without pharyngeal or lingual weakness "seemed to be prominent." Most notable were three hospitalized patients during an acute exacerbation, initially improving and in no distress but with sudden death ("lobular pneumonia with considerable accumulation of mucous in the bronchi" was found at autopsy).

In 16 patients on a mechanical ventilator, "all but two were cyanotic, comatose or apneic before they were placed in the respirator." The degree of pulmonary insufficiency in some patients could not explain fatality. The paper emphasized "refractoriness to neostigmine" and found it was not simply an inadequate dose. Toxicity was considered "more ominous in the possibility that overdosage may cause neuromuscular block, increasing weakness rather than correcting it." However, the authors stated that "in critical conditions there is a greater likelihood of administering too little rather than too much." The authors emphasized "there is not sufficient evidence to conclude that neostigmine should be completely withdrawn from every respirator patient and it may be advantageous to

Fatalities in Myasthenia Gravis

A Review of 39 Cases with 26 Autopsies

Lewis P. Rowland, M.D., Paul F. A. Hoefer, M.D., Henry Aranow, Jr., M.D. and H. Houston Merritt, M.D.

THE MORTALITY RATE of myasthenia gravis is high, despite the advances in therapy of the past two decades. We have reviewed the records of patients with myasthenia who died at the Columbia-Presbyterian Medical Center, in order to evaluate factors which might be responsible for these fatalities and to describe the clinical and pathologic features of a group of patients in whom the disease has been followed to its end.

CASE MATERIAL

During the period from 1930 to 1955 the diagnosis of myasthenia gravis was established unequivocally in 180 patients,[74] all but 13 of whom were seen after 1940 (figure 1). Fifty-five patients are known to have died, a mortality rate of at least 30 per cent. The actual figure is uncertain, since 49 patients have not been followed.

Thirty-nine fatal cases have been selected for review and are the subject of this report, including all of the 34 patients who died in the hospital, two patients who were dead upon arrival at the hospital, two patients who died at home while under our care, and one patient who died at another hospital but who had been seen on our service initially and whose postmortem examination was performed in our department of pathology; other patients who died elsewhere have been excluded. Knowledge of the terminal events was available for each of the cases included and postmortem examination was performed in 26 cases. Only three patients died prior to 1940 (figure 1).

CLINICAL ANALYSIS — GENERAL FEATURES

Age and sex incidence. Of the 39 patients, 13 were men and 26 were women

From the departments of neurology and medicine, College of Physicians and Surgeons and The Presbyterian Hospital, New York City.

Fig. 4.19 The title page

continue the drug in amounts sufficient to increase cooperation, communication, coughing and swallowing." The paper also pointed out the use and dangerous effects of sedatives in restless patients with hypoxemia and hypercarbia. The paper concluded that the physician should recognize premonitory attacks of respiratory distress, use sedatives with caution, and institute mechanical ventilation and control of infection early—advice that rings true today.

The Message and Acceptance

Myasthenia crisis is a poorly defined illness, and physicians typically now recognize a situation in which the patient may need emergency respiratory care. Often, there is upper airway obstruction with excessive secretions and diaphragmatically weakness [50, 62, 67, 130, 179].

Over several decades, experiences from many medical centers throughout the world have been published [50, 62, 127, 139]. The experience of Mayo Clinic was published by Gracey et al. and involved 22 patients from a series of 288 patients diagnosed in 1978 and 1979. Of the 22 patients requiring mechanical ventilation, 21 survived and were weaned from the ventilator after 1–32 days of respiratory support. In this early Mayo Clinic experience, 4 of 22 patients had myasthenic crises, but respiratory failure was provoked by a surgical procedure in 11 patients [69]. Two patients in cholinergic crises were found. (A cholinergic crisis was explained by overdose of anticholinergic drugs causing depolarizing blockade and progressive weakness, fasciculations, and diarrhea.) Others also reported their experiences with patients deteriorating after thymectomy [136].

An important work appeared in 1981 that analyzed the outcome of myasthenic crises between 1960 and 1980 at the Neurological Institute Columbia-Presbyterian Medical Center [50]. Most notable was their policy of discontinuation of anticholinergic drugs while on the ventilator. The incidence of crisis was constant over two decades and was 16%, but with a mortality of 33% in the 1960s. The median onset of MG and first crises was 21 months but could be as early as 1 month and as late as 27 years after diagnosis. Cohen emphasized that the overwhelming proportion of patients had dysarthria and dysphagia before their crisis, suggesting aspiration or pneumonia in some of them. The duration of respiratory support lasted 2 weeks but with a range of several hours to 1 year. Most patients received a tracheostomy. Plasma exchange was used in patients after the first successful description in MG and gradually became an important first intervention in myasthenic crises [140].

A follow-up study from Neurological Institute Columbia-Presbyterian Medical Center appeared in 1997 and included the widespread use of immunotherapies such as intravenous immunoglobulin and plasma exchange. However, mortality declined but remained around 4% as a result of medical complications [181]. More recent published experience continues to emphasize the challenges with respiratory care. In one series, extubation failure was 44%, and a prolonged stay in the intensive care unit was very common [170]. Aggressive respiratory care and prevention of atelectasis may shorten the weaning period, but care of the myasthenic patient in crisis remains extraordinary difficult.

Short Historical Note 29

ACUTE BACTERIAL MENINGITIS

The Title of the Paper

Carpenter RR, Petersdorf RG. The clinical spectrum of bacterial meningitis. Am J Med. 1962;33:262–75.

The Paper and the Times

The syndromes of otitis, sinusitis, pneumonitis, and meningitis have been known since antiquity, but acute meningitis became better characterized presumably first by the Scottish physician John Abercrombie who, in 1829, in his classic textbook of neurology, described inflammation of the arachnoid and pia mater [2]. Abercrombie described the underlying pathology, pointed out inflammation of the arachnoid, pia, and dura mater membranes and called it *meningitis*. Most notably, Abercrombie found that "the brain in other respect was healthy" and there was no "effusion in the ventricles." According to Tyler in a recent review on the history of bacterial meningitis, the term came in general usage after this introduction [182].

The abnormal cerebrospinal fluid (CSF) formula became more detailed after lumbar puncture was introduced as a procedure by Quincke in 1891. Earlier studies in the early 1900s documented a low CSF glucose and pleocytosis. At the end of the nineteenth century, CSF examination became more routine, and this resulted in laboratory characterization of *Pneumococcus*, *Neisseria meningitidis*, and *Haemophilus influenzae*. Important contributions are from Houston Merritt and Feremont-Smith and their textbook, includes analysis of CSF specimens in 152 patients with bacterial meningitis [112].

Although the use of penicillin for meningitis in the early 1940s reduced mortality with roughly 20%, the mortality remained substantial. The propensity for some microorganisms to cause epidemics also was soon recognized. After Weichselbaum discovered gram-negative *diplococci* in meningococcus meningitis, Kuhns, in 1943, found that sulfadiazine prevented outbreaks [33]. Vaccinations—particularly in high-risk groups such as the military and college freshman—were first performed in the early 1970s.

Many clinicians were distinctly aware that bacterial meningitis could present rapidly with little time to make an accurate diagnosis intravitam. Many only saw the ravaging destruction at autopsy with accumulation of pus into the ventricles confirming the fulminant nature of the process.

The most comprehensive review in the modern area, defined as when penicillin therapy became available [178], is from Carpenter and Petersdorf.

The Details of the Paper

The authors reported a series of 209 patients with meningitis largely caused by *Neisseria meningitidis* and *Haemophilus influenzae* (Fig. 4.20). Three patterns were identified: rapid onset with loss of consciousness without any manifesting respiratory infection, slower progression with signs of respiratory infection at the same time of meningitis, and patients with an antecedent infection weeks before the initial symptoms.

The level of consciousness was considered an important prognostic sign with very few patients alert. The clinical characteristics identified in their study are shown in their table (Fig. 4.21). The paper warned that "toxic depression" of the central nervous system could in fact represent the beginning of a meningitis. The series emphasized that meningococcal disease may present with a fulminant irreversible course and found that endotoxic shock accounted for early mortality. The high mortality in meningitis caused by less commonly identified microorganisms was explained by more serious conditions such as bacterial endocarditis and ruptured brain abscesses. The use of corticosteroids with concomitant use of antibiotics was stressed, but the series found no evidence of improved outcome.

The Message and Acceptance

The paper set the tone for further detailed studies in bacterial meningitis [27].

Many descriptive studies appeared later and focused on neurologic recognition of the disorder, as well as on interpretation of CSF. Management of bacterial meningitis mostly concentrated on the best choice of antibiotics. Soon, articles appeared

Fig. 4.20 The title page

The Clinical Spectrum of Bacterial Meningitis*

ROBERT R. CARPENTER, M.D.† and ROBERT G. PETERSDORF, M.D.
Seattle, Washington

EPIDEMIC meningitis with a rash of "purple spots" was clearly described by Vieusseux following an outbreak in Geneva in 1805 [1]. In the era before diagnostic bacteriology, meningitis was known to be an occasional complication of pneumonia and tuberculosis. In 1886 Frankel as well as Foa and Bondoni-Uffreduzzi demonstrated the pneumococcus in human spinal fluid. The following year Weichselbaum noted gram-negative diplococci in six cases of acute meningitis. Hemophilus influenza meningitis was described by Slawyk in 1899 [2]. During the ensuing thirty years many of the less common etiologic agents were isolated, including the staphylococcus and a number of coliform organisms. More recently Mima polymorpha [3–5] and Listeria monocytogenes [6,7] have received attention as occasional causes of bacterial meningitis.

Although clinical interest in meningeal infection has remained high, few advances have been made in understanding its pathogenesis [8]. This retrospective study of non-tuberculous bacterial meningitis at the King County Hospital during the decade from 1950 to 1960 represents an attempt to gain some insight into the mechanisms of meningeal infection. We were particularly interested in assessing the effects of antimicrobial agents and delineating the factors influencing prognosis. Two hundred and nine patients, who presented with bacterial meningitis during the period of study, comprise the basis for this report.

ETIOLOGY

Diplococcus pneumoniae, Neisseria meningitidis and H. influenza were the most common pathogens. In 173 of the 209 patients the etiologic diagnosis was established by culture of the cerebrospinal fluid. (Table I.) In eight cases the causative organism grew in blood cultures and was seen in the gram stain of the cerebrospinal fluid sediment. In six cases the diagnosis of meningococcal meningitis was made in patients with a purpuric rash and sterile cerebrospinal fluid containing typical gram-negative diplococci.

In twenty-two cases the etiologic agent was unknown. In twelve of these, definite organisms were seen in the sediment of the cerebrospinal fluid. In two additional cases the diagnosis of purulent meningitis was confirmed at autopsy. The remaining patients recovered promptly from a clinically typical illness; in each instance the sugar in the cerebrospinal fluid was less than

TABLE I
CAUSATIVE PATHOGENS IN BACTERIAL MENINGITIS

Etiologic Agent	No. Cases	No. Positive Cerebrospinal Fluid Culture	No. Fatal Cases
Meningococcus	53	46	7 (13%)
Pneumococcus	63	59	37 (59%)
Hemophilus influenza	35	34	6 (18%)
Other	58	34	33 (57%)
Unknown agent	22	...	6
Mixed infections	9	9	9
Escherichia coli	9	9	7
Staphylococcus	8	6	5
Pseudomonas	3	3	1
Streptococcus	3	3	1
Paracolon	2	2	2
"Diphtheroid"	2	2	2

* From the Department of Medicine, University of Washington School of Medicine and King County Hospital, Seattle, Washington. Manuscript received August 8, 1961.

† Present address: National Institute of Allergy and Infectious Diseases, National Institutes of Health, Bethesda, Maryland.

TABLE V
NEUROLOGIC SIGNS IN BACTERIAL MENINGITIS

Signs	No. Patients	No. Deaths
Signs of diffuse damage*	23	12
Hemiparesis	32	21
Cranial nerve damage		
IV	3	2
VI	11	3
VII	5	1
VIII	6	1
Nystagmus	4	1
Head or eyes deviated	10	6
Convulsions	40	29
Pupillary abnormality	13	9
Tremor	3	1
Total with one or more signs	107	61
Total with neurologic signs	102	17

* Bilateral Babinski, absent "doll's head" movements, fixed, mid-stage pupils.

Fig. 4.21 Patient characteristics

that described complications such as subdural effusions, vascular occlusions, thrombophlebitis of the cerebral venous sinus, and long standing neurologic sequelae [161, 162, 183]. Only in the early 1970s, when computed tomography scans became available, was hydrocephalus recognized and the benefits of shunting.

Antibiotic therapy also has evolved over time. Sulfonamide drugs were highly effective in meningococcal meningitis, but not for most other microorganisms. With the introduction of intra venous penicillin, most patients were initially treated with high doses and mortality decreased dramatically. A rapid increase in the prevalence of *pneumococcal* isolates resistant to penicillin occurred in the United States during the late 1980s. Several epidemiologic studies have shown that prophylactic use of antibiotics was associated with drug-resistant *pneumococcal* carriage. Drug-resistant *pneumococci* nowadays may be present in up to one in three patients with meningitis and that development prompted change in empirical treatment. Increasing resistant bacteria and reducing the prevalence of *Haemophylus influenzae* and meningococcal meningitis as a result of vaccinations in vulnerable groups also changed the clinical spectrum. Underreporting and antibiotic prescribing practices bias epidemiologic studies in many countries around the world, but it is clear that a worldwide emergence of antibiotic resistance among *Streptococcus pneumoniae* has complicated treatment. Initial treatment for pneumococcal meningitis now involves vancomycin and expanded-spectrum cephalosporin.

Most of the early discoveries focused on the bacterial inflammation. Later work did redirect attention to immunologic pathways and the neurologic and systemic complications. Although there was initially less enthusiasm, there is compelling evidence that corticosteroids used early in the clinical course improve outcome, and most recent information shows a 10% reduction in mortality [18]. There is uncertainty about the duration of administration, dose, and why corticosteroids reduce mortality. It may reduce inflammation, vasculitis and improve septic shock.

Although a Cochrane analysis found no benefit, a more recent study found considerable benefit from corticosteroids (using historical controls) in meningitis caused by *Streptococcus pneumoniae* [35]. Its benefit in meningococcal meningitis in adults remains uncertain.

Short Historical Note 30

PITUITARY APOPLEXY

The Title of the Paper

Brougham M, Heusner P, Adams RD. Acute degenerative changes in adenomas of the pituitary body – with special reference to pituitary apoplexy. J Neurosurgery. 1950;7: 421–39.

The Paper and the Times

Pituitary apoplexy has been recognized as a rare and potentially fatal disorder. Around the turn of the century, there was mention of old hemorrhages in patients with acromegaly who came to autopsy [13, 59, 87]. Bailey – cofounder of the Neurological Institute in New York – and Bleibtreu neuropathologist from Munich were among the first to describe cases in acromegaly [13, 22, 25]. Subsequent clinical case reports noted acute ophthalmoplegia and stupor progressing to coma associated with a gross hemorrhage into a pituitary adenoma. None of the cases had detailed neurologic findings or an explanation of why it occurred. The nature of the pathologic process was unexplained. The highlighted paper in this short historical note would go all the way in trying to explain the mechanism of this disorder. Over the years, asymptomatic pituitary hemorrhage became more noticed on magnetic resonance imaging (MRI) and, in many instances, was not followed by a clinical presentation of pituitary apoplexy.

The Details of the Paper

The nature of the pathologic process led to the term *pituitary apoplexy* and was first mentioned in this paper. Five cases were reported from Boston City Hospital (Fig. 4.22). Infarction of the pituitary was related to the tumor, which had "outgrown its blood supply." Acute swelling of the tumor led to compression of the optic chiasm and optic nerves. The ophthalmoplegia was understood as a result of compression of the cranial oculomotor nerves in the cavernous sinus. Stupor was explained from acute compression of the hypothalamus or due to acute Addison's disease. In one case, a ruptured aneurysm was considered because blood had extended to the sylvian fissures and was confined to the subarachnoid spaces, but none was found at autopsy. The pathology suggested tumor swelling with further compression of feeding arteries leading to massive necrosis of all the clinical features. Impaired consciousness was emphasized, but other mechanisms were suggested such as acute adrenal insufficiency or a temporal lobe pressure cone due to extension of the tumor or convulsions. Hypoglycemia and hypotension from Addison's disease could mimic pituitary apoplexy. The dangers of lumbar puncture in a patient causing a temporal lobe shift were mentioned.

> It is important to emphasize that if the acute symptoms here described overtake a patient who shows either the stigmata of acromegaly or those of pituitary insufficiency, the diagnosis of adenomatous apoplexy is tenable but only presumptive. In either instance the acute features of the illness might with equal plausibility be ascribed to the occurrence of a meningocerebral hemorrhage stemming, for example, from the rupture of a berry aneurysm. Therefore, for the certainty of diagnosis which is requisite for operative treatment, intracranial vascular malformations should be excluded by angiography. This study might also provide valuable data regarding the suspected extrasellar extension of the pituitary lesion.

The authors also emphasized that surgery was imperative:

> Unfortunately, our pathological material suggests that few patients will make spontaneous improvement beyond a condition of partial and temporary betterment. An extensive though largely circumscribed extravasation of blood at the infundibular region, or a post-infarction swelling of the extrasellar portion of the adenoma would doubtless give rise, in most cases, either to paralytic effects upon adjacent parts of the brain, or to blockage of CSF [cerebrospinal fluid] pathways and progressive internal hydrocephalus. Operation would then become necessary not in any prophylactic sense, but for relief of chronic headache, hemiparesis, impending stupor, papilledema or threatened optic atrophy. The principal objective would be that of evacuating necrotic and hemorrhagic material so as to remove the pressure from neural elements and/or the obstruction to the free flow of CSF.

ACUTE DEGENERATIVE CHANGES IN ADENOMAS OF THE PITUITARY BODY—WITH SPECIAL REFERENCE TO PITUITARY APOPLEXY

MILTON BROUGHAM, M.D., A. PRICE HEUSNER, M.D.,
AND RAYMOND D. ADAMS, M.D.

Neurological Unit and Neurosurgical Service, Boston City Hospital, and Department of Neurology, Harvard Medical School, Boston, Massachusetts

(Received for publication February 13, 1950)

DEGENERATIVE changes in pituitary adenomas and their attendant clinical manifestations occur not infrequently yet they have been mentioned in only a few of the more complete descriptions of these tumors. These changes usually consist of small hemorrhages and areas of necrosis with "cyst" formation, reparative fibrosis and sometimes calcification. Some writers relate such lesions to the apparent arrest of acromegaly or to the rapid development of dyspituitarism. However, in most instances these degenerative changes are regarded as unimportant findings without precise relationship to symptoms and without significant effect on the growth of the adenoma.

In the routine examination of the brains of individuals who have died unexpectedly we have several times discovered tumors of the pituitary gland in which widespread necrosis and/or extensive hemorrhage had occurred. Clinically, these changes were associated with a sudden onset of neurological symptoms such as ophthalmoplegia, blindness, stupor or coma and they have resulted in death within a few hours to days. Extensive lesions of this type have seldom been described. In fact, a review of the literature disclosed only 5 cases showing similar symptomatology and pathological findings. The following cases are presented, therefore, in order to call attention to these severe retrogressive pituitary lesions.

REPORT OF CASES

Case 1. (B.C.H. 115140, A 44–421) This patient, a 65-year-old negro, was hospitalized because of epigastric pains of 7 weeks' duration. Investigation revealed nothing of importance except a low blood pressure (100/70) and a slight reduction of blood chlorides. A diagnosis of adrenal insufficiency was made and treatment with sodium chloride and desoxycorticosterone was instituted.

On the night of the 16th hospital-day the patient complained of severe frontal headache, and the next morning he was found semicomatose. Temperature was 105°F. and the neck was very stiff. The right pupil measured 6 mm., the left 4 mm. and neither reacted to light or on convergence; there was a complete right ophthalmoplegia. No other abnormal signs were elicited. CSF was xanthochromic and under a pressure of 180 mm.; it contained 155 RBC, 55 neutrophilic leucocytes and 295 lymphocytes/c.mm.; total protein 182 mg., and sugar 55 mg./100 cc.

On the 21st hospital-day there was definite improvement in that the patient was able to respond to simple questions. However, he remained confused and the

Fig. 4.22 Title page

The Message and Acceptance

This clinical entity commonly is seen in a patient with no established diagnosis of a pituitary tumor and thus should be considered in any patient with new cranial nerve deficit and headache. Surgery is usually preferred within 1 week of symptom onset. When compression of the optic chiasm impacts vision, either severely reducing visual acuity or deteriorating visual fields, pituitary apoplexy becomes a neurosurgical emergency.

Pituitary apoplexy may occur in any tumor, although most commonly in a patient with stigmata of acromegaly. The incidence may be higher in the MRI era, and small hemorrhages can be recognized without the clinical "apoplexy." Moreover MRIs have demonstrated smaller hemorrhages without clinical correlates. Multiple precipitating factors have been linked to acute hemorrhage within the tumor and include general surgical procedures, administration of bromocriptine, anticoagulation, estrogen therapy, diabetic ketoacidosis, radiation, and hypertensive crises [104]. Pituitary apoplexy may be the first presentation of the tumor and may become quickly life-threatening, owing to glucocorticoid deficiency [32, 46, 104]. It is common for the patient to experience a thunderclap retro-orbital headache that is similar to the headache in aneurysmal subarachnoid hemorrhage and is followed by visual field deficits or oculomotor abnormalities [12]. Hypopituitarism occurs in a large proportion of patients and may make it a critical illness.

Short Historical Note 31

CRITICAL ILLNESS POLYNEUROPATHY

The Title of the Paper

Roelofs RI, Cerra F, Bielka N, Rosenberg L, Delaney J. Prolonged respiratory insufficiency due to acute motor neuropathy: a new syndrome? Neurology. 1983;33:240.
Bolton CF, Gilbert JJ, Hahn AF, Sibbald WJ. Polyneuropathy in critically ill patients. J Neurol Neurosurg Psychiatry. 1984;47:1223–31.

The Paper and the Times

In the early 1980s, when these novel observations were published, medical and surgical intensive care units (ICUs) were well established. Many patients with sepsis and multiorgan failure were admitted to medical ICUs. In surgical ICUs, major surgeries could become more complicated after a systemic infection. Often, these patients, after surviving such an ordeal, were ventilator dependent and continued to be dependent despite marked improvement in pulmonary parameters and radiologic studies. For many intensivists and surgeons, this was a reason to consult neurologists with the specific question whether there was a neuromuscular respiratory failure that would prevent the patient from coming off the ventilator. In some patients, there were additional complaints of numbness, tingling, and burning of the hands and feet. In others, there was more profound weakness and atrophy that could not be attributed to prolonged illness, neuromuscular junction blockers, or a combination of the two.

In 1983, two abstracts by Roelofs and Bolton appeared at the annual meeting of the American Academy of Neurology. Both authors described an axonal polyneuropathy, and Roelofs suggested it may represent a possible new syndrome. Their patients had sepsis and multiorgan failure and had developed profound weakness and "prolonged respiratory insufficiency" [152].

The Details of the Paper

Roelofs and associates published an abstract that included four patients weaned off the ventilator after several months and electrodiagnostic studies showing active denervation. No explanation for respiratory insufficiency was provided [152]. In Bolton's series the polyneuropathy developed soon after admission to the ICU and likely at the onset of infection. The electromyography findings included fibrillation potentials, positive sharp waves, normal or mildly prolonged motor nerve conduction velocities, and muscle biopsies, which showed mostly type II fiber atrophy. The clinical setting was uniformly sepsis often in association with severe pulmonary disease, which included acute pulmonary edema, empyema, and bilateral lobar pneumonia. Systemic illness always evolved into a multiorgan dysfunction. Cerebrospinal fluid was unremarkable in most patients, making Guillain-Barré syndrome much less likely. This was also supported by demonstrating an axonal injury rather than demyelination after examination of the sural nerve biopsy. Both studies speculated about the origin of this neuropathy and included causes such as nutritional deficiencies, toxicity from antibiotics, or toxins associated with a bacterial infection. Obviously, it could not be determined whether the nerve was just one of the many tissues directly damaged by sepsis or if the treatment of sepsis could be implicated.

Pathology of the patients who died showed normal cranial nerves, but there was moderate to severe loss of large and small myelinated fibers in the median and lateral cutaneous, sciatic, common peroneal, superficial, and deep peroneal and sural nerves. Mostly macrophages containing lipid debris were found, but occasional clusters of mononuclear inflammatory cells were seen. Outcome in survivors was good, but recovery could be prolonged.

The Message and Acceptance

The term *critical illness polyneuropathy* was proposed, linking it to stays in the ICU and not to a specific illness [128]. Several years later, in 1985, Op de Coul et al. published a similar article on neuromuscular complications in patients given pancuronium bromide during mechanical ventilation. This was followed by a larger study by Zochodne and colleagues from Bolton's group who saw 5 patients in a 4-year period and then 14 patients in the next 2 years, suggesting increased recognition of the disorder [206, 209].

Prolonged Respiratory Insufficiency Due to Acute Motor Neuropathy: A New Syndrome? *11:00 AM* 9

R.I. Roelofs, F. Cerra, N. Bielka, Minneapolis, MN; L. Rosenberg, Canton, OH and J. Delaney, Minneapolis

Four patients (2 men, aged 68 and 74; 2 women, aged 67 and 58), during the course of a septic illness, developed respiratory insufficiency requiring prolonged ventilatory support. Neurologic exam, while respirator-dependent, revealed proximal weakness, decreased to absent reflexes, normal sensation, and normal cranial nerve function. CSF studies were normal in two patients. EMG findings included fibrillation potentials, positive sharp waves, normal or slightly prolonged motor-nerve conduction velocities, and prolonged F-wave latencies. Muscle biopsy findings included Type II fiber atrophy; small dark angular fibers with the NADH-TR reaction; spread of acetylcholinesterase activity around the sarcolemma of atrophic fibers; and mild fiber type grouping in one biopsy. Two patients eventually improved and were weaned off the respirator after 2 to 3 months of ventilator support; two patients died after 1 to 3 months of intensive care. The EMG and biopsy findings of active denervation, with normal NCVs and CSF findings, suggest an acute, axonal motor neuropathy, and separate this entity from the Guillain-Barré syndrome. Possible etiologic factors include multiple antibiotic therapy, sepsis due to multiple organisms, or associated metabolic disorders.

Fig. 4.23 Title page

Polyneuropathy in critically ill patients

CHARLES F BOLTON, JOSEPH J GILBERT, ANGELIKA F HAHN, WILLIAM J SIBBALD

From Departments of Clinical Neurological Sciences, Pathology and Medicine, and The Critical Care/Trauma Unit, Victoria Hospital, University of Western Ontario, London, Ontario, Canada

SUMMARY Five patients developed a severe motor and sensory polyneuropathy at the peak of critical illness (sepsis and multiorgan dysfunction complicating a variety of primary illnesses). Difficulties in weaning from the ventilator as the critical illness subsided and the development of flaccid and areflexic limbs were early clinical signs. However, electrophysiological studies, especially needle electrode examination of skeletal muscle, provided the definite evidence of polyneuropathy. The cause is uncertain, but the electrophysiological and morphological features indicate a primary axonal polyneuropathy with sparing of the central nervous system. Nutritional factors may have played a role, since the polyneuropathy improved in all five patients after total parenteral nutrition had been started, including the three patients who later died of unrelated causes. The features allow diagnosis during life, and encourage continued intensive management since recovery from the polyneuropathy may occur.

Fig. 4.24 Title page

For many of us, critical illness polyneuropathy has been an accepted complication of patients who have been admitted with severe sepsis and were treated with sedation and neuromuscular blockers. Most intensivists recognize severe weakness, although failure to wean from the ventilator has not been definitively linked to phrenic nerve involvement or any of the nerve or muscle injury. It is far more likely these patients with severe nerve injury and severe pulmonary injury represent one end of the spectrum. Clinical illness polyneuropathy has now been recognized as patients who have variable muscle weakness and fasciculations, often severe quadriplegia and muscle wasting. Most muscle biopsies show neurogenic atrophy and muscle involvement, suggesting a secondary injury to the muscle rather than the nerve or neuromuscular junction.

Management has remained supportive with no specific treatment available. The cause has not been elucidated since the original description almost 30 years ago [19, 29, 30, 55, 84, 102, 109, 199, 206]. Bolton has speculated that impaired microvascular supply to the endoneurium was a major factor [29, 30]. Cytokines activated in the sepsis cascade could be neurotoxic. A nutritional factor has always been put forward as a major candidate, but whether supplements are useful has not been established. Most recently aggressive glucose control has been linked to a markedly reduced incidence of critical illness polyneuropathy, but confirmation of this tentative association is awaited [78]. Many of the same mechanisms in diabetic polyneuropathy may play a role, and in critical illness these damaging factors may be enhanced. Some recent work has suggested that changes in the axon excitability could be a result of hyperglycemia induced sodium–potassium pump malfunction. Improvement, at least under experimental conditions, could be observed with glycemic control [95]. Whether this translates to the clinical setting is not known—and considering the severity of axonal injury—unlikely.

Short Historical Note 32

CYCLOSPORINE NEUROTOXICITY

The Title of the Paper

Joss DV, Barrett AJ, Kendra JR, et al. Hypertension and convulsions in children receiving cyclosporin A. Lancet. 1982;1:906.

Thompson CB, June CH, Sullivan KM, et al. Association between cyclosporin neurotoxicity and hypomagnesemia. Lancet. 1984:1116–9.

The Paper and the Times

The immunosuppressive drug cyclosporine was discovered by a multidisciplinary team of scientists in the 1970s in the laboratories of Sandoz in Basel, Switzerland [34]. Azathioprine and prednisone already had dramatically improved survival after organ and bone marrow transplantation, but cyclosporine would make a much bigger impact and revolutionize transplantation outcome. Calne's group earlier reported nephrotoxicity with cyclosporine A, but in this report, 34 patients treated with cyclosporine A received a variety of organ allografts (kidney, pancreas, and liver). The authors noted tremor in most patients with severe manifestations in three patients [39]. Calne and his colleagues concluded, "We are still ignorant of the pharmacodynamics of cyclosporine A in man. … from our limited experience, we feel that 10 mg/kg/day may be too little and 25 mg/kg/day too much."

Cyclosporine neurotoxicity also brought the neurologist into the transplant unit [23, 54, 60, 74, 204]. Neurotoxicity became first known in the bone marrow transplantation population, but reports in liver transplantation soon followed [15, 195]. Cyclosporine remained a major immunosuppressant drug until the introduction of FK506 (Tacrolimus) [82].

The Details of the Paper

One of the first reports of seizures involved 26 patients with bone marrow transplantation. Seven patients developed seizures, and in all, diastolic blood pressure was increased (Fig. 4.25). Nephrotoxicity was considered the cause for fluid retention and hypertension. The convulsions were described as "grand mal" and treated with diazoxide, mannitol and furosemide to control fluid retention. Soon after, case reports appeared with seizures in cardiac and liver transplants [5, 74].

A detailed study of 12 patients with cyclosporine neurotoxicity suggested that hypomagnesemia was a major cause and noted improvement after normalization of serum magnesium levels. Hypomagnesemia was considered a manifestation of toxic effect of cyclosporine on the tubular function of the kidney (Fig. 4.26). For the first time, this study described neurotoxicity in sufficient detail. Seizures occurred early during the course of cyclosporine therapy (median of 12 days) Other seizure risk factors were identified and included hypertension and corticosteroid therapy. None of the patients had severe hyponatremia, hypoglycemia, or severe hypoxemia. Phenytoin and phenobarbital were used as antiepileptic drugs, but seizures reoccurred if hypomagnesemia was not corrected. Seizures did not return after magnesium replacement. The authors also described cerebellar ataxia, tremor, and depression. The tremor was diagnosed as "cerebellar" after a neurologist consultation. One neurologist noted, "muscular tetany" in one patient. Two patients developed a transient aphasia. In all patients, computed tomography (CT) scan of the brain was normal and electroencephalogram (EEG) was unrevealing.

The Message and Acceptance

Soon after these initial observations, a major paper appeared on neurologic complications in liver transplant, implicating cyclosporine neurotoxicity. Adams and colleagues described serious neurologic complications in one-third of 52 patients, mostly seizures and occurring within the first week after transplantation [5]. Cyclosporine was titrated to whole blood levels using a radioimmunoassay. A connection of seizures with cyclosporine neurotoxicity was suggested after several patients had high cyclosporin levels and in particular because seizures occurred during the infusion of cyclosporine. Hypertension and fluid retention did not appear as a major cofactor. Most interesting were the focal EEG abnormalities in the posterior parietal regions, but CT scans were

HYPERTENSION AND CONVULSIONS IN CHILDREN RECEIVING CYCLOSPORIN A

SIR,—Cyclosporin A (CyA) can reduce the severity of graft-versus-host disease after transplantation, but renal toxicity has been reported as a significant side-effect.[1,2] Since 1980 we have used CyA in 36 bone-marrow transplant patients, and report here new side-effects in children previously undescribed.

The patients given bone-marrow transplants were 26 with acute lymphoblastic leukaemia in remission, 5 with aplastic anaemia, and 5 with inborn errors of metabolism (4 mucopolysaccharidoses, 1 metachromatic leucodystrophy). CyA was given orally from at least the day before the graft at a dose of 12·5 mg/kg twice daily (30 patients) or 25 mg/kg twice daily for the first ten days and 12·5 mg/kg twice daily thereafter, until a hundred days post graft. Some degree of renal impairment occurred in every patient, as shown by a rise in blood urea and creatinine in the two weeks of treatment. This effect was reversible in all but 4 patients in whom oliguric renal failure developed. 2 of these patients died with multiple problems.

In addition, and particularly in children, we observed fluid retention and hypertension associated with convulsions in 7 children (figure). Body weight increase due to fluid retention was frequently insidious, but diastolic blood pressure often rose rapidly in the space of 48 h. Only 4 out of 29 patients under the age of 17 remained normotensive; 16 (55%) had a diastolic blood pressure of greater than 100 mm Hg at some stage after transplantation, and most of these children were less than 12 years of age. 6 of the 7 children who had grand mal convulsions had a diastolic blood pressure of over 120 mm Hg, and only 2 patients with blood pressure over 120 mm Hg did not convulse. Hypertension and convulsions were successfully treated with a combination of diazoxide and diuresis with mannitol and frusemide. We have subsequently monitored blood pressure regularly in patients on CyA, and have avoided severe hypertension by missing one dose of CyA when diastolic blood pressure rises, and reintroducing it at a lower dose.

Fig. 4.25 Title page

ASSOCIATION BETWEEN CYCLOSPORIN NEUROTOXICITY AND HYPOMAGNESAEMIA

CRAIG B. THOMPSON CARL H. JUNE
KEITH M. SULLIVAN E. DONNALL THOMAS

Division of Oncology, Fred Hutchinson Cancer Research Center and University of Washington School of Medicine, Seattle, Washington, USA

Summary The serum magnesium levels of all 12 allogeneic bone-marrow transplant recipients who experienced the neurotoxic effects of cyclosporin (CyA) were more than two standard deviations below the normal range. The neurological events seemed to segregate into three separate syndromes. 7 patients had grand-mal seizures, which occurred within the first several weeks of CyA therapy (median onset 12 days). At the time of their first seizure all 7 patients had hypomagnesaemia, which had developed rapidly over the preceding 1–3 weeks. 3 patients had four episodes of cerebellar ataxia, tremor, and depression. These subacute episodes developed after prolonged CyA therapy (median onset 67 days). Each episode was associated with hypomagnesaemia. 2 patients had a transient episode of expressive aphasia following a long period of hypomagnesaemia. In all cases symptoms resolved or did not recur with adequate magnesium replacement. These data suggest that CyA neurotoxicity is associated with hypomagnesaemia and may be treated or prevented with magnesium replacement.

Fig. 4.26 Title Page

not performed. Another landmark paper would show dramatic white matter lesions and suggested low cholesterol was at play [54]. In this situation, unique for liver transplant recipients, it was speculated that cyclosporine was transported into neurons by the low-density lipoprotein receptor.

Cyclosporine neurotoxicity has been further characterized over the years, but severe manifestations (cortical blindness or status epilepticus) have become less common due to better dosing schedules and the introduction of other immunosuppressive drugs with lower incidences of neurotoxicity (e.g., sirolimus).

The similarity of the white matter lesions with posterior reversible encephalopathy syndrome (PRES) is striking, and if PRES is interpreted as a brain capillary leak syndrome with disruption of the blood–brain syndrome, it likely is the same entity. Hypertension, the most common reason for PRES, however is rarely implicated in this patient population. A sudden high doses of exposure to cyclosporin may cause endothelial damage and vasogenic edema. The clinical manifestations even if severe and leading to coma are fully reversible and the same applies to the magnetic resonance abnormalities.

Neurotoxicity due to immunosuppressive agents remains a common reason for neurologists to see patients who have had a recent organ transplantation. This area of acute neurology is specialized and the neurologist must remain informed about the complexity of transplantation in order to be helpful. Over the years, several publications have documented the spectrum of neurologic complications, but in this field, new problems will emerge. The more severe manifestations are now history.

Short Historical Note 33

CEREBRAL EDEMA AND FULMINANT HEPATIC FAILURE

The Title of the Paper

Ware AJ, D'Agostino AN, Combes B. Cerebral edema: a major complication of massive hepatic necrosis. Gastroenterology. 1971;61:877–84

The Paper and the Times

Liver failure may make patients drowsy, inattentive, and nonchalant. Most cases of liver failure have been attributed to the toxic effects of ammonia. Whether a structural injury exists was a matter of debate for pathologists, but when patients with acutely worsening chronic liver failure came to autopsy, changes were found that included large Alzheimer type II astrocytes, neuronal loss in cerebellar cortex and basal ganglia, and glycogen-staining inclusions in astrocytes [3]. First reports of cerebral edema in acute liver failure emerged in the early 1970s, and fulminant hepatic failure ("massive liver cell necrosis") was defined as a separate entity from acute worsening chronic liver disease. Boston City Hospital published the largest series with 18 patients seen in a decade but representing less than 0.2% of all autopsies [151]. Most patients "became hypotensive and died in hepatic coma." "Terminally these patients developed generalized bleeding with hemorrhages into the skin, lungs, or gastrointestinal tract." Causes were considered viral or much less common a hepatotoxin (i.e., halothane), and vasopressors were considered. None of the autopsy studies examined brain tissue [44, 49, 113].

In the late 1960s, liver transplantation became a possible option for patients with usually fatal liver failure and mostly through the pioneering work of Roger Williams over a 7-year period, at King's College Hospital in London. In William's early experience, he found that about one-third of the patients had cerebral edema [143]. The observations made in this series also suggested for the first time that cerebral herniation was a direct cause of death. Both dexamethasone and mannitol were considered, but fear of gastrointestinal hemorrhage and possible rebound of intracranial pressure (ICP) with mannitol restricted its use (Williams' group would revisit this issue in a clinical trial later).

Acceptance of cerebral edema as a phenomenon in fulminant hepatic failure by neurologists was slow and the finding was considered controversial. In Plum and Posner's text, the autopsies were considered insufficiently detailed. "None of the reports included descriptions of the brain by experienced neuropathologists," or the observation was possibly considered "a terminal complication [142]."

The Details of the Paper

Case materials of 48 patients with massive hepatic necrosis were reviewed from 1958 to 1970 (Fig. 4.27). Cerebral edema was found in 16 of 32 patients who had a detailed examination of the brain. Macroscopically, there was flattening of the gyri, compression of the ventricles, and poor differentiation of white or gray matter. Herniation of cerebellar tonsils was seen in three patients, and uncal herniation was seen in two. Microscopically, edema was seen with prominent large swollen glia cells in the gray matter in 14 patients.

Clinical neurologic examination and clinicopathologic correlation were incomplete. Twelve of 16 patients were in stage IV hepatic encephalopathy (coma) for more than 48 h. Three illustrative cases were described with patients developing "grand mal seizure" and deteriorating to deep coma with "decerebrate opisthotonic movements." Lumbar puncture showed marked increased opening pressure (>300 mm saline). Papilledema was noted in one patient with development of light-fixed pupils followed by sudden respiratory arrest. Another patient with increased cerebrospinal fluid pressure was treated with corticosteroids and a combination of mannitol with furosemide, but with no success. The authors noted that shock, infection, or hemorrhage were not confounding factors. Acidosis and renal failure also were not commonly found in patients who developed cerebral edema.

The Message and Acceptance

One of the first indications that cerebral edema in fulminant hepatic failure could be treatable came with a series of five patients with fulminant hepatic failure and deterioration to

LIVER PHYSIOLOGY AND DISEASE

CEREBRAL EDEMA: A MAJOR COMPLICATION OF MASSIVE HEPATIC NECROSIS

ATHOL J. WARE, M.B.B.S., M.R.A.C.P., ANTHONY N. D'AGOSTINO, M.D., AND BURTON COMBES, M.D.

Liver-Gastrointestinal Unit, The Department of Internal Medicine, and the Department of Pathology, The University of Texas Southwestern Medical School at Dallas, Texas

A review was conducted of 32 patients dying of massive hepatic necrosis and subject to complete autopsy examination. Sixteen of the 32 patients were found to have cerebral edema and 4 of these had evidence of cerebellar and/or uncal herniation. Those patients with cerebral edema were younger, had a more prolonged period of stage IV coma, and were less likely to have terminal azotemia and acidosis than the patients without cerebral edema. The pathogenesis of the cerebral edema in these patients is unknown but it does not appear to be related to secondary complications causing cerebral hypoxia nor to any specific form of therapy.

Massive hepatic necrosis is a serious disorder with a very high mortality rate.[1] Major complications frequently occur in patients with this illness and these potentially reversible lesions are often responsible for the patient's death. In the absence of specific therapy for the underlying disease, much of our therapeutic effort is aimed at preventing such complications or treating them as they occur. Infection, bleeding, renal failure, acute gastrointestinal ulceration, and pancreatitis are all well established sequelae of this syndrome.[1, 2] Less well recognized is the occurrence of cerebral edema and raised intracranial pressure. We have been impressed by the frequency with which this phenomenon has been present in our patients dying with massive necrosis of the liver and have reviewed the experience of this unit since 1958 with respect to the neuropathology of these patients.

Fig. 4.27 Title page

deep unresponsive coma (grade 4 hepatic encephalopathy). The patients were treated with loading doses of glycerol, but intravascular hemolysis occurred. Lower doses of glycerol (50 g/day) were ineffective [44]. A later study using both dexamethasone and mannitol decreased ICP in patients with mildly increased ICPs [40].

Other options included high doses of barbiturates, propofol, and hypertonic saline—all traditional measures for treatment of ICP [63, 73, 106, 119]. The effect of indomethacin and induced hypothermia has been currently investigated [49, 156]. Risk factors for cerebral edema have been recognized and included high serum ammonia concentrations, hyperacute progression of liver injury, renal replacement therapy and infections, and in particular, the development of a systemic inflammatory response [20, 123, 176, 207].

The mechanism of brain edema has always been considered astroglial swelling from the toxic effects of ammonia, but inflammatory pathways are of recent interest, and minocycline has resulting in inhibition of microglial activation [38, 153]. Survival of fulminant hepatic failure is determined by many factors, but treatment and early recognition of hepatic encephalopathy converting into cerebral edema has become an important part of management and ongoing research. Currently, ICP monitor placement is standard management in the more severe cases, and the coagulopathy can be temporarily controlled with use of factor VII or prothrombin complex [101].

References

1. A definition of irreversible coma. Report of the Ad Hoc Committee of the Harvard Medical School to Examine the Definition of Brain Death. JAMA. 1968;205:337–40.
2. Abercrombie J. Pathological and practical researches on diseases of the brain and the spinal cord. Edinburgh: Waugh and Innes; 1834.
3. Adams R, Foley J. Neurological disorder associated with liver disease. Res Publ Assoc Res Nerv Ment Dis. 1953;32:198–237.
4. Adams JH, Graham DI, Jennett B. The neuropathology of the vegetative state after an acute brain insult. Brain. 2000;123:1327–38.
5. Adams DH, Gunson B, Honigberger L, et al. Neurological complications following liver transplantation. Lancet. 1987;1:949–51.
6. Adams JH, Jennett B, Murray LS et al. Neuropathological finidings in disabled survivors of a head injury. J Neurotrauma 2011;28:701–709.
7. Adams RD, Jéquier M. The brain death syndrome: hypoxemic panencephalopathy. Schweiz Med Wochenschr. 1969;99:65–73.
8. An appraisal of the criteria of cerebral death, a summary statement of a collaborative study. JAMA. 1977;237:982–6.
9. Andrews K, Murphy L, Munday R, et al. Misdiagnosis of the persistent vegetative state: retrospective study in a rehabilitation unit. BMJ. 1996;313:13–6.
10. Annas G. Worst Case Bioethics. Oxford University Press New York; 2010.
11. Asbury AK, Arnason BG, Adams RD. The inflammatory lesion in idiopathic polyneuritis. Medicine. 1969;48:173–215.
12. Ayuk J, McGregor EJ, Mitchell RD, et al. Acute management of pituitary apoplexy–surgery or conservative management? Clin Endocrinol. 2004; 61: 747–52.
13. Bailey P. Pathological report of a case of acromegaly, with special reference to the lesions in the hypophysis cerebri and in the thyroid gland; and a case of hemorrhage into the pituitary. Philadelphia Med J. 1898;1:789–92.
14. Bauby J-D, editor. The Diving Bell and the Butterfly (French translation by Jermy Leggatt). New York: Knopf; 1997.
15. Bechstein WO. Neurotoxicity of calcineurin inhibitors: impact and clinical management. Transpl Int. 2000;5:313–26.
16. Bedlack RS, Sanders DB. On the concept of myasthenic crisis. J Clin Neuromuscul Dis. 2002;4:40–2.
17. Bell JA, Hodgson HJF. Coma after cardiac arrest. Brain. 1974;97:361–72.
18. Belsey MA, Hoffpauir CW, Smith MH. Dexamethasone in the treatment of acute bacterial meningitis: the effect of study design on the interpretation of results. Pediatrics. 1969;44:503–13.
19. Berek K, Margreiter J, Willeit J, et al. Polyneuropathies in critically ill patients: a prospective evaluation. Intensive Care Med. 1996;22:849–55.
20. Bernal W, Hall C, Karvellas CJ, et al. Arterial ammonia and clinical risk factors for encephalopathy and intracranial hypertension in acute liver failure. Hepatology. 2007;46:1844–52.
21. Bernat JL, Rottenberg DA. Conscious awareness in PVS and MCS: the borderlands of neurology. Neurology. 2007;68:885–6.
22. Bills DC, Meyer FB, Laws Jr ER, et al. A retrospective analysis of pituitary apoplexy. Neurosurgery. 1993;33:602–8; discussion 608–9.
23. Bird GL, Meadows J, Goka J, et al. Cyclosporine-associated akinetic mutism and extrapyramidal syndrome after liver transplantation. J Neurol Neurosurg Psychiatry. 1990;53:1068–71.

24. Bivins D, Biller J, Laster DW, et al. Recovery from posttraumatic locked-in syndrome with basilar artery occlusion. Surg Neurol. 1981;16:230–4.
25. Bleibtreu L. Ein fall von akromegalie (zerstorung der hypophysis durch blutung). Munch Med Wschr. 1905;52:2079–80.
26. Blunt SB, Boulton J, Wise R, et al. Locked-in syndrome in fulminant demyelinating disease. J Neurol Neurosurg Psychiatry. 1994;57:504–5.
27. Bohr V, Rasmussen N, Hansen B, et al. Pneumococcal meningitis: an evaluation of prognostic factors in 164 cases based on mortality and on a study of lasting sequelae. J Infect. 1985;10:143–57.
28. Bollinger O. Ueber traumatische spät-apoplexie. Ein beitrag zur lehre von der hirneschutterung. Internationale Beitrage zur Wissenschaftlichen Medicin. Festschrift, Rudlof Virchow. Berlin A, Hirschwald. 1891;2:457–70.
29. Bolton CF. Sepsis and the systemic inflammatory response syndrome: neuromuscular manifestations. Crit Care Med. 1996;24:1408–16.
30. Bolton CF. Neuromuscular manifestations of critical illness. Muscle Nerve. 2005;32:140–63.
31. Boly M, Faymonville ME, Schnakers C, et al. Perception of pain in the minimally conscious state with PET activation: an observational study. Lancet Neurol. 2008;11:1013–20.
32. Bonicki W, Kasperlik-Zaluska A, Koszewski W, et al. Pituitary apoplexy: endocrine, surgical and oncological emergency. Incidence, clinical course and treatment with reference to 799 cases of pituitary adenomas. Acta Neurochir (Wien). 1993;120:118–22.
33. Borchardt JK. The history of bacterial meningitis treatment. Drug News Perspect. 2004;17:219–24.
34. Borel JF, Kis ZL. The discovery and development of cyclosporine (Sandimmune). Transplant Proc. 1991;2:1867–74.
35. Brouwer MC, Heckenberg SGB, de Gans J, et al. Nationwide implementation of adjunctive dexamethasone therapy for pneumococcal meningitis. Neurology. 2010;75:1533–9.
36. Buchman AS, Wichter MD. Recovery following the "locked-in" syndrome. Stroke. 1986;17:558.
37. Burns JD, Rabinstein AA, Cloft H, Lanzino G, Daniels DJ, Wijdicks EFM. Minimally conscious state after ruptured giant basilar aneurysm. Arch Neurol. 2009; 66:786–8.
38. Butterworth RF. Hepatic encephalopathy: a central neuroinflammatory disorder? Hepatology. 2011;53: 1372–6.
39. Calne RY, Rolles K, Thiru S, et al. Cyclosporine initially as the only immunosuppressant in 34 recipients of cadaveric organs: 32 kidneys, 2 pancreases, and 2 livers. Lancet. 1979;2:1033–6.
40. Canalese J, Gimson AE, Davis C, et al. Controlled trial of dexamethasone and mannitol for the cerebral edema of fulminant hepatic failure. Gut. 1982;23: 625–9.
41. Caplan LR. Charles Foix, the first modern stroke neurologist. Stroke. 1990;21:348–56.
42. Caplan LR, Wityk RJ, Glass TA, et al. New England Medical Center posterior circulation registry. Ann Neurol. 2004;56:389–98.
43. Cappa SF, Vignolo LA. Locked-in syndrome for 12 years with preserved intelligence. Ann Neurol. 1982;11:545.
44. Caravati CM, Wooton P. Acute massive hepatic necrosis with fatal liver failure. South Med J. 1962;55:1268–77.
45. Cardiopulmonary resuscitation: statement by the Ad Hoc Committee on Cardiopulmonary Resuscitation of the Division of Medical Sciences NAoS-NRC. JAMA. 1966;198:372–9.
46. Cardoso ER, Peterson EW. Pituitary apoplexy: a review. Neurosurgery. 1984;14:363–73.
47. Caronna J, Finkestein S. Neurological syndromes after cardiac arrest. Stroke. 1978;9:517–20.
48. Chase TN, Moretti L, Prensky AL. Clinical and electroencephalographic manifestations of vascular lesions of the Pons. Neurology. 1968;18:357–68.
49. Clemmesen JO, Hansen BA, Larsen FS. Indomethacin normalizes intracranial pressure in acute liver failure: a twenty-three-year-old woman treated with indomethacin. Hepatology. 1997;26:1423–5.
50. Cohen MS, Younger D. Aspects of the natural history of myasthenia gravis: crises and death. Ann N Y Acad Sci. 1981;377:670–7.
51. Conference of Medical Royal Colleges and Faculties of the United Kingdom. Diagnosis of brain death. BMJ. 1976;2:1187–8.
52. Courville CB, Blomquist OA. Traumatic intracerebral hemorrhage with particular reference to its pathogenesis and its relation to 'delayed traumatic apoplexy. Arch Surg. 1940;41:1–28.
53. Davis LE, Wesley RB, Juan D, et al. "Locked-in syndrome" from diazepam toxicity in a patient with tetanus. Lancet. 1972;1:101.
54. de Groen PC, Aksamit AJ, Rakela J, et al. Central nervous system toxicity after liver transplantation. The role of cyclosporine and cholesterol. N Engl J Med. 1987;317:861–6.
55. de Seze M, Petit H, Wiart L, et al. Critical illness polyneuropathy. A 2-year follow-up study in 19 severe cases. Eur Neurol. 2000;43:61–9.
56. Dejerine J. Semiologie des affections du systeme nerveux. 2nd ed. Paris: Masson; 1914. p. 1219.
57. Denny-Brown D. The treatment of recurrent cerebrovascular symptoms and the question of vasospasm. Med Clin North Am. 1951;35:1457–74.
58. Dieleman J, Romio S, Johansen K, et al. Sturkenboom M, VAESCO-GBS Case–control Study Group. Guillain-barre syndrome and adjuvanted pandemic influenza a (H1N1) 2009 vaccine: multinational case–control study in Europe. BMJ. 2011;343:d3908.
59. Dingley LA. Sudden death due to a tumor of the pituitary gland. Lancet. 1932;2:183–4.
60. Drachman BM, DeNofrio D, Acker MA, et al. Cortical blindness secondary to cyclosporine after orthotopic heart transplantation: a case report and review of the literature. J Heart Lung Transplant. 1996;15: 1158–64.

61. Duménil L. Paralysie peripherigue du mouvement et du sentiment portant sur les quatres members. Atrophie des rameaux nervous des parties paralysees. Gazette Hebdomadaire de Médicine. 1864; 1:203–6.
62. Eaton LM. Care of the patient who has myasthenia gravis. Med Clin North Am. 1947;31:907–23.
63. Evans JP, Scheinker IM. Histologic studies of the brain following head trauma. II. Post-traumatic petechial and massive intracerebral hemorrhage. J Neurosurg. 1946;3:101–13.
64. Foix C, Hillemand P. Les syndromes de l'artère cerebrale anterieure. Encéphale. 1925;20:209–32.
65. Foix C, Masson A. Le syndrome de l'artère cerebrale posterieure. Presse Med. 1923;31:361–5.
66. Forbes A, Alexander GJ, O'Grady JG, et al. Thiopental infusion in the treatment of intracranial hypertension complicating fulminant hepatic failure. Hepatology. 1989;10:306–10.
67. Genkins G, Kornfeld P, Papatestas AE, et al. Clinical experience in more than 2000 patients with myasthenia gravis. Ann N Y Acad Sci. 1987;505:500–13.
68. Giacino JT, Whyte J, Bagiella E, et al. Placebo-controlled trial of amantadine for severe traumatic Brain Injury N Engl J Med 2012;366:819–26.
69. Gracey DR, Divertie MB, Howard FM. Mechanical ventilation for respiratory failure in myasthenia gravis. Two year experience with 22 patients. Mayo Clin Proc. 1983;58:597–602.
70. Guillain G. Radiculoneuritis with acellular hyperalbuminosis of the cerebrospinal fluid. Arch Neurol Psychiatry. 1936;36:975–90.
71. Guillain G. Considerations sur le syndrome de Guillain et Barré. Ann Med. 1953;54:81–149.
72. Haig AJ, Katz RT, Sahgal V. Mortality and complications of the locked-in syndrome. Arch Phys Med Rehabil. 1987;68:24–7.
73. Hanid MA, Davis M, Mellon PJ, et al. Clinical monitoring of intracranial pressure in fulminant hepatic failure. Gut. 1980;21:866–9.
74. Hardesty RL, Griffith BP, Debaski RF, Bahnson HT. Experience with cyclosporin in cardiac transplantation. Transplant Proc. 1983;15:2553–8.
75. Hawkes CH. "Locked-in" syndrome: report of seven cases. BMJ. 1974;4:379–82.
76. Hawkes CH, Bryan-Smyth L. The electroencephalogram in the locked in syndrome. Neurology. 1974;24: 1015–8.
77. Haymaker W, Kernohan JW. The Landry-Guillain-Barré syndrome. A clinicopathologic report of fifty fatal cases and a critique of the literature. Medicine. 1949;28:59–141.
78. Hermans G, De Jonghe B, Bruyninckx F, et al. Interventions for preventing critical illness polyneuropathy and critical illness myopathy. Cochrane Database Syst Rev. 2009;1:CD006832.
79. Hirsh LF. Delayed traumatic intracerebral hematomas after surgical decompression. Neurosurgery. 1979;5: 653–5.
80. Hochberg FH, Fisher CM, Robertson GH. Subarachnoid hemorrhage caused by rupture of a small superficial artery. Neurology. 1974;24:319–21.
81. Holzer M. Targeted temperature management for comatose survivors of cardiac arrest. N Engl J Med. 2010;363:1256–64.
82. Hooks MA. Tacrolimus, a new immunosuppressant: a review of the literature. Ann Pharmacother. 1994; 28:501–11.
83. Horowitz SH. The idiopathic polyradiculoneuropathies: a historical guide to an understanding of the clinical syndromes. Acta Neurol Scand. 1989;80:369–86.
84. Hund EF, Fogel W, Krieger D, et al. Critical illness polyneuropathy: clinical findings and outcomes of a frequent cause of neuromuscular weaning failure. Crit Care Med. 1996;24:1328–33.
85. Huneidi AH, Afshar F. Delayed intracerebral hematomas in moderate to severe head injuries in young adults. Ann R Coll Surg Engl. 1992;74:345–9.
86. Hyland HH. Thrombosis of the basilar artery. Arch Neurol Psychiatry. 1933;30:342–56.
87. Jefferson G. Extrasellar extensions of pituitary adenoma. Proc R Soc Med. 1940;33:433–58.
88. Jennett B. The Vegetative State. Medical facts, ethical and legal dilemmas. Cambridge: Cambridge University Press; 2002.
89. Jennett B. Thirty years of the vegetative state: clinical, ethical and legal problems. Prog Brain Res. 2005;150:537–43.
90. Jolly F. Pseudoparalysis myasthenica. Neurol Centralbl. 1895;14:34.
91. Kaufman HH, Moake JL, Olson JD, et al. Delayed and recurrent intracranial hematomas related to disseminated intravascular clotting and fibrinolysis in head injury. Neurosurgery. 1980;7:445–9.
92. Keesey JC. Contemporary opinions about Mary Walker, a shy pioneer of therapeutic neurology. Neurology. 1998;51:1433–9.
93. Keesey JC. "Crisis" in myasthenia gravis: an historical perspective. Muscle Nerve. 2002;26:1–3.
94. Khan S, Khan N, Masood S, et al. Evolution of traumatic intracerebral hemorrhage captured with CT imaging: report of a case and the role of serial CT scans. Emerg Radiol. 2010;17:493–6.
95. Kitano Y, Kuwabara S, Misawa S, et al. The acute effects of glycemic control on axonalexcitability in human diabetics. Ann Neurol. 2004;56:462–7.
96. Kompagne EJ, Walgaard C, de Groot YJ, et al. Historical sources of basilar artery occlusion. Neurology. 2011;76:1520–3.
97. Krings T, Noelchen D, Mull M. A hyperdense posterior cerebral artery sign. Stroke. 2006;37:399–403.
98. Landry O. Note sur la paralysie ascendante aigué. Gaz Hebd Méd. 1859;6:472–4.
99. Laureno R. Raymond Adams: a life of mind and muscle. New York: Oxford University Press; 2009.
100. Laureys S, Celesia GG, Cohadon F, et al. Unresponsive wakefulness syndrome: a new name for the vegetative state or apallic syndrome. BMC Med. 2010;8:68.
101. Le TV, Rumbak MJ, Liu SS, et al. van Loveren H, Agazzi S. Insertion of intracranial pressure monitors in fulminant hepatic failure patients: early experience using recombinant factor VII. Neurosurgery. 2010;66:455–8.

102. Leijten FS, Harinck-de-Weerd JR, Poortvliet DC, de Weerd AW. The role of polyneuropathy in motor convalescence after prolonged mechanical ventilation. JAMA. 1995;274:1221–5.
103. Levine S. Anoxic-ischemic encephalopathy in rats. Am J Pathol. 1960;36:1–17.
104. Levy A. Pituitary disease: presentation, diagnosis, and management. J Neurol Neurosurg Psychiatry. 2004;75 Suppl 3:iii 45–7.
105. Levy D, Bates D, Caronna J, et al. Prognosis in nontraumatic coma. Ann Intern Med. 1981;94: 293–301.
106. Lidofsky SD, Bass NM, Prager MC, Washington DE, Read AE, Wright TL, et al. Intracranial pressure monitoring and liver transplantation for fulminant hepatic failure. Hepatology. 1992;16:1–7.
107. Lofstedt S, von Reis G. Intracranial lesions with abolished passage of x-ray contrast throughout the internal carotid arteries. PACE. 1956;8:99–202.
108. Luauté J, Maucort-Boulch D, Tell L, et al. Long-term outcomes of chronic minimally conscious and vegetative states. Neurology. 2010;75:246–52.
109. Maramattom BV, Wijdicks EFM. Acute neuromuscular weakness in the intensive care unit. Crit Care Med. 2006;34:2835–41.
110. Marie P, Chatelin C. Note sur un syndrome de paralysie flasque plus ou moins généralisée avec abolition des reflexes, hyperalbuminose massive et xanthochromie du liquide céphalorachidien, évoluant spontanément vers la guérison et de nature indéterminée. Rev Neurol (Paris). 1916;23:564–5.
111. McKhann GM, Cornblath DR, Ho T, et al. Clinical and electrophysiological aspects of acute paralytic disease of children and young adults in North China. Lancet. 1991;338:593–7.
112. Merritt HH, Feremont-Smith M. The cerebrospinal fluid. Philadelphia: WB Saunders; 1937.
113. Miyai K, Ruebner BH. Acute yellow atrophy, cirrhosis and hepatoma. Arch Pathol. 1963;75:609–17.
114. Mohandas A, Chou SN. Brain death-a clinical and pathologic study. J Neurosurg. 1971;35:211–8.
115. Mollison WM. Case of heart failure during an operation for the removal of tonsils and adenoids; heart massage through an abdominal incision; recovery. Proc R Soc Med. 1917;10:1–7.
116. Monti MM, Vanhaudenhuyse A, Coleman MR, et al. Willful modulation of brain activity in disorders of consciousness. N Engl J Med. 2010;362:579–89.
117. Morrison L. Histopathologic effect of anoxia on the central nervous system. Arch Neurol Psychiatry. 1946;55:1–34.
118. Multi-Society Task Force on PVS. Medical aspects of the persistent vegetative state: second of two parts. N Engl J Med. 1994;330:1572–9.
119. Murphy N, Auzinger G, Bernel W, et al. The effect of hypertonic sodium chloride on intracranial pressure in patients with acute liver failure. Hepatology. 2004;39:464–70.
120. Nakase-Richardson R, Yablon SA, Sherer M, et al. Emergence from minimally conscious state. Neurology. 2009;73:1120–6.
121. Negovsky V. The second step in resuscitation-the treatment of the 'post-resuscitation' disease. Resuscitation. 1972;1:1–7.
122. Nichoji T, Uemura K, Shimoyama I, et al. Traumatic intracerebral hematomas of delayed onset. Acta Neurochir (Wien). 1984;71:69–90.
123. O'Grady JG, Schlam SW, Williams R. Acute liver failure: redefining the syndromes. Lancet. 1993;342: 73–275.
124. Oertel M, Kelly DF, McArthur D, et al. Progressive hemorrhage after head trauma: predictors and consequences of the evolving injury. J Neurosurg. 2002;96:109–16.
125. Ohry A. The locked-in syndrome and related states. Paraplegia. 1990;28:73–5.
126. Oksenberg A, Soroker N, Solzi P, et al. Polysomnography in locked-in syndrome. Electroencephalogr Clin Neurophysiol. 1991;78:314–7.
127. Oosterhuis HJ. The natural course of myasthenia gravis: a long term follow up study. J Neurol Neurosurg Psychiatry. 1989;52:1121–7.
128. Op de Coul AA, Lambregts PC, Koeman J, et al. Neuromuscular complications in patients given pavulon (pancuronium bromide) during artificial ventilation. Clin Neurol Neurosurg. 1985;87: 17–22.
129. Osserman KE. Myasthenia gravis. New York: Grune & Stratton; 1958.
130. Osserman KE, Genkins G. Studies in myasthenia gravis: reduction in mortality rate after crisis. JAMA. 1963;183:97–101.
131. Osserman KE, Kornfeld P, Cohen E, et al. Studies in myasthenia gravis; review of two hundred eighty-two cases at the mount Sinai hospital, New York city. AMA Arch Intern Med. 1958;102:72–81.
132. Pallis C. Diagnosis of brain death. Br Med J. 1980;281:1491–2.
133. Pallis C. The ABC of brainstem death. London: British Medical Journal Publishing Group; 1983.
134. Pallis C. Brainstem death. In: Braakman R, ed. Handbook of Clinical Neurology, Head Injury. Revised series, vol. 57. Amsterdam: Elsevier; 1990.
135. Patterson JR, Grabois M. Locked-in syndrome: a review of 139 cases. Stroke. 1986;17:758–64.
136. Payne WS. Postoperative respiratory care after transsternal thymectomy in myasthenia gravis: a 3-year experience in 53 patients. Chest. 1984;86: 67–71.
137. Pearce JM. The locked in syndrome. BMJ. 1987;294: 197–9.
138. Pearce JMS. Fragments of neurological history. London: Imperial College Press; 2003.
139. Perlo VP, Poskanzer DC, Schwab RS, et al. Myasthenia gravis: evaluation of treatment in 1,355 patients. Neurology. 1966;16:431–9.
140. Pinching AJ, Peters DK, Davis JN. Remission of myasthenia gravis following plasma exchange. Lancet. 1976;2:1373–6.
141. Pines L, Gilinsky E. Thrombosis of the basilar artery and the vascularization of the pons. Arch Psychiatry. 1932;97:380–7.

142. Plum F, Posner J. The diagnosis of stupor and coma. 3rd ed. Philadelphia: FA Davis Company; 1980.
143. Record CO, Chase KA, Hughes RO, et al. Glycerol therapy for cerebral edema complicating fulminant hepatic failure. BMJ. 1975;2:540.
144. Reilly PL, Graham DI, Adams JH,et al. Patients with head injury who talk and die. Lancet. 1975;2:375–7.
145. Rider JA, Pickett WH, Harrison AW. Myasthenia gravis: report of case receiving unusual dosage of neostigmine. Ann Intern Med. 1951;35:463–8.
146. Rinkel GJE. Perimesencephalic nonaneurysmal hemorrhage [thesis]. Utrecht: University of Utrecht; 1991.
147. Rinkel GJE, Wijdicks EFM, Hasan D, et al. Outcome in patients with subarachnoid hemorrhage on computed tomography. Lancet. 1991;338:964–8.
148. Rinkel GJE, Wijdicks EFM, Vermeulen M, et al. The clinical course of perimesencephalic nonaneurysmal subarachnoid hemorrhage. Ann Neurol. 1991;29: 463–8.
149. Rinkel GJE, Wijdicks EFM, Vermeulen M, et al. Nonaneurysmal perimesencephalic subarachnoid hemorrhage: CT and MR patterns that differ from aneurysmal rupture. AJNR. 1991;12:829–34.
150. Rockswold GL, Leonard PR, Nagib MG. Analysis of management in thirty-three closed head injury patients who "talked and deteriorated". Neurosurgery. 1987;21:51–5.
151. Rodgers JB, Mallory GK, Davidson CS. Massive liver cell necrosis: a retrospective study. Arch Intern Med. 1964;114:637–45.
152. Roelofs RI, Cerra F, Bielka N, Rosenberg L, Delaney J. Prolonged respiratory insufficiency due to acute motor neuropathy: a new syndrome? Neurology. 1983;33:240.
153. Rolando N, Wade J, Davalos M, et al. The systemic inflammatory response syndrome in acute liver failure. Hepatology. 2000;32:734–9.
154. Ronnov-Jensen V. The death of Porthos, or the first description of vertebrobasilar insufficiency in fiction. BMJ. 1988;297:1658.
155. Ropper AH. Unusual clinical variants and signs in Guillain-Barré syndrome. Arch Neurol. 1986; 43:1150–2.
156. Rose C, Michalak A, Pannuzio M, et al. Mild hypothermia delays the onset of coma and prevents brain edema and extracellular brain glutamate accumulation in rats with acute liver failure. Hepatology. 2000;31:872–7.
157. Rottenberg DA, Hochberg FH. Neurologic Classics in Modern Translation. New York: Hafner Press; 1977. p. 309–10, translated by Hochberg by permission of the McMillan Publishing.
158. Safar P. Community-wide cardiopulmonary resuscitation. J Iowa Med Soc. 1964;54:629–35.
159. Safar P, Behringer W, Böttiger BW, et al. Cerebral resuscitation potentials for cardiac arrest. Crit Care Med. 2002;30(4 Suppl):S140–4.
160. Safar PJ, Kochanek PM. Therapeutic hypothermia after cardiac arrest. N Engl J Med. 2002;346:612–3.
161. Salmon JH. *H. influenzae* meningitis: associated ventriculitis. N Engl J Med. 1972;287:1203–4.
162. Salmon JH. Ventriculitis complicating meningitis. Am J Dis Child. 1972;124:35–40.
163. Schievink WI, Wijdicks EFM. Origin of pretruncal nonaneurysmal subarachnoid hemorrhage: ruptured vein, perforating artery, or intramural hematoma? Mayo Clin Proc. 2000;75:1169–73.
164. Schiff ND, Giacino JT, Fins JJ. Deep brain stimulation, neuroethics, and the minimally conscious state: moving beyond proof of principle. Arch Neurol. 2009;66:697–702.
165. Schiff ND, Giacino JT, Kalmar K, et al. Behavioral improvements with thalamic stimulation after severe traumatic brain injury. Nature. 2007;448:600–3.
166. Schiff ND, Rodriguez-Moreno D, Kamal A, et al. FMRI reveals large-scale network activation in minimally conscious patients. Neurology. 2005;64:514–23.
167. Scholz W. Selective neuronal necrosis and its topistic patterns in hypoxemia and oligemia. J Neuropathol Exp Neurol. 1953;12:249–61.
168. Schwab RS, Potts F, Mathis P. EEG as an aid in determining death in the presence of cardiac activity. Electroencephalogr Clin Neurophysiol. 1963;15:147.
169. Scott M, Lennon HC. Decerebrate tonic extensor convulsions as a sign of the basilar artery: report of a case with autopsy. Arch Neurol Psychiatry. 1940;44: 1102–8.
170. Seneviratne J, Mandrekar J, Wijdicks EFM, et al. Predictors of extubation failure in myasthenic crisis. Arch Neurol. 2008;65:929–33.
171. Shafey S, Scheinblum A, Schienberg P. The ventral Pontine syndrome. Trans Am Neurol Assoc. 1968; 93:21–4.
172. Snyder B, Ramirez-Lassepas M, Lippert D. Neurological status and prognosis after cardiopulmonary arrest. Neurology. 1977;27:807–11.
173. Soloniuk D, Pitts LH, Lovely M, et al. Traumatic intracerebral hematomas: timing of appearance and indications for operative removal. J Trauma. 1986; 26:787–94.
174. Stein SC, Spettell C, Young G, et al. Delayed and progressive brain injury in closed-head trauma: radiological demonstration. Neurosurgery. 1993;32:25–31.
175. Stone CT, Rider JA. Treatment of myasthenia gravis. JAMA. 1949;141:107–11.
176. Stravitz RT, Lee WM, Kramer AH, et al. Therapeutic hypothermia for acute liver failure: toward a randomized, controlled trial in patients with advanced hepatic encephalopathy. Neurocrit Care. 2008; 9:90–6.
177. Sulkava R, Kovanen J. Locked-in syndrome with rapid recovery: a manifestation of basilar artery migraine? Headache. 1983;23:238–9.
178. Täuber MG, Sande MA. Landmark perspective: the impact of penicillin on the treatment of meningitis. JAMA. 1984;251:1877–80.
179. Tether JE. Management of myasthenic and cholinergic crises. Am J Med. 1955;19:740–2.

180. Thadani VM, Rimm DL, Urquhart L, et al. "Locked-in syndrome" for 27 years following a viral illness: clinical and pathologic findings. Neurology. 1991;41: 498–500.
181. Thomas CE, Mayer SA, Gungor Y, et al. Myasthenic crisis: clinical features, mortality, complications, and risk factors for prolonged intubation. Neurology. 1997;48:1253–60.
182. Tyler KL. A history of bacterial meningitis, Chapter 28. In: Handbook of Clinical Neurology. 3rd ed., vol. 94, History of neurology. 2010. Elsevier Publishing.
183. van de Beek D, de Gans J, Tunkel AR, et al. Community-acquired bacterial meningitis in adults. N Engl J Med. 2006;354:44–53.
184. Van Gijn J. Lijf en Leed, Geneeskunde voor iedereen. Amsterdam: Atlas; 2011.
185. Van Gijn J, van Dongen KJ. Computerized tomography in subarachnoid hemorrhage: difference between patients with and without aneurysms on angiography. Neurology. 1980;30:538–9.
186. Viets HR. Myasthenia gravis treated with large doses of neostigmine methylsulfate, intramuscularly and intravenously, and with neostigmine bromide orally. Am J Med Sci. 1944;208:701–8.
187. Viets HR. Myasthenia gravis. JAMA. 1945;127: 1089–96.
188. Viets HR. The emergency treatment of myasthenia gravis. Med Clin North Am. 1946;30:1035–41.
189. Voetsch B, DeWitt LD, Pessin MS, et al. Basilar artery occlusive disease in the New England medical center posterior circulation registry. Arch Neurol. 2004;61:496–504.
190. Voss HV, Uluç AM, Dyke JP, et al. Possible axonal regrowth in late recovery from the minimally conscious state. J Clin Invest. 2006;116:2005–11.
191. Wade DT. Ethical issues in diagnosis and management of patients in the permanent vegetative state. BMJ. 2001;322:352–4.
192. Waxman SG, Brill MH, Geshrind N, et al. Probability of conduction deficit as related to fiber length in random distribution models of peripheral neuropathy. J Neurol Sci. 1976;29:39–53.
193. Wertheimer P, Jouvet M, Descotes J. A propos due diagnostic de la mort du système nerveux dans les comas avec arrêt respiratoire traités par respiration artificielle. Presse Med. 1959;67:87–8.
194. White JB, Wijdicks EFM, Cloft HJ, et al. Vanishing aneurysm in pretruncal nonaneurysmal subarachnoid hemorrhage. Neurology. 2008;71:1375.
195. Wijdicks EFM. Neurotoxicity of immunosuppressive drugs. Liver Transpl. 2001;7:937–42.
196. Wijdicks EFM. The neurologist and Harvard criteria for brain death. Neurology. 2003;61:970–6.
197. Wijdicks EFM. Minimally conscious state vs persistent vegetative state: the case of terry (Wallis) vs the case of Terri (Schiavo). Mayo Clin Proc. 2006; 81:1155–8.
198. Wijdicks EFM. The comatose patient. New York: Oxford University Press; 2008.
199. Wijdicks EFM, Litchy WJ, Harrison BA, Gracey DR. The clinical spectrum of critical illness polyneuropathy. Mayo Clin Proc. 1994;69:955–9.
200. Wijdicks EFM, Miller GM. Transient locked-in syndrome after uncal herniation. Neurology. 1999;52: 1296–7.
201. Wijdicks EFM, Schievink WI. Perimesencephalic nonaneurysmal subarachnoid hemorrhage: first hint of a cause? Neurology. 1997;49:634–6.
202. Wijdicks EFM, Schievink WI, Miller GM. Pretruncal nonaneurysmal subarachnoid hemorrhage. Mayo Clin Proc. 1998;73:745–52.
203. Wijdicks EFM, Varelas PN, Gronseth GS, et al. Evidence based guideline update: determining brain death in adults. Report of the quality standards subcommittee of the American Academy of Neurology. Neurology. 2010;74:1911–8.
204. Wijdicks EFM, Wiesner RH, Krom RAF. Neurotoxicity in liver transplant recipients with cyclosporin immunosuppression. Neurology. 1995;45:1962–4.
205. Willoughby J, Leach B. Relation of neurological findings after cardiac arrest to outcome. Br Med J. 1974;3:437–9.
206. Witt NJ, Zochodne DW, Bolton CF, et al. Peripheral nerve function in sepsis and multiple organ failure. Chest. 1991;99:176–84.
207. Yaquero J, Polson J, Chung C, et al. Infection and the progression of hepatic encephalopathy in acute liver failure. Gastroenterology. 2003;125:755–64.
208. Young HA, Gleeve JR, Schmidek HH, et al. Delayed traumatic intracerebral hematoma: report of 15 cases operatively treated. Neurosurgery. 1984;14:22–5.
209. Zochodne DW, Bolton CF, Wells GA, et al. Critical illness polyneuropathy: a complication of sepsis and multiple organ failure. Brain. 1987;110:819–41.

First Descriptions of Initial Management

5

E.F.M. Wijdicks, *Famous First Papers for the Neurointensivist*,
DOI 10.1007/978-1-4614-3182-4_5, © Springer Science+Business Media New York 2013

Short Historical Note 34

INCREASED INTRACRANIAL PRESSURE AND HYPERVENTILATION

The Title of the Paper

Gibbs FA, Gibbs EL, Lennox WG. Changes in human cerebral blood flow consequent on alterations in blood gases. Am J Physiol. 1935;111:557–63.

The Paper and the Times

For quite some time, physiologists felt that cerebral blood flow was entirely dependent on systemic arterial blood pressure and passively followed any fluctuation in pressure. Even distinguished physiologists such as Sherrington, Bayliss, and Hill were unconvinced that a specific vasomotor regulation existed that was controlled by cerebral vasomotor nerves.

However, earlier studies, most prominently by Forbes and Wolff in 1928, found in experiments with cats that brain circulation was not regulated from a distance but that arteries constricted after direct application of epinephrine or stimulation of the cervical sympathetic nerves. The experiments also showed dilatation following stimulation of the vagus nerve [18].

There also was interest in whether cerebral blood flow could be altered by changes in blood gases [35]. Animal experiments showed that cerebral blood flow was dependent on carbon dioxide (CO_2) or oxygen tension of blood and brain tissue and that cerebral blood flow could vary with the CO_2 tension of arterial blood. Gibbs and Lennox from the Neurologic Unit of Boston City Hospital, the Department of Neurology of Harvard Medical School and Laboratory of Physiology of Yale University School of Medicine did one of the first experiments in healthy volunteers [20] (Fig. 5.1).

The Details of the Paper

The experiment involved normal volunteers who agreed to have a fine stylet introduced into the jugular vein. The tip was heated by means of a constant electrical current to a temperature that was slightly higher than the blood. The assumption was that if blood flowed faster past the tip, the tip would be become cooler; if the blood flow slowed down, the tip would become warmer. Volunteers were asked to breathe deeply and exhale forcibly for several minutes. This resulted in a sudden and pronounced decrease in blood flow through the internal jugular vein. Additionally, the CO_2 content of the blood was increased from a tank containing a gas mixture of 10% CO_2 and 90% oxygen that resulted in a marked increase in cerebral blood flow. Systemic arterial blood pressure remained largely constant, which then would allow the experiment to demonstrate that cerebral blood vessels change in caliber due to changes in concentration of these parameters. Increase of blood CO_2 resulted in dilatation and decrease resulted in constriction of the arterioles of the brain. The effect of hyperventilation on a normal volunteer is shown in Fig. 5.2.

The authors concluded:

> We find that "blowing off" CO2 from the alveoli of the lungs and from the blood caused a decrease in cerebral blood flow, whereas breathing a high concentration of CO2 caused an increase. The interesting question arises concerning the mechanism responsible for these changes in flow. Alterations in systemic arterial blood pressure may play a part, but lack of any close correlation of blood flow and blood pressure curves requires another explanation. The explanation lies, we believe, in alterations in caliber of the cerebral blood vessels in response to changes in the concentration of the blood gases. Increase of the blood CO2 results in a dilatation and decrease results in a constriction of the arterioles of the brain.

The Message and Acceptance

These experiments were followed by studies of situations where there was documented increase in intracranial pressure (ICP). Most noticeable was Lundberg's paper that documented a reduction of increased ICP using hyperventilation [39] (Fig. 5.3). Lundberg's paper reported on 18 patients with mostly glioblastomas, in whom hyperventilation markedly reduced ICP. Lundberg's paper clearly defined the clinical practice of hyperventilation using the ventilator to manipulate blood CO_2. Changes in respiratory minute volume induced rapid change in ventricular fluid pressure in the opposite direction. Other observations were

CHANGES IN HUMAN CEREBRAL BLOOD FLOW CONSEQUENT ON ALTERATIONS IN BLOOD GASES[1]

F. A. GIBBS, E. L. GIBBS AND W. G. LENNOX

From the Neurological Unit of the Boston City Hospital, Boston, Massachusetts

Received for publication December 27, 1934

Although the cerebral circulation of man is of the utmost interest and importance, observations in this field have been fragmentary or indirect. The following procedures have been used: inspection of the vessels of the retina, or of the meninges at operation, measurements of changes in the pressure of the spinal fluid or of the arterial blood, and measurements of the alterations in the gases of blood drawn from an internal jugular vein. An instrument has recently been developed by one of us (1) which makes it possible to obtain a running record of the changes occurring in the flow of blood through an internal jugular vein of unanesthetized human subjects. By means of this device, we have completed observations of the cerebral blood flow in human subjects with respect to seizures (2), syncope (3) and sleep (4), the injection of ergotamine (5), and of various drugs known to influence circulation (6). In the present communication, we report the effect of changes in the composition of respired air.

Fig. 5.1 Title page

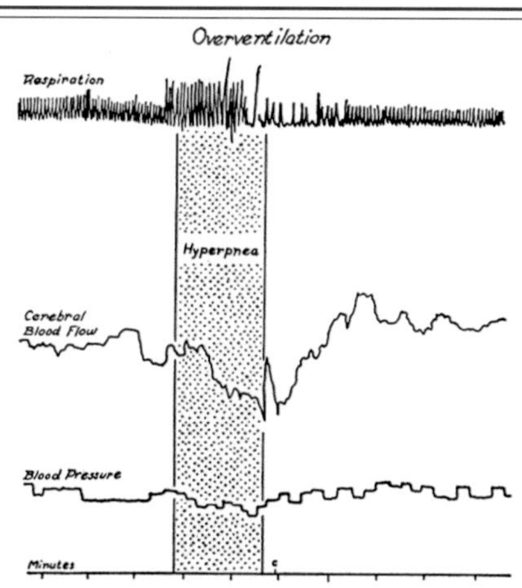

Fig. 1. Effect on cerebral blood flow of voluntary hyperpnea.

The tracings from above downward are: the respiratory movements; the blood flow through an internal jugular vein; the systolic blood pressure (taken by auscultatory method) and, at the bottom, the time recorded in minutes.

During the period marked overventilation, the subject breathed deeply and at an increased rate. At *C* he coughed.

Fig. 5.2 The effects of hyperventilation

made that showed that the flow of cerebrospinal fluid on open drainage was greater during spontaneous breathing than during hyperventilation.

Over the years, the induction of respiratory alkalosis through hyperventilation has remained a rapid and fairly reliable method for controlling ICP during neurosurgical procedures and in the intensive care unit. As a corollary, these findings also demonstrated that CO_2 retention could potentially result in increased ICP. More recently, evidence has been presented that hyperoxemia could further induce vasoconstriction in hyperventilated patients with traumatic brain injury [57].

Acute hyperventilation remains a very effective way of reducing ICP. The effects of hyperventilation on cerebral blood flow and ICP are not that significant after several hours and the prolonged use of hyperventilation has been criticized for its potential adverse effects [55]. In one prospective study, patients with severe traumatic brain injury (TBI) were randomized to prophylactic hyperventilation for 5 days with an average arterial PCO_2 of 25 mmHg or to management without hyperventilation with an average arterial PCO_2 goal of 35 mmHg. At 3 and 6 months, comatose patients in the hyperventilation group had significantly worse outcomes [48]. A recent study that monitored brain tissue oxygen found that even a small reduction in arterial PCO_2 caused a decrease in cerebral oxygenation in comatose patients with TBI, but found that there was minimal cerebral vessel reactivity to arterial PCO_2 changes several days from the insult. It appears that aggressive hyperventilation can cause cerebral blood flow to closely approach an ischemic threshold, and this may explain a potentially more harmful outcome [31].

The neurometabolic changes with acute hyperventilation in the setting of severe traumatic brain injuries have also been studied, but there are contradictory results and comparatively few patients have been reported [9, 13]. When measured, both brain tissue CO_2 and the jugular vein oxygenation are reduced with hyperventilation. Other studies have found that moderate hyperventilation may significantly increase accumulation of lactate.

REDUCTION OF INCREASED INTRACRANIAL PRESSURE BY HYPERVENTILATION

A THERAPEUTIC AID IN NEUROLOGICAL SURGERY

BY

NILS LUNDBERG, ÅKE KJÄLLQUIST
DEPARTMENT OF NEUROSURGERY II

AND CHUAN BIEN
DEPARTMENT OF PULMONARY DISEASES

UNIVERSITY HOSPITAL, LUND, SWEDEN

Fig. 5.3 Lundberg's monograph on hyperventilation

Short Historical Note 35

INCREASED INTRACRANIAL PRESSURE AND OSMOTIC AGENTS

The Title of the Paper

Faye T. Administration of hypertonic salt solution for relief of intracranial pressure. JAMA. 1923;80:1445–8.
Haden RL. Therapeutic applications of the alteration of brain volume. JAMA. 1919;73:983–4.

The Paper and the Times

Reducing the intracranial volume of the brain by extracting water was of paramount interest to neurosurgeons. Relief of increased intracranial pressure (ICP) in patients with a mass and headache and vomiting resulted in improvement of symptoms before surgery and also could reduce swelling seen during surgery.

Neurosurgeons Lewis Weed and Paul McKibben were among the first to study the effects of IV salt solutions on cerebrospinal fluid (CSF) pressure in cats in their Army Neurosurgery Laboratory at Johns Hopkins Medical School. They found that hypertonic solutions lowered the CSF pressure—and vice versa—hypotonic solutions increased CSF pressure [74]. These hypertonic solutions were 30% sodium chloride or saturated sodium bicarbonate. They compared its effect to Ringer's solution (NaCl 0.9%, KCL 0.04%, CaCl 0.025%) and to distilled water. In some cats, trephine openings were added to observe the changes after administration of a hypertonic or hypotonic solution—a shrunken or swollen brain. No changes were seen with Ringer's solution. The investigators could only conclude that changes in the osmotic value of blood were responsible for changes in brain tissue. The investigators surmised that CSF pressure reflected intracranial volume.

Cushing and Foley also tested 2% sodium chloride solution introduced into the duodenum or rectum of a cat. They could document significant reduction of CSF pressure [12]. They found little change in blood pressure and found no changes in pulse or respiration. Cushing and Foley, to use IV injection of 35% sodium chloride solution during neurosurgical procedures [12] and to use it in patients with brain tumor and "cerebral hernias" before a decompression operation. Using hypertonic saline by mouth could result in "occasionally striking results … in which case the tense convex protrusion became a soft concave area over the decompression site" [12].

The simple physics of salt and sugar were applied in the early 1920s, and many physicians became familiar with the fact that both concentrated salt and glucose solutions could create an osmotic effect that would draw water out of the brain [29, 64]. Hypotonic solutions would have the opposite effect, and isotonic solutions had no such effect.

The Details of the Paper

Faye initially used magnesium sulfate by rectum and demonstrated its usefulness—a marked decrease in ICP in 16 patients (Fig. 5.4). The authors used magnesium sulfate because they found that sodium chloride solution by mouth often was associated with vomiting and significant distress such as thirst and gastritis. Additionally, they reported a series of 15 patients undergoing surgery for brain tumor who were treated with IV hypertonic sodium chloride solution and found marked reduction of pressure using a variety of salt solutions varying from 15% to 35%. They also documented that the most marked dehydrating effects were seen in patients with hydrocephalus and recommended its use in exploratory craniotomies.

Haden used 25% concentrated glucose to increase the osmotic value in blood and cause a diuretic effect (Fig. 5.5):

> The one medical condition in which we are most interested in intracranial pressure is cerebrospinal meningitis. The marked increase in pressure in this disease is certainly one of its most serious aspects. There is an increase both in the amount of spinal fluid and in the direct volume of the brain. The increased pressure is often the factor determining the outcome of the disease [29].

THE ADMINISTRATION OF HYPERTONIC SALT SOLUTIONS FOR THE RELIEF OF INTRACRANIAL PRESSURE*

TEMPLE FAY, M.D.
PHILADELPHIA

The use of magnesium sulphate to assist in controlling intracranial tension was first introduced into this clinic a little more than two years ago. During this time, certain observations as to its effects and mode of administration have been recorded, and the conditions in which its use is beneficial will be noted. It was adopted by the neurosurgical service as a means of reducing intracranial pressure and volume, following my observation that infants showed a marked retraction of the fontanels after its use, because of the dehydration that it produces throughout the cerebral system.

At the time a method brought forward by Cushing and Foley[1] of the intravenous injection of 35 per cent. sodium chlorid solution was in use, but since that time this method has been replaced in the majority of cases by the easier and more satisfactory administration of magnesium sulphate solution, either by rectum or by mouth. The intravenous method of sodium chlorid administration is still found to be of great value in cases in which rapid reduction of intracranial pressure and volume is necessary on the operating table.

Magnesium sulphate has been found of decided value in the preoperative study of cases presenting intracranial pressure. The patients have been relieved of headache, vomiting, choke disk, medullary depression and coma. Their symptoms and responses could be more carefully observed when the intracranial tension was relieved, and they could be kept in comfort for several days previous to operation. Dangerous medullary symptoms may be relieved long enough to permit time for the proper localization of a lesion before an operation is undertaken (Chart 1). The use of magnesium sulphate as a routine measure before operation in cases of suspected intracranial tension has permitted exposure of the cortex otherwise unsafe in the presence of decided pressure.

In the postoperative treatment of the so-called medullary edema, magnesium sulphate had been found indispensable. Cases in which stupor supervenes following intracranial exploration, with marked fall in respiration and pulse, rapid dehydration will check the pressure on the basal centers and allow a return of the respiration and pulse to normal (Chart 2).

In cases of traumatic injuries to the brain in which fracture of the skull or concussion is associated with marked stupor, respiratory and cardiac depression due to intracranial pressure and "medullary edema," dehydration by magnesium sulphate is followed by marked relief of these symptoms (Chart 3).

Fig. 5.4 Title page

THERAPEUTIC APPLICATION OF THE ALTERATION OF BRAIN VOLUME

BY THE INTRAVENOUS INJECTION OF GLUCOSE

RUSSELL L. HADEN, M.D. (Detroit)
Lieutenant, M. C., U. S. Army
CAMP LEE, PETERSBURG, VA.

The brain and spinal cord lie within a space of fixed capacity formed by the closed cranium and the spinal canal. The pressure within the meninges is determined by two factors, the amount of cerebrospinal fluid present and the volume of the brain. The removal of spinal fluid by lumbar puncture is commonly employed in controlling intraspinal pressure in a large number of conditions. If there is a very marked increase in the bulk of the brain, however, the intraspinal pressure may still be high, even after the maximum amount of spinal fluid has been drained off. It is also true that the withdrawal, when the high pressure is due to the increased volume of the brain, may cause a herniation of the base of the brain through the foramen magnum, with resulting collapse and death.

The one medical condition in which we are most interested in intracranial pressure is cerebrospinal meningitis. The marked increase in pressure in this disease is certainly one of its most serious aspects. There is an increase both in the amount of spinal fluid and in the direct volume of the brain. The increased pressure is often the factor determining the outcome of the disease.

It has long been recognized that lumbar puncture and drainage of the spinal fluid cause, alone, a marked decrease in the mortality rate. This is unusually well shown in the recent report by Olitsky[1] of an epidemic in China in which only a small amount of immune serum was available for treatment. In 104 cases, in which no treatment of any kind was given, the mortality was 84.6 per cent.; in 346 cases in which lumbar puncture and drainage of the spinal fluid were the only treatment, only 54.1 per cent. of the patients died. The removal of bacteria and toxic material must certainly have had some effect, but it seems most probable that the greatest good was due to the necessary fall of intracranial pressure resulting from the withdrawal of spinal fluid.

The power to control the volume of the brain should be of the greatest help in the treatment of meningitis. The spinal fluid removed must be replaced, in part at least, by immune serum, thus nullifying the good effects of the reduced pressure resulting from the removal of the fluid. In those cases of meningitis in which patients develop block, either at the base of the brain or at some point along the spinal cord, they quickly show the effect of increased intracranial pressure, and we have had no way of decreasing the pressure except by occipito-atlantoid puncture.

Recently, some experiments have been reported by Weed and McKibben[2] which show that the bulk of the brain can be controlled by a change in the concentration of certain elements in the blood stream. These observers have shown that the intravenous injection of hypertonic solutions of certain electrolytes and

1. Olitsky, P. K.: Experiences with a Recent Epidemic of Meningococcic Meningitis Among a Chinese Civil Population, Arch. Int. Med. **23**: 380 (March) 1919.
2. Weed, L. H., and McKibben, P. S.: Am. J. Physiol. **48**: 512 (May) 1919.

Fig. 5.5 Title page

The patient was a 21-year-old man with "epidemic cerebrospinal meningitis." When he deteriorated and became comatose, a marked improvement was noted after 200 mL of 25% IV glucose solution and even more the next day when an additional dose of 550 mL was administered. Another case of "pulmonary consolidation, high fever and stupor" was described as "measles toxemia with cerebral edema," but without much details other than a marked improvement in responsiveness. Haden suggested to use the glucose infusion slowly—1 h—and to repeat it in 12 h.

The Message and Acceptance

At the time, salt solutions were commonly used in operative settings. Morrissey—after Fay's example—published several cases of improvement of CSF pressure using oral magnesium sulfate crystals dissolved in water but was not impressed by its pressure-lowering effect. Morrisey confirmed in his experiments that IV hypertonic saline was quite effective [46].

However, in the 1960s, urea and glycerol were on the radar [8, 32, 80]. Glycerol increased plasma concentration, and therefore its effect would be to draw liquids from the tissues. Glycerol was found to promote diuresis, but it became apparent that the drug effects in nephrectomized animals did not differ from those in animals with normal kidney junction.

Cantore and associates from the Neurological Institute of Rome University in Italy reported on animal experiments and patients and successfully used oral glycerol for the reduction of ICP [10]. Few clinical patient data were provided, but in the scheme of things, it became just another important observation that would push the use of glycerol in neurosurgical practices. Oral glycerol lacked the toxic effects of intravenously applied glycerol.

And so, the salt versus sugar dilemma started. Mannitol replaced glycerol and hypertonic saline eventually may replace mannitol [14, 67, 73, 77]. Mannitol continues to be the first line of treatment and is most favored because of ease of use—rapid administration without the need of central access—and a substantial clinical experience. There is an unsubstantialed concern that excessive administration of mannitol may be harmful as a result of accumulation in brain parenchyma and potentially worsening edema due to reverse osmotic shift.

Hypertonic saline is now more commonly used for treatment of increased ICP [45, 53]. The osmolality of hypertonic saline in the higher concentrations is several folds higher than mannitol and therefore may draw more water. Hypertonic solutions shift fluid from the intracellular space to the extracellular space, and there is little intravascular expansion. Prospective comparisons between hypertonic solutions may be helpful. Concerns about adverse effects are real and involve volume overload, phlebitis at the infusion site, and hyperchloremic acidosis [53].

Short Historical Note 36

CARE OF THE COMATOSE PATIENT

The Title of the Paper

Eckenhoff JE. The care of the unconscious patient. JAMA. 1963;186:541–3.

The Paper and the Times

Treatment of coma—as it is now—was disease specific and took quite some time to evolve. Most physicians understood the need to treat increased intracranial pressure (ICP) after trauma. Around the turn of the century, physicians confronted with coma after traumatic brain injury would consider trepanation to prevent "mortal danger." Marburg—a neurologist from Vienna—mentioned that the two most important issues to consider in comatose patients were increased intracranial pressure and regulation of circulation and respiration. Drugs to be used in hypotension included atropine, strychnine, ergotin, ephedrine, and caffeine [41].

In the second half of the twentieth century, publications were still mostly concerned with management of specific systemic disorders causing coma, often diabetes [16, 37]. Specific treatment of diabetic, hepatic, and thyrotoxic coma or other endocrine crisis dominated the literature [34, 59, 66].

In the neurologic literature and textbooks, very little was written on care of the comatose patient. Depending on the severity of coma, these patients were mostly under the care of anesthesiologists or internists. Neurologists would consult and assess the cause and chances of recovery. Before neurologists Fred Plum and Jerry Posner would write their original textbook on the diagnosis of coma and stupor—as the title implied with less focus on care—other specialists authored papers on management. One paper concerned itself with the nursing care of the comatose patient, but a systematic approach to the comatose patient was only briefly mentioned in textbooks without sufficient attention to detail. Some review articles mentioned use of oxygen, water depletion, and nursing position [3, 43, 44, 58, 47, 78]. Care at the time was mostly directed toward general patient care and avoidance of hypotension and hypoxemia—the precursors of the ABC of resuscitation.

The Details of the Paper

Anesthesiologist Eckenhoff published one of the first comprehensive papers on care of the comatose patient in 1963 (Fig. 5.6). This review was read before the section on Nervous and Mental Diseases during the 112th annual meeting of the American Medical Association. The major theme was induced hypothermia, airway, and pulmonary care. Eckenhoff emphasized the disappearance of normal respiratory protective mechanisms in coma. "In sleeping man, the protective respiratory reflexes are active. Olfactory nerves warn of offending odors and tracheal reflexes react to the presence of foreign material. Respiratory cilia beat secretions toward the bronchi and trachea whence their presence precipitates coughing."… "It is only when alcohol, drugs or disease block the reception of the danger signals…." The paper discussed airway management (lateral position placement, endotracheal tube, or tracheotomy) and adequate oxygenation, but also warned for a rise in arterial carbon dioxide. Eckenhoff remarked:

> It is probably wise to increase the inspired O2 content of all comatose patients, but the need for supplemental oxygen can only be determined accurately by analysis of the arterial blood. If the PO2 is below 90 mm Hg assuming a normal hemoglobin content, then the concentration of inhaled oxygen should be increased. A properly placed nasopharyngeal catheter with oxygen flowing at six liters per minute will increase inspired oxygen concentration to 35%. The highest oxygen concentration likely with an oxygen tent is 50% with careful application. Oxygen hoods or masks offer higher concentrations, but these are seldom needed.

Comments were made on the tracheostomy timing ("there should be no urgency in doing this procedure") and benefits due to reducing respiratory dead space and increasing alveoli ventilation, easy removal of respiratory secretions, and improved mechanical ventilation. The review mentioned a diminished sympathetic tone and predisposition to severe hypotension while turning the patient.

The Care of the Unconscious Patient

James E. Eckenhoff, MD, Philadelphia

The patient who is unconscious from cerebral catastrophe must depend upon others to detect or anticipate his needs and to institute the appropriate measures to assure his recovery if the pathological insult can be overcome. Adequate pulmonary ventilation must be provided by verification of the minute volume of respiration, by respiratory assistance if required, by tracheostomy if indicated, and by periodic analysis of arterial blood for pO_2, pCO_2, and pH. The latter method is the most reliable index since an increased physiological dead space may vitiate a seemingly sufficient respiratory exchange. Arterial blood gas analysis will also reveal hypercarbia which can exist without concomitant cyanosis, and enhance coma. Tracheostomy will reduce respiratory dead space and facilitate removal of respiratory tract secretions; however the respiratory tract usually becomes infected due to poor aseptic technique. Hypothermia to 86 to 88 F (30.0 to 31.1 C) may increase survival from strokes.

THE POSSIBILITIES of complete recovery of patients who have been unconscious from trauma or cerebral catastrophe for long periods of time have improved greatly in the last decade. This was sharply emphasized recently in an interview with a young college student who had suffered critical brain damage in an automobile accident, whose body temperature had been lowered to 88 F (31.1 C) for a week, who did not recover consciousness for three additional weeks, yet who had returned to his college studies and was doing well five months later. While not previously unknown, such recoveries are becoming commonplace. They are only possible with medical attendants who are aware of the body's normal protective mechanisms and have knowledge of how to substitute for them during unconsciousness.

Normal Protective Mechanisms

First let us consider the protective mechanisms of the body during normal sleep, since this most closely approximates the unconscious state. Few persons, if any, remain motionless during sleep, the majority changing their body position often. The purpose of this is probably twofold: (1) for the benefit of circulation, to prevent pooling of blood in dependent portions of the body; and (2) for the benefit of respiration, to counteract the tendency for patchy areas of pulmonary atelectasis to develop. By changing position, one improves muscle tone temporarily, thereby facilitating blood flow. The splinting of chest muscles that occurs with turning is always followed by a deep inspiration which opens up alveolae. Sighing serves similar purposes when one is awake. Recent evidence suggests that the anesthetist should artificially sigh for his patient during general anesthesia.[1]

An additional protection to assure adequacy of ventilation during sleep is the prevention of respiratory obstruction. Few people sleep on their backs for more than short periods. In this position the lower jaw relaxes, the tongue falls against the posterior pharyngeal wall, partial obstruction of the airway occurs, and snoring results. Occasionally a snorer will evince complete airway obstruction, but the normal person never succumbs to this because his pCO_2 rises to stimulate the respiratory center, his pO_2 falls to stimulate his chemoreceptors, and he "fights through" the obstruction usually followed by a change of body position. It should be obvious that the safest body position for preserving the airway is the lateral position.

In sleeping man, the protective respiratory reflexes are active. Olfactory nerves warn of offending odors and tracheal reflexes react to the presence of foreign material. Respiratory cilia beat secretions toward the bronchi and trachea whence their presence precipitates coughing. However, cilia only work well in proper conditions of moisture.

Finally, the brain of the sleeping individual can receive and interpret peripheral stimuli. Pain or discomfort break through his somnolence, awaken him, and cause him to change to a more comfortable position. It is only when alcohol, drugs, or disease block the reception of the danger signals that nerve palsies or pressure necrosis occurs.

Pulmonary Ventilation

The unconscious patient will have lost most if not all his normal protective devices. He must depend upon others to detect or anticipate his needs and to institute appropriate measures to assure his recovery if he himself can survive the immediate accidental or pathological insult. Unfortunately, often attendants of the unconscious fail in their responsibility so that reparative processes of the individual are futile.

The most important task in caring for the un-

From the Department of Anesthesia, University of Pennsylvania Schools of Medicine.

Read before the Section on Nervous and Mental Diseases during the Symposium on Strokes at the 112th Annual Meeting of the American Medical Association, Atlantic City, NJ, June 19, 1963.

Fig. 5.6 Title page

A specific note was made of temperature management:

> Brain damage after trauma can be minimized by lowering body temperature to 86 to 88 F (30.0 to 31.1 degrees of Celsius) for several days after the injury. While this is now a common technique in the treatment of trauma and cerebral aneurysm, it is only beginning to receive trial in the treatment of stroke per se. Theoretically, it could be of value and deserves further exploration.

Accumulation of carbon dioxide and its consequences—increase in cerebrospinal fluid pressure and increase in catecholamines—resulting in peripheral vasostriction, hypertension, increase in brain volume, and cerebral edema was also mentioned.

The Message and Acceptance

Another major work appeared as a chapter and involved more specifics. Rosomoff and Safar's chapter clearly spells out most of the concerns and elaborates on management of fever and the benefits of cooling [63]. Most attention was directed to airway and pulmonary care, but recommendations on fluid management included use of 5% in Ringer's solution or 5% glucose in 0.2% saline in patients with increased ICP. However, Rosomoff and Safar warned that IV solution without solutes could increase ICP and suggested approximately 2,500 mL of fluids.

In a remarkable statement on generalized convulsions and antiepileptic drugs, the author warned against the use of phenobarbital, and other convulsants as acute management interventions. "Suppression of the cortical electrical hyperactivity does not seem to be essential for emergency management, so long as the respiratory manifestations are controlled."

The paper was influential in further elaborating on the treatment of hypothermia. Cooling was achieved with wrapping patients in a cooling mattress and using a "shivering cocktail" (meperidine, promethazine, and phenobarbital).

Why it took so long to organize and teach the management of comatose patients remains unclear. A simple, although inadequate, answer is that neurology was a more a "diagnostic specialty". Care of the comatose patient became more standardized only in the third edition of Plum and Posner's text on the diagnosis of stupor and coma. They suggested that the treatment should involve the following steps: adequate oxygenation, maintenance of circulation, glucose administration if strong suspicion of hypoglycemia, reduction of ICP, treatment of seizures, treatment of any infection, correction of acid–base balance, normalization of body temperature, administration of thiamine, consideration of antidotes, control of agitation, and protection of the eyes.

Short Historical Note 37

MECHANICAL VENTILATION IN NEUROLOGIC DISEASE

The Title of the Paper

Lassen HC. A preliminary report on the 1952 epidemic of poliomyelitis in Copenhagen with special reference to the treatment of acute respiratory insufficiency. Lancet. 1953;1:37–41.

The Paper and the Times

The history of ventilation goes back many centuries with experiments by Galen, Paracelsus, Vesalius, and Harvey. According to Westhorpe and Ball, the first description of airway management was by Arab physician Ibn Sina, also known as Canon of Medicine, and was published in the first half of the eleventh century [75]. "When necessary a cannula of gold or silver or other suitable material is advanced down the throat to support inspiration" [15].

Interestingly, modern mechanical ventilation started with a devastating neurologic disease. Mechanical ventilation has its origins in the early 1800s with negative pressure ventilation and tank respirators. The Drinker–Shaw and the Emerson "iron lungs" are best known. Poliomyelitis was very much on Philip Drinker's mind when he worked on his device:

> A number of patients have come under our observation who have shown intercostal paralysis and considerable weakness of the diaphragm early in the paralytic stage of anterior poliomyelitis; yet the accessory muscles and the diaphragm have been able to support sufficient respiratory movements to keep the patient alive until, in the course of a few days, the paralyzed intercostal muscles began to improve and the patient went on to almost complete recovery [15].

He would invent a machine that incorporated electrically driven blowers and create inspiration with negative pressures and expiration with positive pressures. Within the chamber—sealing the patient at the neck—a negative pressure caused the abdomen and thorax to expand with air flowing in. A cycle was produced by returning to atmospheric pressure or after some positive pressure recoil of the chest and abdomen occurred. Although they maintained support in patients in an often decrepitude state—and many could be liberated from the device—the long term problems with these monstrous devices were well known and included technical difficulties and inability to secure the airway.

In the 1950s, these negative pressure ventilators were the only available ventilators and its dramatic shortage during the zenith of the polio epidemic necessitated other ways of ventilatory support. Positive pressure ventilation (PPV) and tracheostomy became commonplace after the poliomyelitis epidemics.

The most notorious epidemic was in 1952 in Copenhagen [2, 75]. Between July and December, the Blegdam Hospital received 2,722 patients with poliomyelitis; 316 had respiratory insufficiency of varying degree. Most medical historians consider this event and the emergence of respiratory care units soon thereafter the beginnings of critical care (Chapter 2).

The Details of the Paper

The paper vividly describes that the hospital was overwhelmed with only one iron lung and six cuirass respirators available (Fig. 5.7). Lassen said the hospital was in "a state of war." The report describes the use of tracheostomy and manual ventilation, and with this approach the care of patients became much more organized. The new approach included early tracheostomy just below the larynx, suctioning and bronchoscopy via the tracheostomy, aggressive postural drainage, and PPV via a cuffed tube. A tracheostomy was performed with excision of a square opening in the anterior wall of trachea, and the widest possible rubber tube with inflatable cuff was inserted. Repeat suction of the trachea and postural drainage and bag ventilation with insufflation of a mixture of 50% oxygen and 50% nitrogen was next.

This equipment was used in over 150 patients, but initial mortality rates remained high, reaching 80%. Of 55 men treated with tracheostomy and bag ventilation, 31 died; of 43 women, 17 died; and of 74 children, 29 died.

THE LANCET] [JAN. 3, 1953 37

Special Articles

A PRELIMINARY REPORT ON THE 1952 EPIDEMIC OF POLIOMYELITIS IN COPENHAGEN WITH SPECIAL REFERENCE TO THE TREATMENT OF ACUTE RESPIRATORY INSUFFICIENCY

H. C. A. LASSEN
M.D. Copenhagen
PROFESSOR OF EPIDEMIOLOGY IN THE UNIVERSITY OF COPENHAGEN; CHIEF PHYSICIAN, DEPARTMENT FOR COMMUNICABLE DISEASES, BLEGDAM HOSPITAL, COPENHAGEN

THE 1952 epidemic of poliomyelitis in Greater Copenhagen has been the largest and most severe local epidemic ever recorded in Denmark.

ADMISSIONS

The metropolitan area of Copenhagen has a population of 1,200,000 people served by a single hospital for communicable diseases, the Blegdam Hospital. Between July 24 and Dec. 3 2722 patients with poliomyelitis were admitted to this hospital—866 with paralysis and 1856 without. In 316 of the 866 paralytic cases we had to resort to special measures, such as tracheotomy, artificial respiration, postural drainage, or combinations of these. The enormous load of severely ill patients is well illustrated by the fact that in four months we treated three times as many cases with respiratory insufficiency, paralysis of the ninth, tenth, and twelfth cranial nerves, and involvement of the bulbar respiratory and vasomotor centres as in the preceding ten years. At times we had 70 patients requiring artificial respiration, and we still have from 50 to 60 requiring it. To my knowledge nothing comparable has ever been seen in Europe.

The great number of severely ill patients pouring in made therapeutic improvisations necessary. During these months we have in fact been in a state of war, and at the beginning we were not nearly adequately equipped to meet an emergency of such vast proportions.

Fig. 1 shows that the epidemic culminated about Sept. 1. During the week Aug. 28–Sept. 3 our hospital admitted 335 patients or nearly 50 cases daily. The descending branch of the epidemic curve is, as usual, less steep than the ascending branch. At the time of writing, Dec. 7, the epidemic seems to be nearing its

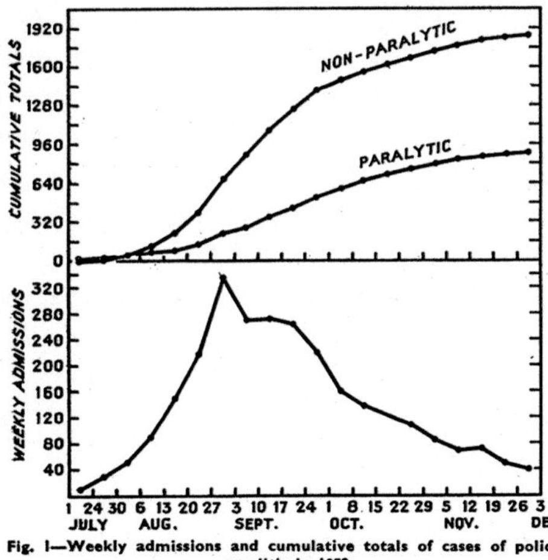

Fig. 1—Weekly admissions and cumulative totals of cases of poliomyelitis in 1952.

end. During the last two months the proportion of paralytic in relation to non-paralytic cases has grown steadily, but as a whole the ratio is 1 : 2. Naturally the number of patients admitted with non-paralytic poliomyelitis does not give an accurate picture of the true incidence of such cases in the epidemic area.

TREATMENT OF RESPIRATORY INSUFFICIENCY AND BULBAR DISEASE

In former years our therapeutic results in cases with respiratory insufficiency and involvement of the lower cranial nerves and the bulbar centres have always been very bad.

During the eleven years 1934–44 respirator treatment was used in 76 cases with a mean mortality-rate of 80%. Only cuirass respirators were used.

It is generally agreed that respiratory insufficiency of spinal origin is far easier to treat than respiratory insufficiency due to the involvement of the lower cranial nerves and the bulbar centres. Table I shows clearly the extremely grave prognosis of the pure bulbar and combined forms of respiratory insufficiency. With very few exceptions all our patients belonging to these groups died.

In 1948 we started using tracheotomy in all cases where it proved impossible to maintain an open airway because of pooling of secretions and aspiration into the lungs. In the U.S.A. this procedure seems to have had

TABLE I—RESULTS OF RESPIRATOR TREATMENT OF POLIOMYELITIS 1934–44

Type of disease	No. of cases	No. of deaths
Respiratory paralysis without bulbar involvement	17	5 (*28%*)
Respiratory paralysis with bulbar involvement	51	48 (*94%*)
Respiratory paralysis of undetermined type	8	8 (*100%*)

a beneficial influence on prognosis. In our hands this has not been so.

Table II shows that all the patients treated by tracheotomy and with respirators died, whereas treatment with respirators alone had a somewhat better prognosis, 1 man and 4 children surviving. Of these 5 patients 4 had respiratory insufficiency of purely spinal origin, and 1 patient had transient slight impairment of swallowing.

Thus the prognosis of poliomyelitis with respiratory insufficiency was rather gloomy at the outbreak of the present epidemic in Copenhagen. At our disposal we had one tank respirator (Emerson) and six cuirass respirators. This equipment proved wholly insufficient when the epidemic developed into a major catastrophe.

Fig. 2 shows the admission dates of the 316 poliomyelitis patients requiring special treatment—i.e., tracheotomy, artificial respiration, postural drainage, and combinations of these forms of treatment. The chart exclusively comprises patients with respiratory insufficiency, paralysis of the lower cranial nerves, the respiratory or vasomotor bulbar centres or combinations of these forms of paralysis. During the epidemic tracheotomy was performed in about 250 cases. The indication for this operation was invariably stagnation of secretions in the upper airway, leading to inadequate ventilation. By far the greater number of the patients had simultaneously paralysis of the respiratory muscles. The 316 cases did not all come from the metropolitan area, because in recent years we have done much to centralise the treatment of such patients. Consequently fig. 2 includes 75 cases brought in from localities outside our usual area. These admissions account for the three peaks of the curve.

Until the last week of August we used the therapeutic methods practised in 1948–50, but during these terrible weeks the situation became increasingly critical. The

Fig. 5.7 Title page

The paper stated, "During the several weeks we had 40–70 patients in our hospital requiring continuous or intermittent bag ventilation. To do this we have employed about 200 medical students daily."

There were enormous challenges to manage a large number of patients with poliomyelitis at the same time (75 patients under manual ventilation requiring next to the medical students, 260 nurses to provide care, and 27 technicians to control the machinery). Early tracheostomy with bag ventilation and repeated suctioning and positioning could bring mortality down from 80% to 40%. The anesthesiologists also recognized that with PPV, pulmonary edema could occur. The patient, therefore, was kept relatively dry, and there was specific attention to the presence of a "too high" pressure during ventilation that was recognized as inciting pulmonary edema.

Lassen also anticipated future problems such as a negative effect of PPV on cardiac output, difficulty with weaning and patient–ventilator asynchrony.

The Message and Acceptance

More experiences in using mechanical ventilation of patients with neurologic disease were published from newly organized respiratory care units, and they could accommodate neurologic patients with a variety of neurologic diseases, most notable the Batten Respiratory Unit in National Hospital, Queen Square, London.

This respiratory unit admitted patients with acute polyneuritis (Guillain–Barré syndrome), myasthenia gravis, obstruction of the airway in deeply unconscious patients after traumatic brain injury, barbiturate poisoning, and patients with impairment of the movement of the chest wall from muscle spasm of tetanus, transverse myelitis, but also acute brainstem lesions associated with multiple sclerosis [42].

There was a concern about its consequences in certain neurologic diseases. Marshall stated:

> The institution of respiratory aid permits an accurate diagnosis to be made. It is rare for the outcome to be a matter of regret, because when the primary lesion is irreversible the patient does not usually survive as a chronic respiratory invalid. But when the primary lesion does not present acutely, as in motor neuron disease, the institution of respiratory aid is usually regretted as the patient may survive for many months in a distressing condition.

The development of an effective vaccine against poliomyelitis reduced requirements of respiratory care in poliomyelitis. However, tracheostomy and PPV became more technically advanced and led to the emergence of a diverse selection of mechanical ventilators [19, 22, 33]. In Tobin's words: "with advances in computer and electronic technology ventilators have changed markedly in appearance and there is an array of options that is increasingly intimidating" [70].

The use of noninvasive mechanical ventilation is a major development in neurologic disease associated with respiratory failure [1, 7, 65]. It has a place in mostly chronic neuromuscular disorders. Bilevel positive airway pressure (BiPAP) however is useful in myasthenia gravis exacerbation with respiratory failure and as a weaning device. Patients with worsening myasthenia gravis may considerably benefit from noninvasive ventilation using a BiPAP trial if there is no severe carbon dioxide retention. BiPAP could be used while the patient is undergoing plasma exchange that often leads to fairly rapid improvement in muscle and respiratory weakness.

Finally, management of the mechanical ventilator is different in neurologic critical illness. Patients in the neurosciences ICU have often normal baseline pulmonary function, and mechanical ventilation is needed to assist with respiratory drive or to protect the upper airway from collapse.

Short Historical Note 38

THERAPEUTIC HYPOTHERMIA

The Title of the Paper

Sedzimir CB, Jacobs D, Dundee JW. Induced hypothermia as a therapeutic measure in neurology; a clinical study of a hopeless case. Br J Anaesth. 1955;27:93–100.

The Paper and the Times

Induced hypothermia—as a measure to protect tissue—has been known for centuries.

Hypothermia was used to preserve injured limbs in the Napoleon wars in the 1800s, and in Russia, victims of cardiac arrest would be covered in snow. Wartime observations mentioned that injured soldiers would better tolerate pain when exposed to cold and injuries rubbed with ice would bleed less. Exposure to cold also taught physicians that gradual warming may have a better physiologic effect than rapid rewarming. In the nineteenth century, most experience with hypothermia was in the battlefield.

In the 1940s and 1950s, therapeutic hypothermia entered hospital practice. Cooling the patient was occasionally used during surgery, and most of the time it was applied to patients undergoing cardiac surgery and to patients undergoing a major general surgical procedure with an expected poor outcome. Hypothermia also was used to protect the brain in cardiac resuscitation and was advocated in many authoritative reviews, but without a good understanding of how it could possibly work.

The potential therapeutic use of hypothermia in neurologic disorders—as with so many other therapies—had a clinical beginning followed by multiple laboratory experiments and a return to the intensive care setting for clinical trials. Experimental studies in the 1950s found that therapeutic hyperthermia could reduce cerebral oxygen consumption and metabolic rate. In 1954, Woringer et al. described hypothermia to manage marked hyperthermia in midbrain lesions after head injury [79].

Neurosurgeons would apply hypothermia in complex surgeries. One paper specifically describes the challenges of managing a patient with hypothermia (Fig. 5.8).

The Details of the Paper

The authors describe the use of hypothermia in a severe subarachnoid hemorrhage. A 40-year-old woman was admitted with sudden headache and became rapidly unconscious. The patient underwent a cerebral angiogram and a fronto-temporal craniotomy to clip a middle cerebral artery aneurysm. During surgery, hypothermia was applied. The patient had multiple periods of deterioration but also developed significant tachycardia and hyperthermia that required further control with hypothermia. She was treated with ice packs as well as chlorpromazine, pethidine, and methorphinan; hexamethonium was used to improve shivering. The therapeutic hypothermia was used "in the hope that reducing local tissue metabolism the patient might be tided over to the acute phase of vascular embarrassment."

It can be deduced from Fig. 5.9 that the effect of hypothermia was not entirely satisfactory. Shivering occurred frequently and prevented the lowering of temperature to hypothermic levels. The respiratory and pulse rate, however, were rapidly controlled, and soon, the temperature was reduced to normal. An increase in responsiveness and movement in the limbs was again observed. The authors concluded that "despite the considerable cerebral destruction and by clipping of the middle cerebral artery, the rapidly recovery of consciousness and degree to which the hemisphere retained its physiological function during the immediate postoperative period can only be described by hypothermia." The authors said that being in extreme hypothermia "saved her life and in fact, before she died from what is presumed to be a pulmonary embolus, she was nodding and recognizing her husband." The authors noted that the striking significant improvement with hypothermia could indicate that two groups of patients would lend themselves to this form of therapy: patients with ischemic lesions where hypothermia can lower the brain metabolism while the blood pressure is maintained to open up collateral circulation and those who experience significant pyrexias of hypothalamic and brainstem origin.

Fig. 5.8 The title page

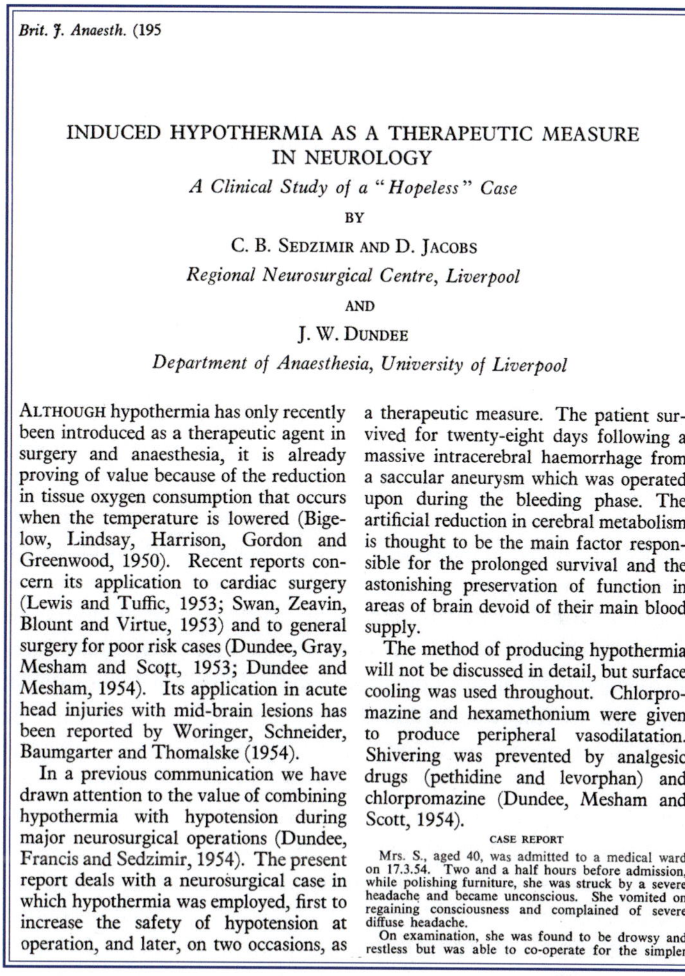

Brit. J. Anaesth. (195

INDUCED HYPOTHERMIA AS A THERAPEUTIC MEASURE IN NEUROLOGY

A Clinical Study of a "Hopeless" Case

BY

C. B. SEDZIMIR AND D. JACOBS

Regional Neurosurgical Centre, Liverpool

AND

J. W. DUNDEE

Department of Anaesthesia, University of Liverpool

ALTHOUGH hypothermia has only recently been introduced as a therapeutic agent in surgery and anaesthesia, it is already proving of value because of the reduction in tissue oxygen consumption that occurs when the temperature is lowered (Bigelow, Lindsay, Harrison, Gordon and Greenwood, 1950). Recent reports concern its application to cardiac surgery (Lewis and Tuffic, 1953; Swan, Zeavin, Blount and Virtue, 1953) and to general surgery for poor risk cases (Dundee, Gray, Mesham and Scott, 1953; Dundee and Mesham, 1954). Its application in acute head injuries with mid-brain lesions has been reported by Woringer, Schneider, Baumgarter and Thomalske (1954).

In a previous communication we have drawn attention to the value of combining hypothermia with hypotension during major neurosurgical operations (Dundee, Francis and Sedzimir, 1954). The present report deals with a neurosurgical case in which hypothermia was employed, first to increase the safety of hypotension at operation, and later, on two occasions, as a therapeutic measure. The patient survived for twenty-eight days following a massive intracerebral haemorrhage from a saccular aneurysm which was operated upon during the bleeding phase. The artificial reduction in cerebral metabolism is thought to be the main factor responsible for the prolonged survival and the astonishing preservation of function in areas of brain devoid of their main blood supply.

The method of producing hypothermia will not be discussed in detail, but surface cooling was used throughout. Chlorpromazine and hexamethonium were given to produce peripheral vasodilatation. Shivering was prevented by analgesic drugs (pethidine and levorphan) and chlorpromazine (Dundee, Mesham and Scott, 1954).

CASE REPORT

Mrs. S., aged 40, was admitted to a medical ward on 17.3.54. Two and a half hours before admission, while polishing furniture, she was struck by a severe headache and became unconscious. She vomited on regaining consciousness and complained of severe diffuse headache.

On examination, she was found to be drowsy and restless but was able to co-operate for the simpler

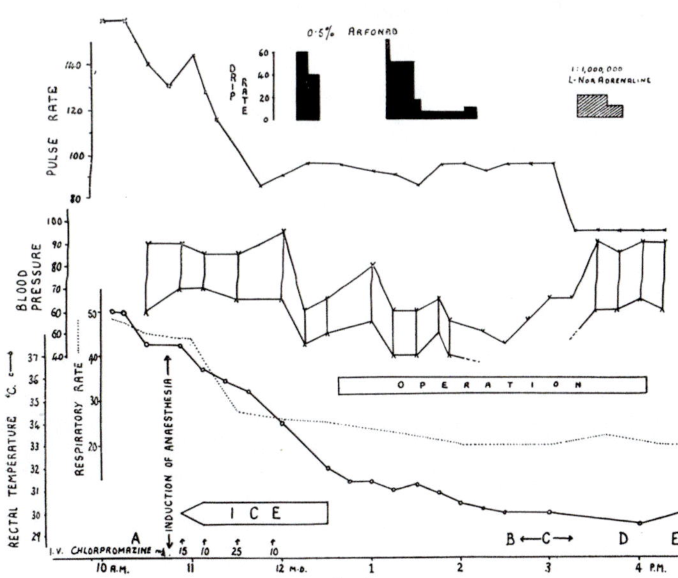

FIG. 1
Details of the first hypothermia and operation.

Fig. 5.9 The patient treated with hypothermia

The Message and Acceptance

The "hypothermia story" is still evolving, but its benefit in some acute neurologic disorders has been accepted by most intensivists. There is no question that induced hypothermia—now named therapeutic hypothermia to distinguish it from other causes of hypothermia—had a sound experimental basis and the discovery is perhaps one of the most celebrated examples of translational neurology. Careful planning by a number of investigators, most notably, Hubert Rosomoff from the Neurologic Institute of New York [54, 60–62], Peter Safar from the University of Pittsburgh [36], and Guy Clifton [11] from the University of Texas Health Science Center in Houston, would result in ways to study hypothermia in animal models and provide a solid basis for clinical studies. As mentioned earlier, Rosomoff, a neurosurgeon, and Safar, an internist, would later collaborate on a book chapter on the management of the comatose patient [63]. According to Kochaneck, this chapter provided the first thoughts on how to use therapeutic hypothermia. For comatose patients, they suggested, "hypothermia seems indicated in any patient who has brain damage severe enough to produce unconsciousness—usually the temperature is kept at 32°C [36]."

Nonetheless, use of hypothermia remained mostly in the operating room [72]. Concerns about a great number of complications such as cardiac irritability and ventricular fibrillation with deep hypothermia reduced the enthusiasm of hypothermia [6, 17, 21, 76, 79]. Between 1960 and 1990, there was little use of hypothermia in daily practice, but after animal models revealed that hypothermia could have an improved neurologic outcome, clinical trials were organized.

The effect of hypothermia in experimental model of traumatic brain injury was first studied by Rosomoff and Holoday [21, 38, 40, 54]. Most importantly, they documented that hypothermia of 25°C would reduce cerebral blood flow and could potentially worsen neurologic injury. Clifton and associates documented reduced mortality and less neurologic damage in rats with lowering core temperature to 33°C.

A recent meta-analysis of studies in traumatic brain injury included eight trials and showed that hypothermia reduced mortality, but differences were not statistically significant [56].

Although there is a good fundamental basis from experimental studies, therapeutic hypothermia for ischemic stroke has not yet been proven by randomized clinical trials.

The most widely accepted use of hypothermia is after cardiac arrest, and series of patients from many institutions around the world are appearing—all invariably claiming success. Any intensive care cohort will have to be carefully judged for selection bias.

Short Historical Note 39

ACUTE SPINAL CORD INJURY AND SPINAL SHOCK

The Title of the Paper

Guttman L. Rehabilitation after injuries of the spinal cord and cauda equina. Br J Phys Med. 1946;9:130–7, 162–71.

Munro D. Rehabilitation of veterans paralyzed as the result of injury to the spinal cord and cauda equina. Am J Surg. 1948;75:3–18.

The Paper and the Times

Care of spinal cord injury became more organized in the early 1900s and in particular after World War I. Two neurosurgeons are responsible for pioneering the care of these devastated patients. One major spinal unit was developed by US neurosurgeon Donald Munro [50]. He established the first Spinal Unit at the Boston City Hospital in 1936. With his comprehensive approach to care, patients survived and were in much better medical condition. He has been called the "father of paraplegia." He was also known as a driven optimist, because he "refused the defeatist attitude of his neurosurgical colleagues."

Another major Spinal Unit was organized by Sir Ludwig Guttmann, a neurologist and neurosurgeon who escaped from Germany to England in 1939 and in 1944 founded a Spinal Unit at Stoke-Mandeville Hospital in Aylesbury [23]. He emulated the work of Munro and he also treated spinal cord injury as a complex disease. This Spine Unit was created in anticipation of casualties of war in the major spring offensive. The objective was to "return most of them in spite of their profound disability to the community as useful and respected citizens."

In developing appropriate care of spinal cord injury, it was logical to understand the pathophysiology. Acute injury to the spinal cord may lead to loss of all function and has been described as "spinal shock." The term *spinal shock* has been attributed to physiologist Marshall Hall who in 1841 introduced the word *shock*: "If, in a frog, spinal marrow be divided…there are for a very short time no diastaltic actions (meaning reflexes) in the extremities, the diastaltic actions speedily return. This phenomenon is shock" [30].

Nearly 100 years earlier, Whytt described a similar phenomenon of spinal shock as a loss of sensation accompanied by motor paralysis and eventually return of reflexes. Confusion has remained about whether spinal shock relates to circulatory disturbances or to a transient hypoexcitability of the spinal cord [4, 52, 68, 71, 81]. Sherrington's work in spinal cord injury focused precisely on this issue and considered spinal shock part of a general concept of diaschisis [68]. Diaschisis has been defined as sudden inhibition of function in a distant area of the brain or spine, but anatomically connected with the primary injury through transsynaptic neural pathways. Diaschisis physiologically may mean hypoperfusion, decreased oxygen consumption, and hypometabolism. Spinal shock could work itself upward or downward, but the more distal segments from the original lesion would last longer to recover.

Other notable experiments with creating the phenomenon of spinal shock were by Tarlow in 1953 who compressed spinal cords with balloons for 15 min to 2 h and found full recovery of function—and minimal neuronal damage—after normalizing pressure [69]. These experiments were interpreted—by some—as an argument for early laminectomy after a contused spinal cord.

Munro published his first major article in 1948 and several years later published a series of articles and eventually reviewing 232 patients with cord transections and 337 patients with a partial cord injury treated over 25 years in Boston City Hospital [49–51]. Another paper describes the management of the acute stage of spinal cord injury in Stoke Mandeville National Spinal Injury Center. Guttmann later published a remarkable series of papers detailing each of his observations [23–28].

The Details of the Paper

Munro's paper included patients admitted to the Cushing Veteran Administration General Hospital from 1946 to 1947 (Fig. 5.10). Ambulation was achieved in many patients. Munro also wrote "of the twenty one that were not ambulatory at dis-

Fig. 5.10 Title page of Munro

REHABILITATION OF VETERANS PARALYZED AS THE RESULT OF INJURY TO THE SPINAL CORD AND CAUDA EQUINA*

DONALD MUNRO, M.D.

Consultant in Neurosurgery at Cushing Veterans' Administration General Hospital, Framingham, Mass.; Formerly National Consultant for Paraplegia to the Veterans' Administration; Surgeon-in-Chief for Neurosurgery at the Boston City Hospital

Boston, Massachusetts

IT is well known that during and immediately after the first world war patients who had been paralyzed as the result of a wound or injury to the spinal cord and cauda equina had a minimal chance of survival and no chance whatever of rehabilitation to a point where they could again lead a normal social and work life. In the following years preceding the second world war, work with civilian prototypes of these patients, together with the development of certain technics for dealing with their peculiar problems, has made it possible to change this deplorable situation. The twenty-four-hour mortality in the author's clinic has been reduced to 8 per cent and the mortality at the end of the first week to 19 per cent. Deaths at the time of discharge from the hospital have been reduced from about 75 to 37 per cent and it is now possible virtually to eliminate all later fatalities. In addition, such patients as will cooperate and have the use of their hands and arms can be promised a normal social and work life limited only by the restrictions made necessary by their enforced use of braces and crutches. This knowledge was first available only just in time for its application to the so-called "paraplegic" soldier.[1] Because of certain characteristics peculiar to the circumstances of their wounding and immediate care, it was possible to study in more detail certain complications of these injuries and to extend the benefits gained by this knowledge to both civilian and service patients. Nutritional problems, for example, that, because of lack of material in the civilian group, could be no more than recognized as in need of treatment, were much more common and required urgent solution in service patients. New ideas and methods of therapy were quickly developed to a high point of efficiency. Bed sores, prevented in civilian patients before methods either could or must needs be devised for their surgical therapy, appeared in service patients in practically every case. They were of such enormous size that surgical closure was not only imperative as a life-saving measure but essential for any degree of rehabilitation as well. Such complications as renal and bladder stones, hypertrophy of the internal urethral sphincter and the effects of prolonged suprapubic and perineal bladder fistulas, could all be studied. Finally, the usefulness of certain surgical procedures[2,3,4] in the treatment of spasm was confirmed and the operations standardized.

* The opinions expressed herewith are those of the author and do not necessarily agree with those of the Veterans' Administration or the United States Army or Navy.

REHABILITATION AFTER INJURIES TO THE SPINAL CORD AND CAUDA EQUINA*

By LUDWIG GUTTMANN, M.D. (Freiburg).

Neurological Surgeon in Charge, Head and Spinal Injuries Centre, Ministry of Pensions' Hospital, Stoke Mandeville, near Aylesbury, Buckinghamshire

PREFATORY NOTE

The physical medicine department of a large general hospital has to provide facilities for the adequate treatment of patients suffering from many different disorders. At Stoke Mandeville Hospital, for patients whose stay in hospital is short (such as those admitted for hernia and appendicectomy, and for medical disorders such as pneumonia, bronchitis and asthma) pre-operative and post-operative exercises, class work and occupational therapy are arranged. There are special orthopaedic and plastic units and a head and spinal injuries centre. In general, patients in these units may be considered as long-term cases, the pattern and management of whose treatment is naturally more complex and detailed than is that of the short-term cases. The medical officer in charge of the rehabilitation unit must appreciate the differing needs of these patients in planning the work of his staff and the use of the equipment. The work must, in great part, be decentralized, so that those on the technical staff, although continuing to work as part of the physical medicine team, are also essential and articulate members of the special unit to which they are seconded.

The physical rehabilitation of persons with head and spinal injuries entails several hours daily, for many weeks and months, of careful, detailed work by the physiotherapist, the sergeant instructor, and the occupational therapist and her technical instructors. In Dr. L. Guttmann, the neurological surgeon in charge of the head and spinal injury unit, we have been fortunate in having a colleague with whom a happy partnership could be formed. His knowledge of the structural and psychological aspects of spinal nerve injuries has enabled him to make a wise and full use of the physical medicine department. As he himself says in his paper, a strong doctor-patient relationship is of first importance in the handling of these patients. The patient and his doctor must create a pattern in the weaving of which each member of the technical staff must play his individual role. Successful management depends upon carefully planned and ably executed team work. The modern treatment of spinal injuries, as practised in this hospital, is an example of the important part that physical medicine plays in helping the sick man to regain his health.

Consultant in Physical Medicine to the Emergency Medical Service, with charge of Physical Medicine Department at Stoke Mandeville Hospital, Ministry of Pensions.

FRANCIS BACH, D.M., D.Phys.Med.

INJURIES TO THE SPINAL CORD: THE MODERN STANDPOINT

A complete lesion of the spinal cord, whether caused by injury, by inflammatory or vascular processes or by other influences, presents a grave problem as one of the most tragic calamities in human life. It always results in one of the most devastating types of disablement, with loss of essential functions from the site of the lesion downwards, paralysis of all motor and sensory functions and loss of control of vasomotor, bladder, intestinal, and sexual functions.

In the past, a man with a complete transverse lesion of the spinal cord was generally considered as a hopeless case, in that death might follow within a short time of his injury. Statistics of World War I on this subject in the British and American Armies show a mortality rate of not less than 80 per cent, the early mortality rate (death within the first few weeks or months after injury) varying from 47 to 65 per cent. Those patients who managed to survive dragged out their lives as useless and hopeless cripples, "unemployable" and unwanted. Many of them were doomed to spend the rest of their lives in an institution or at home, with the poor consolation of, perhaps, a little basket-work as their only hope for the future.

Even during the first years of World War II, most members of the medical profession were still possessed of the old idea that little could be done for these unfortunate sufferers. It was, therefore, not surprising that, in the publications on rehabilitation during these years, the subject of paraplegics was hardly mentioned. Things have changed considerably since then.. Experience during the later stages of World War II has shown that these cases, if treated properly from the start, are by no means as hopeless as was thought previously, and a defeatist attitude towards them, therefore, can no longer be tolerated. The modern principles of rehabilitation, now legalized in the Disabled Persons (Employment) Act 1944—that great charter of humanity—can be applied successfully to most of these men, to prevent their being cast on the human scrap-heap. Indeed, their particular situation, as severely disabled men and long-term hospital patients, is admirably suited to prove that medical rehabilitation, industrial rehabilitation and settlement are closely linked and can go hand in hand.

The installation in Great Britain, during the recent war, of spinal units, and the congregation of spinal cord casualties in a single department, were the first steps forward in the systematic study of the whole problem. Until recently, however, it has not been generally recognized that, in order to prevent such a unit from becoming merely an accumulation of doomed cripples, and to develop at least a few of these units into real rehabilitation centres for spinal cord lesions, certain conditions are indispensable. Although it is not within the scope of this paper to discuss all the details of the set-up of such a centre, a few fundamentals, which have emerged from war-

*A paper read to a meeting of the British Association of Physical Medicine, held at Stoke Mandeville on 12th June 1946.

Fig. 5.11 Title page

charge five were failures because of the untreatable nature of their disease, nine because of patient's peculiarities and seven because the doctor failed to hold interest." Munro's initial 2-year follow up of these spinal cord injury veterans is another landmark observation [49] He reports on 228 patients and describes the results of complex care. He introduces bilateral anterior dorsolumbar rhizotomy for disabling spasm. In his series, 86% had control of bowels and 62% had control of the bladder. Mortality from complications was very low.

Guttmann's paper describes the "principles and objects" of general treatment in 160 patients (141 were war casualties from gunshot injuries or fractures.) (Fig. 5.11). The patients were referred at different intervals and often were in a deplorable state (with "gaping wounds discharging cerebrospinal fluid," "marked extension or flexion contractures," "emaniciation due to ascending urinary infection," "pressure sores or infections of other organs").

The aspects of general treatment are described herein and include avoidance of prolonged recumbency, restoration of nutrition "at the highest possible level," skin care with excision of necrotic portions and plastic surgery, bladder care that included suprapubic drainage in patients with urethral strictures, and care of the bowels.

Guttmann felt the positioning of the patient during spinal shock had an impact on reflex synergy. In his view, prolonged fixation of the paralyzed limbs in adduction and semiflexion—caused by the faulty placement of pillows under the knees—would promote flexor synergy and paraplegia in flexion. Promoting extensor activity could be done with placing limbs in abduction and extension in the hip and knees and keeping feet and toes in dorsiflexion when the patient was supine.

It was recognized that the vital capacity in spinal shock virtually disappeared in cervical lesions. Guttmann claimed that with overdevelopment of the sternomastoid, scaleni, and trapezius, using exercises, an improvement in vital capacity of the lungs could be achieved. The bladder function showed no volitional or reflex function of the bladder due to flaccidity of the detrusor muscle. Overdistention of the bladder during the spinal shock phase resulted in long standing atonicity of the bladder. The duration was estimated 8 weeks followed by delayed development of reflex automatisms. Peristalsis was absent and bowel sounds could disappear resulting in complete fecal retention. Abnormal extension could also interfere with function of the diaphragm and cause respiratory distress.

The autonomic mechanisms were recognized as well. Orthostatic hypotension and measures to treat it with binders are discussed. Finally, there is mention of abnormality of temperature regulation. In high lesions, most of the sweat glands are out of function. All cutaneous and tendon reflexes are abolished. Bulbocavernous and anal reflexes may remain and disappear later.

The Message and Acceptance

The clinical manifestations of spinal shock are neurologic and systemic. Improvement in patients with a complete transverse lesion clinically involves return of the reflexes in a headward direction. No typical pattern was recognized with reappearance of ankle and knee jerk reflexes. The duration of the spinal shock could be defined as ending with appearance of the bulbocavernous reflex, defined as recovery of deep tendon reflexes or even defined as a return of reflexive detrusor function.

Bradyarrhythmias, and hypotension as a result of impaired sympathetic innervations but unopposed vagal parasympathetic action, are common in the first 24 h. In several days to weeks, autonomic function improves and autonomic dysreflexia can emerge and is often triggered by a distended bowel or bladder.

Recognition of a dire need to care for these helpless patients was essential. Munro was very clear in his opinion, and he brought new ideas to the table. His approach was that late complications are "preventable under ordinary circumstances." In comparison, his series showed a reduction of bedsores and an increase in patients never developing bedsores. In a historical view of spinal cord treatment, Munro was cited as stating that [5]:

> House officers and nurses cannot be made to believe that failure to move the patient on schedule, failure to change a wet bed within 15 minutes

of its having become wet and failure to maintain an adequate level of serum protein cause pressure and bed sores and prevent bed sores from healing until the patient has proved it to their satisfaction by dying. Then, having learned their lesson by bitter experience, these trained attendants are transferred to another ward or leave the hospital, and the education process has to be repeated with another untrained group. Constant attention to these apparently trivial details is consequently imperative on the part of the visiting staff if it has any desire to lower the mortality and shorten the hospital stay of these patients.

In a later report, Munro reported on 569 patients and also describes therapeutic options [51]. Munro considered the condition in a state of areflexia. The paper reports on respirator areflexia (increasing anoxia and provision of high oxygen environment), stomach and bowel areflexia (acute paralytic ileus and withholding food and fluids and "patience of the physician" rather than ineffective drugs or even abdominal operations), bladder areflexia (catheter placement), skin–vascular areflexia (correction of hypoproteinemia, frequent turning and meticulous care), and areflexic sweating (creating a constant temperature environment).

References

1. American Association for Respiratory Care. Consensus statement on the essentials of mechanical ventilators. Respir Care. 1992;37:1000–8.
2. Andersen EW, Ibsen B. The anaesthetic management of patients with poliomyelitis and respiratory paralysis. Br Med J. 1954;1:786–8.
3. Atkinson WJ. Posture of the unconscious patient. Lancet. 1970;295:404–5.
4. Atkinson PP, Atkinson JL. Spinal shock. Mayo Clin Proc. 1996;71:384–9.
5. Bedbrook G. Fifty years on fundamentals in spinal cord injury care are still important. Paraplegia. 1992;30:10–3.
6. Benson DW, Williams Jr GR, Spencer FC, et al. The use of hypothermia after cardiac arrest. Anesth Analg. 1959;38:423–8.
7. Bolton CF, Chen R, Wijdicks EFM, Zifko UA. Neurology of breathing. Philadelphia: Butterworth Heinemann; 2004.
8. Buckell M. Effect of glycerol by mouth on raised intracranial pressure in man. Lancet. 1964;284(7370): 1151–2.
9. Bullock R. Hyperventilation. J Neurosurg. 2002;96: 157–8.
10. Cantore G, Guidetti B, Virno M. Oral glycerol for the reduction of intracranial pressure. J Neurosurg. 1964;21:278–83.
11. Clifton GL, Jiang JY, Lyeth BG, et al. Marked protection by moderate hypothermia after experimental traumatic brain injury. J Cereb Blood Flow Metab. 1991;11:114–21.
12. Cushing H, Foley F. Alteration of intracranial tension by salt solutions in the alimentary canal. Proc Soc Exp Biol Med. 1920;17:217–8.
13. Diringer MN, Videen TO, Yundt K, et al. Regional cerebrovascular and metabolic effects of hyperventilation after severe traumatic brain injury. J Neurosurg. 2002;96:103–8.
14. Diringer MN, Zazulia AR. Osmotic therapy: fact and fiction. Neurocrit Care. 2004;1:219–33.
15. Drinker P, McKhann CF. The use of a new apparatus for the prolonged administration of artificial respiration: I. A fatal case of poliomyelitis. JAMA. 1929;92: 1658–60.
16. Duncan GG. Diabetic coma; a therapeutic problem. Ann Intern Med. 1952;37:1188–96.
17. Fay T. Early experiences with local and generalized refrigeration of the human brain. J Neurosurg. 1959; 16:239–60.
18. Forbes HS, Wolff HG. Cerebral circulation. III. The vasomotor control of cerebral vessels. Arch Neurol Psychiatr. 1928;19:1057–86.
19. Frost EA. Tracing the tracheostomy. Ann Otol Rhinol Laryngol. 1976;85:618–24.
20. Gibbs EL, Gibbs FA, Lennox WG, et al. Regulation of cerebral carbon dioxide. Arch Neurol Psychiatr. 1942;47:879–89.
21. Gisvold SE, Safar P, Rao G, et al. Multifaceted therapy after global brain ischemia in monkeys. Stroke. 1984;15:803–12.
22. Grum CM, Chauncey JB. Conventional mechanical ventilation. Clin Chest Med. 1988;1:37–45.
23. Guttmann L. Organization of spinal units. History of the National Spinal Injuries Centre, Stoke Mandeville Hospital, Aylesbury. Paraplegia. 1967;5:115–26.
24. Guttmann L. Spinal cord injuries: comprehensive management and research. 2nd ed. Oxford: Blackwell Scientific Publications; 1976.
25. Guttmann L. Spinal shock and reflex behavior in man. Paraplegia. 1970;8:100–16.
26. Guttmann L. Spinal cord injuries. Comprehensive management and research. Oxford: Blackwell; 1973.
27. Guttmann L, Munro A, Robinson R, Walsh J. Effects of tilting on the cardiovascular responses on plasma catecholamine levels in spinal man. Paraplegia. 1963;1:4–18.
28. Guttmann L, Silver J, Wyndham CH. Thermoregulation in the spinal man. J Physiol. 1958;142:406–18.
29. Haden RL. Therapeutic application of the alteration of brain volume. JAMA. 1919;73:983–4.
30. Hall M. On the diseases and derangement of the nervous system in their primary forms and in their modifications by age, sex, constitution, hereditary disposition. Excesses, general disorder, and organic disease. London: H Bailliere; 1841.

31. Imberti R, Bellinzona G, Langer M. Cerebral tissue PO_2 and $SjvO_2$ changes during moderate hyperventilation in patients with severe traumatic brain injury. J Neurosurg. 2002;96:155–7.
32. Javid M. Urea – new use of an old agent, reduction of intracranial and intraocular pressure. Surg Clin North Am. 1958;38(4):907–28.
33. Kacmarek RM, Meklaus GJ. The new generation of mechanical ventilators. Crit Care Clin. 1990;6: 551–78.
34. Karl MM, Howell RA, Hutchinson JH, et al. Liver coma, with particular reference to management. Arch Intern Med. 1953;91:159–76.
35. Kety SA, Shenkin HA, Schmidt CF. The effects of increased intracranial pressure on cerebral circulatory function in man. J Clin Invest. 1948;27:493–9.
36. Kochanek P, Drabek T, Tisherman SA. Therapeutic hypothermia: the Safar vision. J Neurotrauma. 2009; 26:417–20.
37. Lawrence RD. The treatment of desperate cases of diabetic coma. Br Med J. 1930;1:690–2.
38. Lund LO, Beckwitt HJ, Grover RF, et al. Effect of hyperventilation, hypothermia and urea on circulation and cerebrospinal fluid pressure in the dog. (2). Anesthesiology. 1965;26:45–8.
39. Lundberg N, Kjällquist Å, Bien C. Reduction of increased intracranial pressure by hyperventilation: a therapeutic aid in neurological surgery. Acta Psychiatr Neurol Scand. 1959;34:1–64.
40. Lyeth BG, Jiang JY, Robinson SE, et al. Hypothermia blunts acetylcholine increase in CSF of traumatically brain injured rats. Mol Chem Neuropathol. 1993;18:247–56.
41. Marburg O. Die traumatischen erkrankungen des gehirns und rückenmarks. In: Bumke O, Foerster O, editors. Handbuch der Neurologie, Spezielle neurologie III, vol. 11. Berlin: Springer; 1936. p. 1–177.
42. Marshall J. The work of a respiratory unit in a neurologic hospital. Postgrad Med J. 1961;37:26–30.
43. Meyers ME. Nursing the comatose patient. Am J Nurs. 1954;54:716–8.
44. Meyers R, Meyers ME. Managing the comatose patient. GP. 1951;4:45–52.
45. Mirski MA, Denchev DI, Schnitzer MS, et al. Comparison between hypertonic saline and mannitol in the reduction of elevated intracranial pressure in a rodent model of acute cerebral injury. J Neurosurg Anesthesiol. 2000;12:334–44.
46. Morrissey EJ. The effect of magnesium sulphate on the cerebrospinal fluid pressure and on the brain volume. Arch Surg. 1925;11:778–89.
47. Motley HL. The use of oxygen in comatose states. Bull N Y Acad Med. 1950;7:479–94.
48. Muizelaar JP, van der Poel HG, Li ZC, et al. Pial arteriolar vessel diameter and CO_2 reactivity during prolonged hyperventilation in the rabbit. J Neurosurg. 1988;69:923–7.
49. Munro D. Two-year end results in the total rehabilitation of veterans with spinal cord and cauda equina injuries. N Engl J Med. 1950;242:1–16.
50. Munro D. The rehabilitation of patients totally paralyzed below the waist: with special reference to making them ambulatory and capable of earning their living – an end-result study of 445 cases. N Engl J Med. 1954;250:4–14.
51. Munro D. Management of patients with traumatic paraplegia. N Engl J Med. 1964;270:1167–71.
52. Nacimiento W, Noth J. What, if anything, is spinal shock? Arch Neurol. 1999;56:1033–5.
53. Ogden AT, Mayer SA, Connoly ES. Hyperosmolar agents in neurosurgical practice: the evolving role of hypertonic agents. Neurosurgery. 2005;57:207–15.
54. Onesti ST, Baker CJ, Sun PP, et al. Transient hypothermia reduces focal ischemic brain injury in the rat. Neurosurgery. 1991;29:369–73.
55. Patel PM. Hyperventilation as a therapeutic intervention: do the potential benefits outweigh the known risks? J Neurosurg Anesthesiol. 1993;5:62–5.
56. Peterson K, Carson S, Cairney N. Hypothermia treatment for traumatic brain injury: a systematic review and meta-analysis. J Neurotrauma. 2008;25:62–71.
57. Rangel-Castilla L, Lara LR, Gopinath S, et al. Cerebral hemodynamic effects of acute hyperoxia and hyperventilation after severe traumatic brain injury. J Neurotrauma. 2010;27:1853–63.
58. Reinfrank RF, Mcgee CJ. The early management of the unconscious patient. Med Bull US Army. 1952;9: 341–4.
59. Riddell AG, McDermott WV. Hepatic coma. Lancet. 1954;266:1263–7.
60. Rosomoff HL. The effects of hypothermia on the physiology of the nervous system. Surgery. 1956;40:328–36.
61. Rosomoff HL. Experimental brain injury during hypothermia. J Neurosurg. 1959;16:177–87.
62. Rosomoff HL, Holaday DA. Cerebral blood flow and cerebral oxygen consumption during hypothermia. Am J Physiol. 1954;179:85–8.
63. Rosomoff HL, Safar P. Management of the comatose patient. In: Safar P, editor. Respiratory Therapy. Philadelphia: F.A. Davis Co.; 1965.
64. Sachs E, Belcher GW. Use of saturated salt solution intravenously during intracranial operations, preliminary report. JAMA. 1920;75:667.
65. Shapiro BA. A historical perspective on ventilator management. New Horiz. 1994;2:8–18.
66. Sheehan HL, Summers VK. Treatment of hypopituitary coma. Br Med J. 1952;1:1214–5.
67. Shenkin HA, Goluboff B, Haft H. The use of mannitol for the reduction of intracranial pressure in intracranial surgery. J Neurosurg. 1962;19:897–900.
68. Sherrington CS. The integrative action of the nervous system. London: Constable & Company LTD; 1906.
69. Tarlow IMH, Klinger H, Vitale S. Experimental techniques to produce acute and gradual compression of the spinal cord. Arch Neurol Psychiatry. 1953;70:813–9.
70. Tobin MJ. Mechanical ventilation. N Engl J Med. 1994;330:1056–61.
71. Van Harreveld A, Schadé JP. The course of recovery of the spinal cord from asphyxia. Am J Physiol. 1939;2:101–11.

72. Varon J, Acosta P. Therapeutic hypothermia: past, present and future. Chest. 2008;133:1267–74.
73. Vialet R, Albanese J, Thomachot L, et al. Isovolemic hypertonic solutes Isovolume hypertonic solutes (sodium chloride or mannitol) in the treatment of refractory posttraumatic intracranial hypertension: 2 mL/kg 7.5% saline is more effective than 2 mL/kg 20% mannitol. Crit Care Med. 2003;31:1683–7.
74. Weed LH, McKibbin PR. Experimental alteration of brain bulk. Am J Physiol. 1919;85:55–131.
75. Westhorpe RN, Ball C. The history of emergency airway management. Anesth Intensive care. 2010;38:3.
76. Williams Jr GR, Spencer FC. The clinical use of hypothermia following cardiac arrest. Ann Surg. 1958;148:462–8.
77. Wise BL, Chater N. The value of hypertonic mannitol solution in decreasing brain mass and lowering cerebrospinal-fluid pressure. J Neurosurg. 1962;19: 1038–43.
78. Wolfman EF, Schoch HK. Water depletion in the comatose patient. Med Bull. 1951;17:73–82.
79. Woringer E, Schneider J, Baumgartner J, Thomalske G. Hypothermia. Anesth Analg. 1954;11:1.
80. Zilversmit DB, McCandless EL. Fate of intravenously administered glycerol. Proc Soc Exp Biol Med. 1957;95:755–75.
81. Zipnick RI, Scalea TM, Trooskin SZ, et al. Hemodynamic responses to penetrating spinal cord injuries. J Trauma. 1993;35:578–82.

6 First Clinical Studies and Trials

E.F.M. Wijdicks, *Famous First Papers for the Neurointensivist*,
DOI 10.1007/978-1-4614-3182-4_6, © Springer Science+Business Media New York 2013

Short Historical Note 40

TRIPLE H: HYPERTENSION–HYPERVOLEMIA–HEMODILUTION THERAPY

The Title of the Paper

Kosnik EJ, Hunt WE. Postoperative hypertension and management of patients with intracranial arterial aneurysms. J Neurosurg. 1976;45:148–54.

The Paper and the Times

In the late 1940s, it became clear that cerebral infarcts could occur after a ruptured aneurysm, and in particular situated remotely from the aneurysm. Pressure from hematomas, thrombosis and embolism, hypotension, and arterial vasospasm were considered mechanisms [124]. Decades later, when neurosurgeons tried to grasp the consequences of aneurysmal rupture, the development of cerebral vasospasm was recognized as a major cause of deterioration [67]. The mechanism of cerebral vasospasm remained unsatisfactorily explained, and experimental studies testing the effects of "spasmolytic" drugs in animal models also were not encouraging. Different approaches to treat this complication were considered, and they involved manipulating the blood rheology and arterial pressure.

Thus, in cerebral arteries without autoregulation, increasing cerebral blood flow (CBF) could be achieved by increasing cerebral perfusion pressure (CPP) or by reducing viscosity. This concept became the basis of hypertension, hypervolemia, and hemodilution therapy, better known as "triple-H" therapy.

Neurosurgeons Kosnik and Hunt were the first to describe the use of postoperative hypertension, but in fact, they used a combination of volume augmentation and hypertension. No experimental study had previously investigated the possible effects of this intervention, and experience came directly from clinical observations.

The Details of the Paper

The paper was based on the assumption that increasing the CPP would be the most effective way to overcome the severe and diffuse cerebral vasospasm in these patients (Figs. 6.1). The authors describe seven patients with an aneurysmal subarachnoid hemorrhage (SAH), some with postoperative neurologic signs, and others with a neurologic decline while the aneurysm was unsecured. The patients did well until postoperative day 4 or 5, and then became markedly "obtunded with only semi-purposeful movements in response to pain." Patients were treated with colloids and plasmanate followed by norepinephrine. Norepinephrine was used because of both its powerful peripheral vasoconstriction and its inotropic stimulating effects on cardiac muscle. The investigators developed a regimen that they described as "enough norepinephrine to elevate the blood pressure 40–60 points systolic or to produce unmistakable clinical improvement."

Additionally, they administered plasma followed by whole blood transfusion. After blood volume expansion and observing a rise of the central venous pressure, norepinephrine was weaned to a lower dose. After the neurologic deficit improved, blood pressure was maintained for several more days and then gradually allowed to drift down to pretreatment level.

Equally important, they noted that a reduced blood volume could have been present in some of their patients because there was a rapid response with volume augmentation. Additionally, in one patient with adequate systolic blood pressures in the 140 mmHg range, further blood pressure augmentation was successful, suggesting an unknown ceiling of blood pressure effect. The authors also emphasized the importance of timing of augmentation. "The most serious hazard seems to be the institution of treatment too late, after the cerebrovascular system is so damaged that increasing perfusion pressure only increases brain swelling."

Postoperative hypertension in the management of patients with intracranial arterial aneurysms

Edward J. Kosnik, M.D., and William E. Hunt, M.D.

Department of Surgery, Division of Neurological Surgery, Ohio State University College of Medicine, Columbus, Ohio

✔ Elevation of systemic arterial pressure in seven patients with intracranial arterial aneurysms has been shown to be effective in alleviating ischemic symptoms attributed to cerebral vasospasm. Autoregulation is at least partially lost in patients with cerebral hemodynamic crisis. Blood volume expansion was used to augment vasopressors in maintenance of systemic hypertension. The management of these cases is discussed. Caution in the use of this technique is advised, since the regimen is not without risk.

Key Words · **cerebral vasospasm** · **hypertension, therapeutic** · **hypervolemia, therapeutic** · **intracranial arterial aneurysm** · **cerebral hemodynamic crisis** · **cerebral ischemia**

All neurosurgeons are familiar with the problem of arterial spasm, cerebral ischemia, and infarction after intracranial aneurysm repair. Much work has been done with regard to the nature of vascular response, its etiology and physiology.[1-4,10,11,14-16,24,29,30] Numerous medications have been tried locally and systemically with equivocal results, especially in the clinical situation.[7,8,13,17,20,23,27] The neurological deficit is clearly due to tissue ischemia or infarction, whether secondary to cerebral vasospasm, embolization, or thrombosis. Over the past few years we have treated symptoms of ischemia by means of induced arterial hypertension in several carefully selected cases.

Denny-Brown[5] was the first to describe treatment of cerebral ischemia by increasing arterial blood pressure. Shanbrom and Levy[21] discussed two patients with advanced arteriosclerotic disease of the carotid and basilar systems in whom a critical-level systemic arterial pressure was found necessary to overcome ischemic symptoms. Farhat and Schneider[6] reported four patients with cerebrovascular insufficiency. Two of these patients were treated in the postoperative period, and two were treated for postangiographic complications. These authors raised the systolic pressure 50 to 60 mm Hg with good results. Wise, *et al.*,[28] reported a series of patients with cerebral ischemia in whom raising the systemic arterial blood pressure with vasopressors brought about reversal of neurological deficit. Recently Wernick and Sugar[25] reported a case of postangiographic hemiplegia which was successfully treated with vasopressors.

We have raised the systemic mean arterial pressure in a series of aneurysm patients who were suffering from a postoperative cerebral-flow crisis, with good results in most cases. Some cases with clear-cut clinical response are reported below.

Fig. 6.1 Title page

The authors recognized the potential hazards of increasing perfusion that could potentially result in brain edema. There also was a concern that fluid overload in patients with congestive heart failure could further complicate management.

The Message and Acceptance

In literature reviews, two other important manuscripts are usually mentioned concurrently. One paper by Pritz et al. in 1978 described intravascular volume expansion in four additional patients, and their approach was similar, keeping the patient hypervolemic and additionally using vasopressors or discontinuation of antihypertensive medication (Figs. 6.2 and 6.3) [116]. In 1982, Kassel et al. published their surefooted data on 58 patients who deteriorated neurologically from angiographically confirmed cerebral vasospasm. In this study, 81% of the patients responded favorably to therapy, and failure in the remainder of the patients was related to delay initiating therapy or to development of complications, particularly pulmonary edema from overhydration [80] (Fig. 6.4).

The papers tackled the major issues of timing and target of blood pressure augmentation. Kassel's study was unique because for the first time it introduced Swan-Ganz catheterization to monitor intravascular volume and this approach—until recently—became universal in hemodynamic augmentation of patients with SAH complicated by vasospasm.

Complications of aggressive monitoring also became apparent. One study found catheter-related sepsis in 13%, but less commonly cardiac failure (2%), subclavian vein thrombosis (1%) or pneumothorax (1%) [92].

One other important question emerged. Could prophylactic triple-H therapy—instituted before the onset of symptoms—be more effective?

Solomon et al. studied 47 consecutive patients with ruptured intracranial aneurysms that were treated with prophylactic volume expansion for up to 2 weeks after SAH and found no cases of cerebral infarction. However, another key study revealed no difference in mean global CBF—using 133 xenon clearance—in hypervolemic and normovolemic patients. Symptomatic vasospasm occurred in 20% of patients in each group, despite better intravascular volume parameters [135, 136].

The effect of 5% albumin solution on sodium balance and blood volume after SAH was studied in 43 patients treated with either hypervolemia or normovolemia for 1 week after aneurysm clipping. The hypervolemia group received significantly more total fluids, sodium, and 5% albumin than did the normovolemia group and had higher central venous pressure levels. Supplemental 5% albumin solution prevented sodium and fluid losses but did not have an impact on blood volume [95]. Finally, one study found that an increase in cardiac output without changes in mean arterial pressure can increase CBF in the setting of vasospasm and suggested dobutamine as a first measure [78].

Current published data on the best approach are unconvincing because consistent measurements of relevant clinical and laboratory variables are lacking, with different methods used in each of the cohorts. A randomized blinded study of hemodynamic augmentation in aneurysmal SAH has never been performed. Nonetheless, many neurointensivists and neurosurgeons have seen significant improvement of the patient with aggressive fluid management, and supplemental blood pressure increase started soon after onset of symptoms [90]. But when a patient deteriorates, management now has shifted toward early endovascular management in combination with volume augmentation and vasopressors.

0148-396X/78/0303-0364$02.00/0
NEUROSURGERY
Copyright © 1978 by the Congress of Neurological Surgeons
Vol. 3, No. 3, 1978
Printed in U.S.A.

Treatment of Patients with Neurological Deficits Associated with Cerebral Vasospasm by Intravascular Volume Expansion

Michael B. Pritz, M.D., Ph.D., Steven L. Giannotta, M.D., Glenn W. Kindt, M.D., John E. McGillicuddy, M.D., and Richard L. Prager, M.D.

Department of Surgery, Sections of Neurological Surgery and Thoracic Surgery, University of Michigan Medical Center, Ann Arbor, Michigan

Four patients, including one preoperative patient, developed neurological deficits associated with angiographically proven cerebral vasospasm and were treated with intravascular volume expansion. Indicator dilution techniques were employed to monitor intravascular volume and cardiac functions during treatment. All four patients improved promptly. None of the patients developed cardiac or pulmonary dysfunction despite marked increase in intravascular volume and despite several risk factors such as cardiac symptoms, electrocardiographic abnormalities, and advanced age. The techniques of monitoring and controlling intravascular volume are described. We believe that this is an important therapeutic adjunct for certain aneurysm patients.

Key words: Cerebral vasospasm, Indicator dilution technique, Intracranial aneurysms, Intravascular volume expansion

Fig. 6.2 Title page

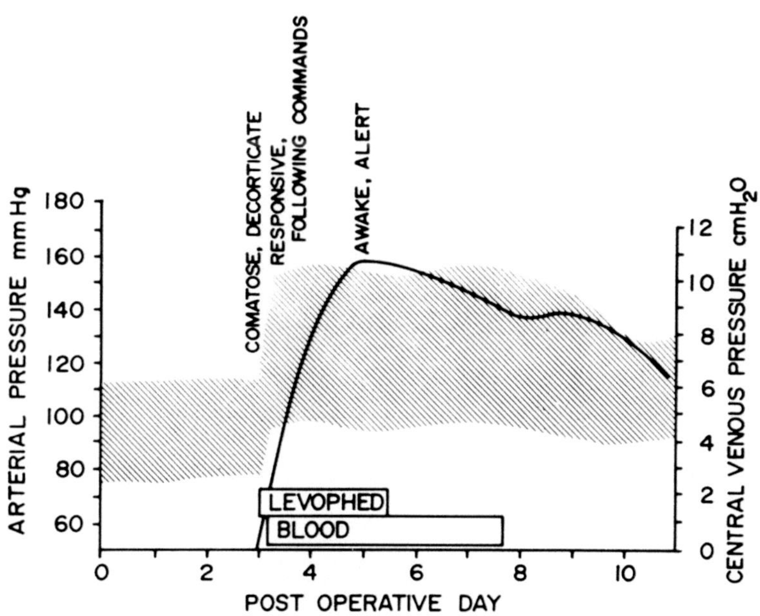

FIG. 1. Postoperative course in Case 1, showing the patient's blood pressure, central venous pressure, and neurological status. Note the improvement occurring with pressure elevation.

Fig. 6.3 Pritz's patient example

Clinical and laboratory reports

Treatment of Ischemic Deficits from Vasospasm with Intravascular Volume Expansion and Induced Arterial Hypertension

Neal F. Kassell, M.D., Sydney J. Peerless, M.D., Quentin J. Durward, M.D., David W. Beck, M.D., Charles G. Drake, M.D., and Harold P. Adams, M.D.

Departments of Neurosurgery (N.F.K., D.W.B.) and Neurology (H.P.A.), University of Iowa Hospitals and Clinics, Iowa City, Iowa, and Departments of Neurosurgery (S.J.P., Q.J.D.) and Surgery (C.G.D.), University of Western Ontario, London, Ontario

In 58 patients with progressive neurological deterioration from angiographically confirmed cerebral vasospasm after spontaneous subarachnoid hemorrhage, arterial hypertension was induced in an attempt to improve their deficits. The most effective regimen consisted of intravascular volume expansion, blockade of the vagal depressor response, and the administration of antidiuretics and vasopressor agents. With this protocol, arterial blood pressure could be sustained at high levels for prolonged periods. Neurological deterioration was reversed in 47 patients, transiently in 4; permanent improvement occurred in 43. Complications experienced during therapy included pulmonary edema, dilutional hyponatremia, aneurysmal rebleeding, coagulopathy, hemothorax, and myocardial infarction. Elevating systemic arterial pressure in states of cerebrovascular insufficiency resulting from vasospasm is safe if meticulous attention is paid to physiological, biochemical, and hematological parameters, with the exception that it may be hazardous in the presence of an untreated ruptured or intact aneurysm. Intravascular volume expansion and induced hypertension are effective in reversing ischemic deficits from vasospasm provided that treatment commences before cerebral infarction and that adequate pressures are maintained for a sufficient period. The production of a hypervolemic state by the use of colloid and crystalloid infusion accompanied by atropine blockade of the vagal depressor response and blunting of the diuresis with vasopressin enables arterial pressure to be elevated for longer than 1 week. (*Neurosurgery* 11:337–343, 1982)

Key words: Arterial hypertension, Cerebral ischemia, Cerebral vasospasm, Hypervolemia, Intracranial aneurysm, Intravascular volume expansion, Subarachnoid hemorrhage

Fig. 6.4 Title page

Short Historical Note 41

TREATMENT OF STATUS EPILEPTICUS

The Title of the Paper

Whitty GWM, Taylor M. Treatment of status epilepticus. Lancet. 1949;2:591–4.

The Paper and the Times

Status epilepticus (SE) was known by the ancient Greek physicians; however, its severity was not always recognized as such, and there was widespread admission to asylums even up to nineteenth century Victorian times [16]. According to Neligan and Shorvon, the first mention of "status epilepticus" was in a translation of Trousseau's classic book on clinical medicine, *Clinique Médicale de l'Hôtel-Dieu de Paris*, 1868 [101].

In the twentieth century in Europe, Bourneville, Westphal, Charcot, and Browne were among physicians who described SE in sufficient detail and often treated it with large doses of Bromides [97, 133]. In the United Kingdom, work done at the National Hospital for the Paralyzed and the Epileptic Queen Square in London—with most notable Gowers as a leading contributor—further elaborated on how to treat SE [57].

Many physicians recognized that once the diagnosis was established, the prognosis could be poor. One of the first descriptive works on SE is by Clark and Prout [31]. They defined SE as a "maximum development" of epilepsy with one seizure after another and with coma in between these seizures. They also recognized tachypnea, tachycardia, and hyperthermia as manifestations. Clark and Prout also purported to show destruction in cortical layers and a relationship with duration of SE, with more severe abnormalities with longer episodes of seizures. This has been considered one of the first documents that emphasized the severity and consequences of this condition and was a novel insight at the time. SE became recognized as following several stages: premonitory, convulsive, and comatose stages [132].

The history of treatment of SE was recently comprehensively summarized by two experts in the field [97, 101]. Before the turn of the century, chloral hydrate and ether were considered for frequent seizures. Phenobarbital was introduced in 1912 [109], paraldehyde in 1914 [34], chloroform anesthesia in 1928 [115], and phenytoin in 1958 [26].

SE—then and now—occurred more often in patients with prior epilepsy. It was also customary at the time to point toward sudden withdrawal of bromides or phenobarbital as a cause of SE. Gradually, it also became quite clear that outcome of the condition could reflect the disorder causing SE in the first place and also that time to resolution of SE was an important factor.

The Details of the Paper

The study involved 36 patients with SE at Radcliffe Infirmary or the head-injury bureau at Wheatley Military Hospital. Seventeen of 36 patients were seen by the authors. The authors emphasized "this condition constitutes a grave medical emergency and may be fatal unless the fits are rapidly controlled." They found evidence that paraldehyde was the drug of choice both because it rapidly controlled seizures and was successful even when barbiturates failed to treat the neurologic emergency. The authors suggested a protocol for the first time.

> As soon as possible 8–10 mL of paraldehyde is injected into the gluteal muscle, and the site of injection is massaged. The paraldehyde need not be sterilised. This treatment usually stops the fits within half an hour.
>
> If the fits continue, 5 mL of paraldehyde intramuscularly is given every half-hour until they cease. The persistence of focal twitching without any tendency to spread does not require further sedation, and attempts to eliminate these entirely may lead to a dangerous level of narcosis.
>
> If the patient's general condition indicates it, an intravenous glucose-saline or plasma drip is given at the rate of one bottle in 3 h. This will also provide a convenient method of continuing the administration of paraldehyde, either by intermittent injections into the drip tubing, or in solution in the drip fluid in any required concentration, since it is soluble 1 in 8 in physiological saline solution.

They also suggested that the patient should be placed on regular anticonvulsant therapy—barbiturates and hydantoins; and anesthetics were described.

TREATMENT OF STATUS EPILEPTICUS

C. W. M. WHITTY
B.M., B.Sc. Oxfd, M.R.C.P.

MARGARET TAYLOR
B.M. Oxfd

From the Department of Neurology, Radcliffe Infirmary, Oxford

STATUS epilepticus, the occurrence of several grand-mal convulsions without recovery of consciousness between each, should be looked on as a grave emergency. If effective measures are not taken promptly to arrest the fits, the patient is likely to die.

The use of modern chemotherapy in the late war allowed the survival of many patients with severe brain wounds which would formerly have proved fatal. Hence there are more traumatic epileptics, and ipso facto cases of status epilepticus, in the community. The subject is inadequately dealt with in standard textbooks ; and the occurrence of several probably avoidable deaths from this cause has prompted us to make this brief review of 25 cases, mostly of the symptomatic group, and to mention one régime which in our experience has proved a safe and usually effective remedy.

Status epilepticus can nearly always be cured if correct treatment is instituted early. Such treatment must not be allowed to obscure the medical or surgical measures required to deal with the underlying lesion in symptomatic epilepsy. However, even in these cases, arresting the fits is generally a life-saving measure and certainly an essential preliminary to further diagnosis and treatment, which may have to be delayed until special facilities are available.

Fig. 6.5 The title page

> If phenobarbitone is used it should be given in doses of 6–12 gr. smaller doses being of little value, and preferably in the "soluble" form by intramuscular or intravenous route. Thiopentone in anesthetic doses may be used, or chloroform anesthesia if no other remedy is at hand. But the effect of these methods is often short-lived, and it may be necessary to establish heavy sedation by other means and to maintain this for twenty-four hours or longer afterwards if the fits tend to recur.

The underlying theme of the paper was that prognosis of SE—in particular the fatal cases—was directly related to the start of treatment. Uncontrolled seizures or late treatment led to a higher probability of fatal outcome. Moreover, the emphasis was on paraldehyde as an important first drug, and they suggested a treatment algorithm—a novel approach to seizures and SE in particular.

The Message and Acceptance

In SE, well defined instructions to manage a persistently seizing patient are helpful, if not essential. Thus, algorithms have dominated the literature on SE, and with more experience, a reasonable acceptable practice evolved. Questions can be raised about initial treatment, which drug and dose, and how to manage refractory SE. Most physicians have now accepted that the first line of treatment should include a combination of a benzodiazepine (i.e., lorazepam or clonazepam) and phenytoin (or fosphenytoin) [159]. Others have advocated the initial use of short-acting midazolam, arguing that when it fails it does not linger [160]. Intramuscular midazolam was effective for prehospital status epilepticus treatment [134]. Second-line drugs have included phenobarbital, midazolam, propofol, valproic acid and there is little consensus among neurologists. How many physicians use a protocol is not known. When asked, many are not even aware of a hospital protocol [158]. Wasterlain and Treiman, in their monograph on SE, wrote a summary of the future ("The status of status epilepticus gives me fits") and emphasized the "snail-like" progress in managing the disorder [160].

Only one major double-blind study [148] has been published in hospitalized patients and thus most of the agents currently used for SE did not go through rigorous efficacy and safety testing. Experiences with newer approaches continue to remain anecdotal (electroconvulsive therapy, hypothermia, levetiracetam), but comparative studies are very difficult to organize. SE has always been major neurocritical illness and not simply a severe manifestation of seizures. Not only is seizure control needed, but control of systemic manifestations is as urgent [28, 29, 115, 147].

Short Historical Note 42

HEMICRANIECTOMY

The Title of the Paper

Rengachary SS, Batnitzky S, Morantz RA, Arjunan K, Jeffries B. Hemicraniectomy for acute massive cerebral infarction. Neurosurgery. 1981;8:321–8.

The Paper and the Times

In ancient times, trepanation—sometimes of considerable size—was performed without a medical objective and more as a result of folkloric belief. It was reintroduced in the 1800s as a treatment for epilepsy.

Decompressive surgery—actually removing bone flaps—developed after the pathophysiology and neuropathology of increased intracranial pressure (ICP) became better understood. Kocher can be credited as one of the first physicians to explain its rationale [85]. Clinical experience may have started with Cushing's paper on decompression in inaccessible brain tumors [36].

In some patients, decompressive surgery was performed with the assumption that the patient harbored a brain tumor, only to find there was a swollen hemispheric infarct [131, 137]. Decompressive surgery was also a last resort in traumatic brain swelling, but the earlier studies reported a circumferential approach—unsuccessful due to damage to the sagittal sinus and upward brain herniation—or a temporal decompression approach with small bone flaps [30].

In the 1970s, decompressive craniectomy—this time involving a large part of the skull—became again of interest to neurosurgeons, and experimental studies of posttraumatic cerebral edema showed survival of animals because the brain could swell through the opening [99]. Hemicraniectomy also was used by some groups in deteriorated patients with a large subdural hematoma who presented with extensor posturing and a dilated pupil. The development of a tight and bulging craniectomy site for a period up to 2 weeks was proof that the surgical decompression was justified. The chance of survival was 40% [122]. Furthermore, radical craniectomy also had been used in patients with severe brain swelling resulting from Reye's syndrome.

Hemicraniectomy again went out of favor, but in the early 1980s was reintroduced as a primary treatment of ischemic brain swelling. Massive acute cerebral infarction—in particular in patients with acute carotid artery occlusion—was considered invariably fatal once cerebral edema developed. Anti-edema agents were rarely successful, and opening of the skull seemed the only option for many patients.

The Details of the Paper

A craniectomy to allow swelling outside the large opening was described. Decompressive craniectomy involved removal of a large bone flap and duraplasty. Generally, the swollen infarct was left intact because removal of necrotic tissue could cause major difficulty with hemostasis. All treated patients were young (ages 15, 27, and 51 years). Patients had a typical deterioration with uncal herniation (unilateral fixed pupil) signs in all three. Outcome was considerable with disability due to hemiplegia in all of the three treated patients. The authors considered the procedure for young patients, stroke involving the nondominant hemisphere, and absence of major comorbidity such as uncontrolled diabetes mellitus or dementing illness, and most importantly, the attitude of the family members to "accept attempts at preservation of life in the face of a severe neurologic deficit." Decompression without temporal lobectomy was considered the best approach.

The Message and Acceptance

The procedure became rarely used in the United States, probably because few neurologists would consider the option in ischemic stroke.

Led by Werner Hacke, the group in Heidelberg reported success in a selected group of patients and further pioneered the procedure. The experience in initially more than 60 surgically treated patients, suggested that mortality is substantially decreased, but still leaving one of four patients with a severe disability. The outcome was poor from aphasia or neglect in addition to a severe hemiparesis [60].

0148-396X/81/0803-0321$02.00/0
NEUROSURGERY
Vol. 8, No. 3, 1981
Printed in U.S.A.

Hemicraniectomy for Acute Massive Cerebral Infarction

Setti S. Rengachary, M.D., Solomon Batnitzky, M.D., Robert A. Morantz, M.D., Kadayampatti Arjunan, M.D., and Barry Jeffries, M.D.

Departments of Surgery (Neurosurgery) (S.S.R., R.A.M., K.A.) and Radiology (S.B., B.J.), Kansas University College of Health Sciences and Hospital, Kansas City, Kansas and Veterans Administration Medical Center, Kansas City, Missouri

Three patients with acute massive multilobar ischemic infarction with uncal herniation and impending death, who were unresponsive to conventional modes of therapy, were treated by ipsilateral hemicraniectomy. All three patients survived, although severe fixed neurological deficit persisted in two. The indication for hemicraniectomy in the management of patients with acute ischemic stroke is reviewed. (*Neurosurgery* 8:321–328, 1981)

Key words: Cerebral infarction, Cerebral ischemia, Hemicraniectomy, Neurological deficit, Stroke, Uncal herniation

INTRODUCTION

Stroke is the third most common cause of death in the United States and is the most common cause of death among diseases of the central nervous system. It is estimated that 200,000 persons die each year from stroke.

A frequent neurological cause of death in patients with an acute ischemic infarct in the carotid distribution is unilateral hemispheric cerebral edema with distortion of the brain resulting in uncal, cingulate, or tonsillar herniation. This phenomenon has been well documented from clinical observations (7, 10, 17–19, 32, 37, 43, 44), autopsy studies (1, 4, 9, 31, 39), and experimental models (21). Although voluminous material has appeared in the recent literature on the experimental evaluation of various antiedema agents in the management of focal cerebral ischemia (including steroids, barbiturates, mannitol, low molecular weight dextran, dimethyl sulfoxide, induced hypertension, hyperventilation, hypothermia, etc.), no one modality or combination of modalities has been shown to be consistently effective in clinical trials (38). With continued effort, a more effective mode of therapy may be discovered, but until that time a viable alternative is necessary to treat patients with massive brain edema from ischemic infarction with uncal herniation and impending death.

CASE REPORTS

Case 1

A 51-year-old man was admitted on February 14, 1980, for cervical radiculopathy. Work-up revealed cervical spondylosis with prominent spondylotic ridges at the C-5, C-6 and the C-6, C-7 levels. While watching television 48 hours before a contemplated operation for cervical spondylosis, the patient suddenly became confused and agitated, wandered around, and fell. This was followed by a brief loss of consciousness. When he regained consciousness, he was unable to move his left arm and leg and was found to be incoherent. Examination at this time revealed a blood pressure of 170/90. He was very drowsy, but responded to his name. A left homonymous hemianopsia was noted. He had a dense hemiplegia and hemianesthesia on the left side. A clinical diagnosis of infarction in the middle cerebral or the internal carotid artery distribution was made. An emergency computed tomogram (Fig. 1*A*) was essentially normal. The patient was started on dexamethasone, 10 mg i.v. followed by 4 mg every 6 hours, and a continuous infusion of low molecular weight dextran at the rate of 50 ml/hour. A Holter monitor (The Holter Co., King of Prussia, Pennsylvania) detected no irregularities in cardiac rhythm. His neurological status stabilized with essentially no change in his fixed deficits. A lumbar puncture yielded clear fluid with an opening pressure of 150 mm of cerebrospinal fluid (CSF). The protein content was 72 mg/100 ml.

Fig. 6.6 Title page

There is now sufficient data that urgently salvaged patients who underwent this dramatic procedure actually may do well despite a fixed hemiparesis. Early decompressive hemicraniectomy (arbitrarily defined as surgery before the first signs of herniation) has been advocated, but under those clinical circumstances, a good result also can be explained by a favorable natural history. Concerns about major morbidity in survivors have been voiced, and the functional outcome in elderly patients is marginal. One study found severe disability more often in patients older than 55 years [118].

The discussion now pertains to selection of patients, timing (early vs. late), age (>55 years), dominance of involved hemisphere and comorbidity [81, 87, 94, 150, 163]. The procedure commonly is refused by family members and mostly performed in younger individuals. Many younger patients, however, eventually become independent [2].

Surgical technique of decompression after traumatic head injury now involves bifrontoparietal decompression [35]. Decompressive craniectomy is more commonly considered in patients with penetrating injury and considered more or less essential to preempt the commonly anticipated cerebral swelling. Complications associated with decompressive craniectomy after traumatic head injury and subsequent cranioplasty are subdural hygroma, relentless progression of contusions in up to 50% of cases, and hydrocephalus in 25% [35].

A new randomized trial performed by Australian New Zealand Intensive Care Society Clinical Trial Group found that outcome was worse in patients treated with decompressive craniectomy [35]. Patients were randomized when their ICP was greater than 20 mmHg after first-tier therapies. Patients in the decompressive surgery group had worse extended Glasgow Outcome Scale scores. Nonetheless, the surgery did reduce ICP and resulted in shorter stay in the intensive care unit. Therefore, there was a beneficiary short-term effect, but worse long-term outcome. The trial has been criticized as being overly aggressive because the design only required increased ICP for more than 15 min despite medical therapy. Many patients had ICP less than 20 mmHg, questioning the "refractory" designation. Moreover, the patients who underwent craniotomy had twice more common fixed pupils than the medically treated group, suggesting a worse neurologic state in the surgically treated patients. Another study—the Randomized Evaluation of Surgery with Craniectomy for Uncontrollable Elevation of ICP (RESCUE *icp*) trial—is under way. In this trial, bilateral craniectomy is considered only after an ICP threshold of 25 mmHg is reached for 1–2 h.

Decompressive craniectomy remains an important procedure. More room under the skull will lead to less damaging mass effect of brain swelling whether caused by trauma, penetrating injury, stroke, or an infectious process.

Short Historical Note 43

FACTOR VII FOR CEREBRAL HEMORRHAGE

The Title of the Paper

Mayer SA, Brun NC, Begtrup K, et al. Recombinant activated factor VII for acute intracerebral hemorrhage. N Engl J Med. 2005;352:777–85.

Mayer SA, Brun NC, Begtrup K, et al. Efficacy and safety of recombinant activated factor VII for acute intracerebral hemorrhage. N Engl J Med. 2008;358:2127–37.

The Paper and the Times

For many years, radiologists—while performing early cerebral angiography in patients with cerebral hematomas—had noted contrast extravasation indicative of continued bleeding. Prior to this observation, a cerebral hemorrhage—without an acquired coagulopathy or anticoagulation treatment—was considered a monophasic event.

Kelley and associates documented for the first time, enlargement of hypertensive hemorrhages [82]. They found significant hypertension (diastolic blood pressures of 140 mmHg) in these patients and considered it a possible factor.

Brott et al. studied 103 patients with computed tomography (CT) scans performed 2–6 h after onset and found 38% of the patients had more than a one-third growth in size within 1 h of admission to the emergency department (mean hematoma volume 26 mL of on initial CT and 32 mL on second CT). Deterioration was captured with scores from the National Institutes of Health Stroke Scale or Glasgow Coma Scale (GCS), and it was noted that not all patients deteriorated, including patients with significant increase in volume [21].

Nevertheless, several studies did document a correlation of outcome with clot volume, with some even suggesting that intracerebral hemorrhage volume of more than 80 mL had a 100% mortality despite intervention [20].

For several years, treatment for cerebral hematoma has remained inadequately studied with mainly a focus on the need for neurosurgical intervention. Blood pressure control also was considered uncertain, with many physicians interpreting a hypertensive surge as a compensatory response. It was argued that aggressive treatment of hypertension could result in worsening ischemia in the perihematoma penumbra.

Efforts to physically control the bleeding started with a pilot study of ε-aminocaproic acid but found continuous bleeding when administered within 12 h of intracerebral hemorrhage [112]. With the availability of recombinant activated factor VII (rFVIIa), it became logical to also study this drug. rFVIIa promotes hemostasis, and through this mechanism it could limit hematoma enlargement. Theoretically, these drugs also could accelerate thrombosis of bleeding, penetrating arteries or arterioles. Two trials were conducted in centers in China, Europe, and United States.

The Details of the Paper

The first rFVIIa trial randomized 399 patients within 3 h of onset into placebo, 40, 80, or 160 mcg/kg within 1 h of admission (Fig. 6.7). Patients who were admitted comatose (GCS score, 3–5), patients with planned surgery within 24 h, patients without spontaneous cerebral hemorrhage, patients on anticoagulation, or patients with known thrombocytopenia among other confounders were excluded. CT scanning was repeated 24 and 72 h after study treatment.

The first trial improved mortality by 38% with the higher (80 and 160 mcg/kg) doses. The reduction in hemorrhage size was stated as follows: "Treatment with rFVIIa resulted in reduced growth in the volume of intracerebral hemorrhage as compared with placebo by approximately 5 ml at 24 h, which translated into a 11-ml reduction in total lesion volume at 72 h." Serious arterial thromboembolic adverse events were found more significantly than in placebo and in the higher doses.

The second clinical trial (Fig. 6.8), FAST (Factor Seven for Acute Hemorrhagic Stroke Trial), initially assigned 841 patients into placebo, 20 or 80 mcg/kg of rFVII within 4 h after onset. Several patients were lost to follow-up, and eventually the analysis included 262 patients who received placebo, 264 patients who received 20 mcg/kg, and 293 received 80 mcg/kg of rfVIIa.

This trial with fairly similar characteristics and execution as the prior trial found no improvement in outcome at 90 days.

Recombinant Activated Factor VII for Acute Intracerebral Hemorrhage

Stephan A. Mayer, M.D., Nikolai C. Brun, M.D., Ph.D., Kamilla Begtrup, M.Sc., Joseph Broderick, M.D., Stephen Davis, M.D., Michael N. Diringer, M.D., Brett E. Skolnick, Ph.D., and Thorsten Steiner, M.D., for the Recombinant Activated Factor VII Intracerebral Hemorrhage Trial Investigators*

ABSTRACT

BACKGROUND

Intracerebral hemorrhage is the least treatable form of stroke and is associated with high mortality. Among patients who undergo computed tomography (CT) within three hours after the onset of intracerebral hemorrhage, one third have an increase in the volume of the hematoma related to subsequent bleeding. We sought to determine whether recombinant activated factor VII (rFVIIa) can reduce hematoma growth after intracerebral hemorrhage.

METHODS

We randomly assigned 399 patients with intracerebral hemorrhage diagnosed by CT within three hours after onset to receive placebo (96 patients) or 40 μg of rFVIIa per kilogram of body weight (108 patients), 80 μg per kilogram (92 patients), or 160 μg per kilogram (103 patients) within one hour after the baseline scan. The primary outcome measure was the percent change in the volume of the intracerebral hemorrhage at 24 hours. Clinical outcomes were assessed at 90 days.

RESULTS

Hematoma volume increased more in the placebo group than in the rFVIIa groups. The mean increase was 29 percent in the placebo group, as compared with 16 percent, 14 percent, and 11 percent in the groups given 40 μg, 80 μg, and 160 μg of rFVIIa per kilogram, respectively ($P=0.01$ for the comparison of the three rFVIIa groups with the placebo group). Growth in the volume of intracerebral hemorrhage was reduced by 3.3 ml, 4.5 ml, and 5.8 ml in the three treatment groups, as compared with that in the placebo group ($P=0.01$). Sixty-nine percent of placebo-treated patients died or were severely disabled (as defined by a modified Rankin Scale score of 4 to 6), as compared with 55 percent, 49 percent, and 54 percent of the patients who were given 40, 80, and 160 μg of rFVIIa, respectively ($P=0.004$ for the comparison of the three rFVIIa groups with the placebo group). Mortality at 90 days was 29 percent for patients who received placebo, as compared with 18 percent in the three rFVIIa groups combined ($P=0.02$). Serious thromboembolic adverse events, mainly myocardial or cerebral infarction, occurred in 7 percent of rFVIIa-treated patients, as compared with 2 percent of those given placebo ($P=0.12$).

CONCLUSIONS

Treatment with rFVIIa within four hours after the onset of intracerebral hemorrhage limits the growth of the hematoma, reduces mortality, and improves functional outcomes at 90 days, despite a small increase in the frequency of thromboembolic adverse events.

From the Departments of Neurology and Neurosurgery, Columbia University College of Physicians and Surgeons, New York (S.A.M.); Novo Nordisk, Bagsvaerd, Denmark (N.C.B., K.B.); the University of Cincinnati Medical Center, Cincinnati (J.B.); Royal Melbourne Hospital, University of Melbourne, Melbourne, Australia (S.D.); Washington University School of Medicine, St. Louis (M.N.D.); Novo Nordisk, Princeton, N.J. (B.E.S.); and the University of Heidelberg, Heidelberg, Germany (T.S.). Address reprint requests to Dr. Mayer at the Neurological Institute, 710 W. 168th St., Box 39, New York, NY 10032, or at sam14@columbia.edu.

*The participating institutions and investigators are listed in the Appendix.

N Engl J Med 2005;352:777-85.

Fig. 6.7 Title page

A similar hemostatic effect of the drug was found with reduction of 29% in the placebo group to 14% in treated patients. The subgroup analysis suggested potential benefit for patients younger than age 70 years, with baseline hematoma volume less than 60 mL, baseline intraventricular hemorrhage volume less than 5 mL, and time from onset less than or equal to 2.5 h.

The Message and Acceptance

The discrepant results between the two studies demanded an explanation, and some differences were immediately evident. First, a higher incidence of intraventricular hemorrhage was present in patients treated with rFVIIa than in patients receiving placebo in the FAST study. Second, there was an increase in arterial thromboembolic events in patients receiving rFVIIa. Third, patients older than age 80 years were included, as were patients with large CT volumes (>60 mL) [42]. There was also a better than expected outcome in the placebo arm of the FAST trial. Tuhrim, in an editorial, noted two lessons that could be learned from these trials:

> First, doses of rFVIIa larger than 80 mcg per kilogram increase the risk of arterial thrombotic events without a corresponding improvement in retarding hematoma growth; lower doses are not as effective. Second, randomization cannot ensure balanced groups, especially in trials of moderate size, and this in turn may affect results. Perhaps most important, these results emphasize two other principles that have emerged from other trials of stroke treatments: a single treatment approach may accomplish its physiological goal but may be insufficient to produce clinical benefit, and an intervention may be helpful to a well-defined subgroup but not to all those who have a particular disease [149].

Enthusiasm for these hemostatic drugs in nonanticoagulation-associated cerebral hemorrhages quickly waned. Hemostatic drugs such as prothrombin complex also became more popular as a result of low cost, longer action, and possibly fewer thromboembolic complications. Other avenues of treatment with rFVIIa were considered, such as its use in patients requiring surgery (to reduce a postoperative clot) and specifically studying its effect in patients with extravasation on contrast CT—indicating ongoing bleeding (the spot sign) [40, 141]. Some answers will come with STOP-IT, a prospective randomized, double-blind trial comparing rFVIIa with placebo for treatment of patients who have a spot sign on CT angiography.

Hemostatic drugs remain useful—if not essential—in rapid reversal of warfarin effect, but despite several studies showing rapid reversal of international normalized ratio, no study has definitively shown an impact on outcome [49, 93, 121, 125, 141]. The side effects of these drugs remain concerning, although a recent study found predominantly deep venous thrombosis usually in patients at risk. Despite use of rFVIIa, the mortality and morbidity of cerebral hemorrhage remain high, and the drug likely does not affect deteriorating patients at presentation.

Efficacy and Safety of Recombinant Activated Factor VII for Acute Intracerebral Hemorrhage

Stephan A. Mayer, M.D., Nikolai C. Brun, M.D., Ph.D., Kamilla Begtrup, M.Sc., Joseph Broderick, M.D., Stephen Davis, M.D., Michael N. Diringer, M.D., Brett E. Skolnick, Ph.D., and Thorsten Steiner, M.D., for the FAST Trial Investigators*

ABSTRACT

BACKGROUND

Intracerebral hemorrhage is the least treatable form of stroke. We performed this phase 3 trial to confirm a previous study in which recombinant activated factor VII (rFVIIa) reduced growth of the hematoma and improved survival and functional outcomes.

METHODS

We randomly assigned 841 patients with intracerebral hemorrhage to receive placebo (268 patients), 20 μg of rFVIIa per kilogram of body weight (276 patients), or 80 μg of rFVIIa per kilogram (297 patients) within 4 hours after the onset of stroke. The primary end point was poor outcome, defined as severe disability or death according to the modified Rankin scale 90 days after the stroke.

RESULTS

Treatment with 80 μg of rFVIIa per kilogram resulted in a significant reduction in growth in volume of the hemorrhage. The mean estimated increase in volume of the intracerebral hemorrhage at 24 hours was 26% in the placebo group, as compared with 18% in the group receiving 20 μg of rFVIIa per kilogram ($P=0.09$) and 11% in the group receiving 80 μg ($P<0.001$). The growth in volume of intracerebral hemorrhage was reduced by 2.6 ml (95% confidence interval [CI], −0.3 to 5.5; $P=0.08$) in the group receiving 20 μg of rFVIIa per kilogram and by 3.8 ml (95% CI, 0.9 to 6.7; $P=0.009$) in the group receiving 80 μg, as compared with the placebo group. Despite this reduction in bleeding, there was no significant difference among the three groups in the proportion of patients with poor clinical outcome (24% in the placebo group, 26% in the group receiving 20 μg of rFVIIa per kilogram, and 29% in the group receiving 80 μg). The overall frequency of thromboembolic serious adverse events was similar in the three groups; however, arterial events were more frequent in the group receiving 80 μg of rFVIIa than in the placebo group (9% vs. 4%, $P=0.04$).

CONCLUSIONS

Hemostatic therapy with rFVIIa reduced growth of the hematoma but did not improve survival or functional outcome after intracerebral hemorrhage. (ClinicalTrials.gov number, NCT00127283.)

From the Departments of Neurology and Neurosurgery, Columbia University College of Physicians and Surgeons, New York (S.A.M.); Novo Nordisk, Bagsvaerd, Denmark (N.C.B., K.B.); the University of Cincinnati Medical Center, Cincinnati (J.B.); the Royal Melbourne Hospital, University of Melbourne, Melbourne, Australia (S.D.); Washington University School of Medicine, St. Louis (M.N.D.); Novo Nordisk, Princeton, NJ (B.E.S.); and the University of Heidelberg, Heidelberg, Germany (T.S.). Address reprint requests to Dr. Mayer at the Neurological Institute, 710 W. 168th St., Box 39, New York, NY 10032, or at saml4@columbia.edu.

*The institutions participating in the Factor Seven for Acute Hemorrhagic Stroke (FAST) trial are listed in the Appendix.

N Engl J Med 2008;358:2127-37.

Fig. 6.8 Title page

Short Historical Note 44

CORTICOSTEROIDS IN CEREBRAL HEMORRHAGE

The Title of the Paper

Poungvarin N, Bhoopat W, Viriyavejakul A, et al. Effects of dexamethasone in primary supratentorial intracerebral hemorrhage. N Engl J Med. 1987;316:1229–33.

The Paper and the Times

Because corticosteroids may reduce brain edema, these drugs have always been of interest to physicians confronted with patients who deteriorate from swelling after a stroke [107, 130]. Corticosteroids also have been used in tumors surrounded by edema and with a major clinical effect. Before computed tomography (CT) scan could differentiate between hemorrhagic and ischemic strokes in the early 1950s, corticosteroids were suggested as the immediate therapy of "apoplectic stroke." Russek et al. reported a preliminary report in 15 patients with apoplectic stroke who were treated with a short course of "cortisone within 48 hours of presentation." The clinical diagnosis in these patients was "cerebral thrombosis or embolism", but there was no later pathologic confirmation. In a follow-up study with more patients, Russek et al. reported dramatic improvement in 21 of 35 patients within 24 h after cortisone therapy.

> There was not only a striking amelioration of paralytic signs and symptoms but also unquestionable benefit from changes in the mental, emotional, sensory and psychomotor status. Conjugate deviation of the eyes, incoherent speech, dysarthria, and aphasia appeared to clear rapidly during cortisone therapy. The greatest effects were noted among those who were somnolent, stuporous, mentally depressed or apathic [107].

The treatment appeared almost a panacea for stroke, and they concluded enthusiastically:

> ...with cortisone therapy rehabilitative measures can be instituted with little difficulty after only one or two days of treatment because of the patient's alertness of mind or euphoria. In a disease that is commonly viewed with a fatalistic philosophy and treated at best with nursing care, cortisone should prove a most valuable addition to therapy and a useful adjunct to rehabilitation.

How to understand these phenomenal results—not seen in later studies of either ischemic or hemorrhagic stroke—has remained unexplained. There are still physicians at conferences who ask the speaker if corticosteroids work in ischemic stroke.

Corticosteroids could potentially have an effect on the disrupted blood–brain barrier. Precisely how is less known, and the operative mechanism often is explained away as "stabilization of the blood–brain barrier." Corticosteroids also may reduce cerebral interstitial edema and then reduce intracranial pressure and damage to the brainstem. Use of corticosteroids seemed random and was influenced by previous claims with very few patient studies done. However, there were two important clinical studies.

First, a 1973 study by Tellez and Bauer included 40 patients with clinical evidence of acute intracerebral hemorrhage due to hypertension, hemorrhagic infarction, or cerebral aneurysm, who were treated with dexamethasone [13, 143]. Impaired consciousness or bloody cerebrospinal fluid was needed for inclusion. There was no CT scan confirmation because in the United States, CT scans were not purchased by hospitals until after 1974. No major differences in outcome were found with 100% mortality in the comatose or stuporous group and 92% in the control group. Only seven patients survived, but better motor function was found in survivors treated with dexamethasone.

Second, a 1986 study by Norris and Hachinski performed a double-blind, controlled trial of high-dose dexamethasone (480 mg over 12 days) in 113 patients with CT-confirmed ischemic stroke [130]. Outcome between the two groups did not differ significantly in mortality or morbidity. The authors warned that widespread use of corticosteroids would expose large numbers of patients with ischemic stroke to serious hazards of corticosteroid treatment.

Additionally, previous clinical trials and cohorts of patients with cerebral hemorrhage did mention the use of corticosteroids, but the decision was left at the discretion of the neurosurgeon. No information could be extracted that could explain the incentive to use corticosteroids, but it is likely that mass effect and visible edema

The New England
Journal of Medicine

Volume 316 MAY 14, 1987 Number 20

EFFECTS OF DEXAMETHASONE IN PRIMARY SUPRATENTORIAL INTRACEREBRAL HEMORRHAGE

Niphon Poungvarin, M.D., Wiyada Bhoopat, M.D., Adulya Viriyavejakul, M.D., Prakit Rodprasert, M.D., Panya Buranasiri, M.D., Sombut Sukondhabhant, M.D., Michael J. Hensley, M.B., B.S., Ph.D., and Brian L. Strom, M.D., M.P.H.

Abstract To evaluate the efficacy of dexamethasone for treatment of primary supratentorial intracerebral hemorrhage, we studied 93 patients 40 to 80 years old, using a double-blind randomized block design. After the subjects were stratified according to their level of consciousness (Glasgow Coma Scale), those with objectively documented primary supratentorial intracerebral hemorrhage were randomly assigned to either dexamethasone or placebo. For ethical reasons, three interim analyses were planned, to permit early termination of the trial if one study group did better than the other.

During the third interim analysis, the death rate at the 21st day was identical in the two groups (dexamethasone vs. placebo, 21 of 46 vs. 21 of 47; chi-square = 0.01, P = 0.93). In contrast, the rate of complications (mostly infections and complications of diabetes) was much higher in the dexamethasone group (chi-square = 10.89, P<0.001), leading to early termination of the study. In the light of the absence of a demonstrable beneficial effect and the presence of a significant harmful effect, current practices of using dexamethasone for treatment of primary supratentorial hemorrhage should be reconsidered. (N Engl J Med 1987; 316:1229-33.)

Fig. 6.9 Title page

on CT scan prompted administration of corticosteroids. Until a study by Poungvarin and associates in Thailand, the validity of the common recommendation to use corticosteroids in intracerebral hemorrhages had never been tested in a large group of patients.

The Details of the Paper

This double blind intention-to-treat study randomized 93 patients with an intracranial hemorrhage and between the ages of 40 and 80 years into dexamethasone versus placebo groups (Fig. 6.9). The study was performed in Siriraj Hospital Medical School in Bangkok, Thailand. The clinical trial, however, prematurely ended when an interim analysis showed important adverse effects. Patients received dexamethasone 10 mg initially followed by 5 mg every 6 h for 6 days, 5 mg every 12 h for 2 days, and 5 mg for 1 day.

The main study results showed no improvement in outcome but with more complications, mostly infections and diabetic complications, in the treatment group than in the placebo group (Fig. 6.9). In clinically less severely affected patients, a benefit could be demonstrated, but only after post hoc analysis of the data. This mostly involved noncomatose patients.

The study had little neurologic details other than a Glasgow Coma Scale score and no measurement of volume of the hematoma. The number of complications in treated patients was significant—ten times higher than controls—with pneumonia, septicemia, urinary tract infection, upper gastrointestinal hemorrhages, and a pronounced diabetogenic effect in almost half of the patients treated with dexamethasone.

The Message and Acceptance

After this landmark trial, another (underpowered) study followed, and data were published as a letter to the editor. Desai and Prasad randomized 26 patients within 5 days of presentation [41] (IV dexamethasone, at a dose of 4 mg every 6 h for 12 days, followed by 4 mg every 12 h for 2 days, and 2 mg every 12 h for 2 days). There were more comatose patients in the dexamethasone-treated group, but again no benefit was found. However, adverse effects were less in this shorter treatment study compared with the Poungvarin study.

The use of corticosteroids since this study has diminished substantially, but the practices are not well known. Some neurosurgeons continue to use corticosteroids in a patient with a large hematoma or hematomas in the brainstem. Others feel there is no proven benefit. No more studies have been sponsored since this randomized study, and perhaps the effect of corticosteroids remains to be explored. A recently published Cochrane analysis found often markedly underpowered clinical trials and no benefit [47]. A recent unusual comparison of two geographically different populations from different centers found a significant difference in outcome in favor of dexamethasone treatment. In the patients treated, the dose of dexamethasone increased with larger size hemorrhages. The authors suggested a new clinical trial [169].

Some continue to argue that the short course of corticosteroids in patients with intracranial hemorrhage might benefit patients, but again there is no good experimental data to support such a claim. Most physicians would be reluctant to use high dose corticosteroids in patients who often have comorbidities, and its administration could lead to exacerbation of diabetes. A modern study using corticosteroids or methylprednisolone may be useful if it would clearly identify the neurologic condition at presentation and delineate the CT scan characteristics.

Currently, corticosteroids are avoided in most neurocritical care or neurosurgical practices, unless hemorrhage occurs in a primary brain tumor or brain metastasis. Corticosteroids also remain indicated in hemorrhages associated with inflammatory processes such as central nervous system vasculitis.

Short Historical Note 45

SURGERY IN CEREBRAL HEMORRHAGE

The Title of the Paper

Mendelow AD, Gregson BA, Fernandes HM, et al. Early surgery versus initial conservative treatment in patients with spontaneous supratentorial intracerebral hematomas in the International Surgical Trial in Intracerebral Hemorrhage (STICH): a randomized trial. Lancet. 2005;365:387–97.

The Paper and the Times

A cerebral hemorrhage may cause mass effect and result in clinical deterioration from compression of critically important brain tissue (i.e., thalamus) and displacement of the brainstem. Relieving this pressure will improve a depressed consciousness, and neurosurgeons and neurointensivists know too well that patients can be much better after surgery. The clot not only may have a mechanical but also a toxic effect on surrounding tissue (i.e., expression of the proinflammatory mediators) that may become irreversibly damaged if the clot is not removed in time.

Removal of a hematoma from the brain—excluding patients with penetrating or closed traumatic head injury—was not commonly entertained in the pre-computed tomography (CT) era. Opinions of neurosurgeons varied widely at the time and still do. Many would only operate in patients progressing to coma or in situations of a worsening neurologic deficit. Neurosurgeons often felt that the immediate preoperative condition of the patient was far more important than the time interval from the ictus. At the time, many neurosurgeons opined that surgery should be delayed for a week.

There was a common understanding that the direction of hematoma advancement and rapidity of clot formation determined outcome. Patients comatose early after onset had a poor outcome.

Surgery for hemorrhages in the brainstem was only considered if the hematoma extended to the fourth ventricle, causing acute hydrocephalus, and successful cases were reported since Dandy's first successful attempt.

One prospective randomized trial by McKissock and colleagues in 1961 showed that the outcome was worse with operative treatment when compared with conservative treatment [96].

When CT scans in the mid-1970s could identify cerebral hematomas, urgent intervention became more in vogue and probably was spurred by the mere sight of a clot. After McKissock's study, clinical trials included studies using endoscopic removal of the hemorrhage, but they showed conflicting results. Most clinical trials involved deep ganglionic hemorrhages. Ultra-early hematoma evacuation also appeared harmful, and a clinical trial testing this strategy had to be terminated because of increased number of deaths among patients operated within hours [100]. Uncertainty about the effects of urgent evacuation eventually led to a large clinical trial and now is considered a benchmark in neurosurgical treatment of cerebral hemorrhage. The trial was organized with the premise that improved surgical techniques, as well as intensive care, could result in a better outcome (Fig. 6.10).

The Details of the Paper

The trial randomized 1,033 patients from 83 centers in 27 countries to early surgery or conservative treatment. Patients were eligible if they had a minimal hematoma diameter of 2 cm and the Glasgow Coma Scale sum score was 5 or more.

Patients were only eligible if they had CT evidence of a spontaneous supratentorial hemorrhage with no evidence of aneurysm or angiographically proven arteriovenous malformation within 72 h.

The clinical trial was based on the "clinical uncertainty principle." This principle implied that if the responsible neurosurgeon was uncertain about the benefits of either treatment—conservative versus surgical—the patient could be randomized. It is unclear from the study results how many patients were rejected for surgery, but neurosurgeons did not feel strongly about it one way or another in more than 1,000 cases. Outcome

Early surgery versus initial conservative treatment in patients with spontaneous supratentorial intracerebral haematomas in the International Surgical Trial in Intracerebral Haemorrhage (STICH): a randomised trial

*A David Mendelow, Barbara A Gregson, Helen M Fernandes, Gordon D Murray, Graham M Teasdale, D Terence Hope, Abbas Karimi, M Donald M Shaw, and David H Barer for the STICH investigators**

Lancet 2005; 365: 387–97

See **Comment** page 361

*Investigators listed at the end of report

Correspondence to:
Prof A David Mendelow, Head of Department of Neurosurgery, Newcastle General Hospital, Newcastle upon Tyne NE4 6BE, UK
a.d.mendelow@ncl.ac.uk

Summary

Background Spontaneous supratentorial intracerebral haemorrhage accounts for 20% of all stroke-related sudden neurological deficits, has the highest morbidity and mortality of all stroke, and the role of surgery remains controversial. We undertook a prospective randomised trial to compare early surgery with initial conservative treatment for patients with intracerebral haemorrhage.

Methods A parallel-group trial design was used. Early surgery combined haematoma evacuation (within 24 h of randomisation) with medical treatment. Initial conservative treatment used medical treatment, although later evacuation was allowed if necessary. We used the eight-point Glasgow outcome scale obtained by postal questionnaires sent directly to patients at 6 months follow-up as the primary outcome measure. We divided the patients into good and poor prognosis groups on the basis of their clinical status at randomisation. For the good prognosis group, a favourable outcome was defined as good recovery or moderate disability on the Glasgow outcome scale. For the poor prognosis group, a favourable outcome also included the upper level of severe disability. Analysis was by intention to treat.

Findings 1033 patients from 83 centres in 27 countries were randomised to early surgery (503) or initial conservative treatment (530). At 6 months, 51 patients were lost to follow-up, and 17 were alive with unknown status. Of 468 patients randomised to early surgery, 122 (26%) had a favourable outcome compared with 118 (24%) of 496 randomised to initial conservative treatment (odds ratio 0·89 [95% CI 0·66–1·19], p=0·414); absolute benefit 2·3% (-3·2 to 7·7), relative benefit 10% (–13 to 33).

Interpretation Patients with spontaneous supratentorial intracerebral haemorrhage in neurosurgical units show no overall benefit from early surgery when compared with initial conservative treatment.

Fig. 6.10 Title page

was determined by the Glasgow Outcome Scale, and other disability scales such as the Barthel Index and Rankin Scale were used. The vast majority of surviving patients were followed for at least 6 months.

Disappointedly, the clinical trial showed no benefit of early surgery versus initial conservative management in patients with a cerebral hemorrhage.

The study included an equal proportion of lobar versus basal ganglia and thalamic hematoma. Volume of the hematoma was on average 40 mL in the early surgery group versus 37 mL in the initial conservative treatment group. Multiple variables were analyzed that included the site of hematoma, volume, depth from cortical surface, deficit of speech or extremity, any thrombolytic or anticoagulant treatment, and also country of origin. The study population had a high mortality, 36% in the early surgery group versus 37% in the initial conservative treatment group. Sixty-seven percent of the early surgery group and 72% of the initial conservation management had an unfavorable Rankin Scale score. The study group had intraventricular hemorrhage (IVH) and acute hydrocephalus in 42%. When a subgroup of patients without IVH or acute hydrocephalus and only superficially (<1 cm from the cortical surface) located lobar hematomas was analyzed, a favorable outcome was found in 39% of conservative group and 49% in surgical group. STICH II (surgical trial in lobar intracerebral hemorrhage) is underway to specifically look at the effect of surgery in such hematomas.

The Message and Acceptance

The STICH trial has reduced any enthusiasm for a preemptive evacuation of deep seated hematomas and, in fact, in any supratentorial cerebral hematoma in a stable patient [114]. Deep seated hematomas do not benefit from evacuation via a traditional open craniotomy that requires dissecting through healthy brain tissue [12, 79, 171]. Some case series and one randomized study indicated that stereotactic surgery could be useful in these cases, but experience in this regard is limited [142].

The STICH study concentrated on initial management of patients who appeared neurologically stable. Deteriorating patients were excluded mostly because they underwent surgery or treatment was not considered. STICH II also is not evaluating the deteriorating patient. We need to keep in mind that trials evaluating surgery in intracerebral hemorrhage typically have not enrolled rapidly deteriorating patients (in fact, "rescue" surgery took place in more than one in four patients randomized to the medical group in STICH). Although outcome is still poor in about 75% of patients, we know that patients with clinical and radiologic signs of brainstem compression or displacement can recover well after emergency evacuation. If those patients have good potential for recovery, surgery should at least be considered.

The STICH investigators were careful to point out that—despite the results of the trial—sizable cerebellar hematomas must be evacuated to avoid obstructive hydrocephalus and brainstem compression, all of which can be fatal or result in irreversible complications. Surgery also is indicated in patients with expanding lobar hematomas and hematomas with underlying vascular anomalies or tumors [117, 119].

Surgical trials in cerebral hematomas may not necessarily impact on practice. Most neurosurgeons will make the arbitrary decision to go ahead with evacuation of the hematoma based on patient's comorbidities, age, coagulation status, neurologic condition at presentation, among other factors. Therefore, if a clinical trial would suggest that a preemptive approach is warranted, the question will remain whether this will be feasible in clinical practice. Most neurosurgeons would want to see some degree of deterioration in order to proceed.

Short Historical Note 46

THERAPEUTIC HYPOTHERMIA AFTER CARDIOPULMONARY RESUSCITATION

The Title of the Paper

The Hypothermia after Cardiac Arrest Study Group. Mild therapeutic hypothermia to improve the neurologic outcome after cardiac arrest. N Engl J Med. 2002; 346:549–56.

Bernard SA, Gray TW, Buist MD, et al. Treatment of comatose survivors of out-of-hospital cardiac arrest with induced hypothermia. N Engl J Med. 2002; 346:557–63.

The Paper and the Times

For many years, little could be done for patients comatose after cardiopulmonary resuscitation (CPR). Not only were earlier trials on neuroprotection unsuccessful, but also the supportive care of the patient following cardiac arrest—often with an acute myocardial infarction—was less clear and not protocolized. One of the first well-organized randomized clinical trials from the Brain Resuscitation Clinical Trial group involved a study on the efficacy of thiopental loading. Presumably, thiopental could lead to a decrease in cerebral metabolic rate or a decrease in cerebral edema. Patients with no purposeful motor response to pain after reestablished systemic circulation were randomly allocated to a thiopental loading dose of 30 mg/kg given intravenously within 10–50 min. Unfortunately, thiopental loading had no benefit on outcome, and high doses resulted in severe hypotension, with many patients thus requiring vasopressors [164].

A second landmark trial was a prehospital IV administration of nimodipine. Again, immediate treatment with calcium channel blockers did not change the neurologic prognosis in patients after out-of-hospital ventricular fibrillation, but recurrent ventricular fibrillation was significantly lower in the nimodipine-treated group [126]. Unfortunately, another trial of the Brain Resuscitation Clinical Trial group using another calcium channel blocker (IV lidoflazine) did not show significant differences in outcome. The future seemed bleak with no potential for improving the often devastating effect of anoxia and ischemia to the brain.

Induced hypothermia has been an age-old treatment for acute brain injury. However, experiments in the 1950s with induced hypothermia showed complications of such intervention, perhaps because temperatures did dip into the 28°C range [14]. A panoply of complications ranged from cardiac arrhythmias (including cardiac arrest) to coagulopathies and infections. Mild hypothermia (33–36°C) did not have these side effects; more easy control of shivering and its use in animal experiments showed still better neurologic outcomes [88, 140]. In hospitals, hypothermia mostly was used to protect the brain during cardiac surgery, but it never reached the intensive care unit (ICU) and even was abandoned from the operating room. A new serious attempt organized in two different centers would appear successful.

The Details of the Paper

Two comparatively small trials were undertaken using superficial cooling of patients for a short period of time (Fig. 6.11 and 6.12). One study coordinated from Vienna and involving nine European hospitals randomized patients into standard intensive care or a hypothermia protocol combined with fentanyl, midazolam, and pancuronium to prevent shivering. Outcome was determined by the Pittsburgh Cerebral Performance Category (a scale almost identical to the Glasgow Outcome Scale, but numbered in reverse), and the investigators decided that favorable outcome was either good recovery or patients with a moderate disability but still able to work. The effect of hypothermia was significant with 55% favorable outcome in the treated group versus 39% in the normothermic group. Mortality also reduced from 55% to 41%. The authors calculated that to prevent one unfavorable outcome, six patients would need treatment, although the confidence interval suggested potentially more patients needed to be treated (i.e., 4 to 25). The second study from Australia, conducted almost in the same time period, was smaller and involved 77 patients in four hospitals, but was not

Fig. 6.11 Title page

The New England Journal of Medicine

VOLUME 346 FEBRUARY 21, 2002 NUMBER 8

MILD THERAPEUTIC HYPOTHERMIA TO IMPROVE THE NEUROLOGIC OUTCOME AFTER CARDIAC ARREST

THE HYPOTHERMIA AFTER CARDIAC ARREST STUDY GROUP*

ABSTRACT

Background Cardiac arrest with widespread cerebral ischemia frequently leads to severe neurologic impairment. We studied whether mild systemic hypothermia increases the rate of neurologic recovery after resuscitation from cardiac arrest due to ventricular fibrillation.

Methods In this multicenter trial with blinded assessment of the outcome, patients who had been resuscitated after cardiac arrest due to ventricular fibrillation were randomly assigned to undergo therapeutic hypothermia (target temperature, 32°C to 34°C, measured in the bladder) over a period of 24 hours or to receive standard treatment with normothermia. The primary end point was a favorable neurologic outcome within six months after cardiac arrest; secondary end points were mortality within six months and the rate of complications within seven days.

Results Seventy-five of the 136 patients in the hypothermia group for whom data were available (55 percent) had a favorable neurologic outcome (cerebral-performance category, 1 [good recovery] or 2 [moderate disability]), as compared with 54 of 137 (39 percent) in the normothermia group (risk ratio, 1.40; 95 percent confidence interval, 1.08 to 1.81). Mortality at six months was 41 percent in the hypothermia group (56 of 137 patients died), as compared with 55 percent in the normothermia group (76 of 138 patients; risk ratio, 0.74; 95 percent confidence interval, 0.58 to 0.95). The complication rate did not differ significantly between the two groups.

Conclusions In patients who have been successfully resuscitated after cardiac arrest due to ventricular fibrillation, therapeutic mild hypothermia increased the rate of a favorable neurologic outcome and reduced mortality. (N Engl J Med 2002;346:549-56.)

An estimated 375,000 people in Europe undergo sudden cardiac arrest yearly.[1] Recovery without residual neurologic damage after cardiac arrest with global cerebral ischemia is rare. After cardiac arrest with no blood flow for more than five minutes, the generation of free radicals, together with other mediators, during reperfusion creates chemical cascades that result in cerebral injury.[2] Until recently, there was no therapy with documented efficacy in preventing brain damage after cardiac arrest.

Several studies have shown that moderate systemic hypothermia (30°C)[3] or mild hypothermia (34°C)[4-8] markedly mitigates brain damage after cardiac arrest in dogs. The exact mechanism for this cerebral resuscitative effect is not clear. A reduction in cerebral oxygen consumption[9,10] and other multifactorial chemical and physical mechanisms during and after ischemia have been postulated.[11-16] These include retardation of destructive enzymatic reactions, suppression of free-radical reactions, protection of the fluidity of lipoprotein membranes, reduction of the oxygen demand in low-flow regions, reduction of intracellular acidosis, and inhibition of the biosynthesis, release, and uptake of excitatory neurotransmitters.

Preliminary clinical studies have shown that patients treated with mild hypothermia after cardiac arrest have an improved neurologic outcome, without important side effects, as compared with the outcome in historical controls.[17-20]

We compared mild hypothermia with standard normothermia in patients who had had cardiac arrest due to ventricular fibrillation. The primary end point

TREATMENT OF COMATOSE SURVIVORS OF OUT-OF-HOSPITAL CARDIAC ARREST WITH INDUCED HYPOTHERMIA

STEPHEN A. BERNARD, M.B., B.S., TIMOTHY W. GRAY, M.B., B.S., MICHAEL D. BUIST, M.B., B.S., BRUCE M. JONES, M.B., B.S., WILLIAM SILVESTER, M.B., B.S., GEOFF GUTTERIDGE, M.B., B.S., AND KAREN SMITH, B.SC.

ABSTRACT

Background Cardiac arrest outside the hospital is common and has a poor outcome. Studies in laboratory animals suggest that hypothermia induced shortly after the restoration of spontaneous circulation may improve neurologic outcome, but there have been no conclusive studies in humans. In a randomized, controlled trial, we compared the effects of moderate hypothermia and normothermia in patients who remained unconscious after resuscitation from out-of-hospital cardiac arrest.

Methods The study subjects were 77 patients who were randomly assigned to treatment with hypothermia (with the core body temperature reduced to 33°C within 2 hours after the return of spontaneous circulation and maintained at that temperature for 12 hours) or normothermia. The primary outcome measure was survival to hospital discharge with sufficiently good neurologic function to be discharged to home or to a rehabilitation facility.

Results The demographic characteristics of the patients were similar in the hypothermia and normothermia groups. Twenty-one of the 43 patients treated with hypothermia (49 percent) survived and had a good outcome — that is, they were discharged home or to a rehabilitation facility — as compared with 9 of the 34 treated with normothermia (26 percent, $P=0.046$). After adjustment for base-line differences in age and time from collapse to the return of spontaneous circulation, the odds ratio for a good outcome with hypothermia as compared with normothermia was 5.25 (95 percent confidence interval, 1.47 to 18.76; $P=0.011$). Hypothermia was associated with a lower cardiac index, higher systemic vascular resistance, and hyperglycemia. There was no difference in the frequency of adverse events.

Conclusions Our preliminary observations suggest that treatment with moderate hypothermia appears to improve outcomes in patients with coma after resuscitation from out-of-hospital cardiac arrest. (N Engl J Med 2002;346:557-63.)

Currently, the treatment of patients with coma after resuscitation from out-of-hospital cardiac arrest is largely supportive. Because cerebral ischemia may persist for some hours after resuscitation,[5] the use of induced hypothermia to decrease cerebral oxygen demand has been proposed as a treatment option.[6] Although this suggestion has been supported by studies in animal models,[7-12] the studies in humans that have been reported to date have been uncontrolled or retrospective.[13-18]

After a pilot study that suggested the feasibility, safety, and possible efficacy of this treatment,[16] we conducted a prospective, controlled trial comparing moderate induced hypothermia with normothermia in comatose survivors of out-of-hospital cardiac arrest.

METHODS

Study Design

The study was performed in Melbourne, Australia, between September 1996 and June 1999. The ambulance service has treatment protocols that follow the recommendations of the Australian Resuscitation Council.[19] Patients were enrolled in the study when the following criteria were fulfilled: an initial cardiac rhythm of ventricular fibrillation at the time of arrival of the ambulance, successful return of spontaneous circulation, persistent coma after the return of spontaneous circulation, and transfer to one of four participating emergency departments. The exclusion criteria were an age of less than 18 years for men, an age of less than 50 years for women (because of the possibility of pregnancy), cardiogenic shock (a systolic blood pressure of less than 90 mm Hg despite epinephrine infusion), or possible causes of coma other than cardiac arrest (drug overdose, head trauma, or cerebrovascular accident). Patients were also excluded if an intensive care bed was not available at a participating institution.

After the return of spontaneous circulation had been accomplished outside the hospital, eligible patients were randomly assigned to hypothermia or normothermia according to the day of the month, with patients assigned to hypothermia on odd-numbered days. For these patients, the paramedics began measures in the field to initiate hypothermia by removing the patient's clothing and applying cold packs (CoolCare, Cheltenham, Victoria, Australia) to the patient's head and torso. The treatment of patients assigned to normothermia followed usual prehospital treatment protocols.

On arrival at a participating emergency department, the patients underwent routine initial assessment and treatment, includ-

Fig. 6.12 Title page

randomized and assigned according to the day of the month with odd numbers for hypothermia. This study found favorable outcome in 26% of the normothermia group and 49% in the hypothermia group. Both studies were not blinded.

The Message and Acceptance

The supportive editorial by Safar and Kochanek—both strong proponents of hypothermia—and general enthusiastic responses in the ICU community created a major surge in this treatment. Endorsement by the International Liaison Committee on Resuscitation and the American Heart Association and the Society of Critical Care Medicine followed [7, 9, 105]. There has been—perhaps surprisingly—very little objection to therapeutic hypothermia, but some problems have been identified. This involved uncertainty whether level of coma was equally distributed and early termination of both trials without power calculations [103, 104].

A recent Cochrane analysis—the authors were principal investigators of the Austrian trial—found sufficient evidence to recommend therapeutic hypothermia in comatose patients after out-of-hospital arrest and CPR for ventricular fibrillation. There has been—in general—an acceptance that short-term hypothermia could help some patients and many critical care units have protocols in place. The treatment spawned an avalanche of papers—mostly reviews with more or less clever titles ("time to chill," "cool new treatment"). Some US states have ambulances that only bring patients after CPR to hospitals with an ICU that have hypothermia protocols.

Patients may benefit from therapeutic hypothermia, but despite recommendation by professional organizations, the practice of therapeutic hypothermia remains underused in academic and tertiary centers. Overall, early on therapeutic hypothermia is applied to possibly only 40% of all patients with out-of-hospital arrests even in hospitals with existing protocols. Nonetheless, studies have shown a steep learning curve with use in up to 85% of patients with shockable rhythms. One possible reason for failure to implement induced hypothermia protocols could be failure to accept published data as conclusive. It has been argued that in the absence of detailed neurologic examination at presentation, the effectiveness of randomization in the hypothermia trials remains unproven, and some institutions could not document improved survival [103, 111]. Another reason may be that the high cost of effective cooling devices and associated services is prohibitive to proceed with such a protocol. The time to reach target temperature of 33–34°C differs between studies and may be important. It was 8 h on average in the European multicenter trial, 2 h in the Australian trial, and 4 h in a large multinational registry study of 982 consecutive patients.

A recent large cohort of therapeutic hypothermia in 1,145 patients with out-of-hospital arrest from multiple hospitals in Paris confirmed better neurologic outcome in patients with shockable rhythms, but not in patients with nonshockable rhythms (asystole and pulseless electrical activity). Even a trend toward worse outcome was noted in this subset of patients [45].

Most cooling techniques employ cooling pads with embedded circulating water tubes. Shivering is suppressed with sedation and paralytic agents. Hypothermia (32–34°C) is maintained for 24 h followed by controlled rewarming at 0.5°C/h.

Postresuscitation encephalopathy often is devastating and results in prolonged coma or severe disability in the majority of patients [104]. There is now encouraging data that outcome can be improved with early hypothermia treatment, but likely only for a few less severely affected patients.

Short Historical Note 47

NIMODIPINE IN ANEURYSMAL SUBARACHNOID HEMORRHAGE

The Title of the Paper

Allen GS, Ahn HS, Preziosi TJ, et al. Cerebral arterial spasm – a controlled trial of nimodipine in patients with subarachnoid hemorrhage. N Engl J Med. 1983;308: 619–24.

Pickard JD, Murray GD, Illingworth R, et al. Effect of oral nimodipine on cerebral infarction and outcome after subarachnoid hemorrhage: British aneurysm nimodipine trial. BMJ. 1989;298:636–42.

The Paper and the Times

Before calcium channel blockers were considered in randomized prospective clinical trials, experimental studies had discovered that calcium antagonists such as nimodipine had a moderate vasodilatory effect [32, 43]. Nimodipine, therefore, became an interesting study drug to investigate for its potential for reducing cerebral infarction after subarachnoid hemorrhage as a result of cerebral vasospasm [43, 64]. When primates were studied, neither the severity of the vasospasm nor the incidence was reduced. But in rats and cats when the drug was given before occlusion of a cerebral artery the size of the infarcts was markedly attenuated.

Most experimental work on calcium antagonists can be credited to neurosurgeon George Allen and his coworkers from the Department of Neurosurgery, University of Minnesota [5, 6]. In dogs, subarachnoid injection of blood produced cerebral vasospasm. Sublingual nifedipine reversed both acute and chronic cerebral vasospasm and even could prevent it when administered preemptively [5]. In cats, IV administration of nimodipine produced 25% dilatation of the pial arteries more prominently in small arteries [10]. Unfortunately, high doses of IV nimodipine caused a marked in blood pressure [5].

Furthermore, it was found that [3H] nimodipine did bind frontal cortex and that the binding site was regulated by calcium [110]. Topically applied nimodipine during clipping of an aneurysm also caused visible vasodilation, but mostly in small vessels [11].

With these data, there was sufficient underpinning for a large-scale clinical trial.

The Details of the Paper

The first study was performed by Allen et al. in 1983 (Fig. 6.13). The trial investigators also were interested in examining whether nimodipine could have an effect on cerebral infarction due to causes other than vasospasm. The study suggested that nimodipine could impact on outcome, but the trial was small and largely a selection of patients with cerebral ischemia from cerebral vasospasm [3]. The study enrolled 125 patients with intracranial aneurysm; patients were enrolled within 96 h after their subarachnoid hemorrhage. The study found that at 21 days of treatment, 8 of the 60 patients given placebo, and 1 of the 56 patients given nimodipine had a neurologic deficit from cerebral arterial spasm. Side effects were not noted. The study also remarkably found that a large amount of subarachnoid blood on computed tomography (CT) scan did not negatively impact on the effect of nimodipine.

Pickard and coinvestigators studied a much larger group of 554 patients recruited in 3 years from multiple British centers (Fig. 6.14). This study confirmed Allen's study that oral nimodipine 60 mg every 4 h was well tolerated and reduced cerebral infarction. Additionally, outcome was better in treated patients. The benefit of nimodipine, however, was relatively small, reducing cerebral infarction on CT scan from 33% to 22%. However, poor outcome was reduced by 40% (poor outcome in 20% of nimodipine-treated placebo and 33% in patients given placebo). The Pickard study noted reduction in blood pressure with the use of nimodipine, but reported no adverse effects.

The Message and Acceptance

Oral nimodipine has become a standard treatment in aneurysmal subarachnoid hemorrhage. Calcium antagonists do not influence rebleeding rate, but studies included patients with clipped aneurysms. Nimodipine may block calcium influx and may act on smaller perforating arteries rather than larger cerebral arteries [110]. Transcranial Doppler and angiography have never found a significant

Fig. 6.13 Title page

CEREBRAL ARTERIAL SPASM — A CONTROLLED TRIAL OF NIMODIPINE IN PATIENTS WITH SUBARACHNOID HEMORRHAGE

George S. Allen, M.D., Ph.D., Hyo S. Ahn, M.D., Thomas J. Preziosi, M.D., Roy Battye, M.B., Ch.B., Stephen C. Boone, M.D., Ph.D., Shelley N. Chou, M.D., Ph.D., David L. Kelly, M.D., Bryce K. Weir, M.D., Ruth A. Crabbe, R.N., M.S.N., Paula J. Lavik, R.N., Shelley B. Rosenbloom, M.D., Frank C. Dorsey, Ph.D., Charles R. Ingram, Ph.D., David E. Mellits, Sc.D., Linda A. Bertsch, R.N., Donald P. J. Boisvert, M.D., Mary B. Hundley, R.N., M.S., Rayetta K. Johnson, R.N., Jo A. Strom, R.N., and Carole R. Transou, R.N.

Abstract We enrolled 125 neurologically normal patients with intracranial aneurysms in a multi-institution, prospective, double-blind, randomized, placebo-controlled trial within 96 hours of their subarachnoid hemorrhage, to determine whether treatment with the calcium blocker nimodipine would prevent or reduce the severity of ischemic neurologic deficits from arterial spasm. A deficit from cerebral arterial spasm that persisted and was severe or caused death by the end of the 21-day treatment period occurred in 8 of 60 patients given placebo and in 1 of 56 given nimodipine ($P = 0.03$, Fisher's exact test). Analysis of the amount of basal subarachnoid blood on pre-entry CAT scans in patients with deficits from spasm showed that an increase in subarachnoid blood was not associated with a worse neurologic outcome among patients who received nimodipine, unlike the situation in patients given a placebo. There were no side effects from nimodipine. We conclude that nimodipine should be given to patients who are neurologically normal after subarachnoid hemorrhage in order to reduce the occurrence of severe neurologic deficits due to cerebral arterial spasm. (N Engl J Med. 1983; 308:619-24.)

THE patient who survives the initial subarachnoid hemorrhage from an intracranial aneurysm remains at risk during the next three weeks because of recurrent hemorrhage and cerebral arterial spasm. Recurrent hemorrhage is effectively treated by clipping the aneurysm. Cerebral arterial spasm is focal or diffuse narrowing of one or more of the large arteries at the base of the brain and is usually demonstrated by angiography. Spasm occurs frequently between 4 and 14 days after the subarachnoid hemorrhage and is thought to cause ischemic neurologic deficits.[1,2] If the initial event in the development of this spasm is the contraction of smooth-muscle cells in the large cerebral arteries, then a drug that inhibits these contractions should prevent these neurologic deficits. To be effective, such a drug must also cross the blood–brain barrier in order to reach the cerebral arterial smooth-muscle cells. Its inhibitory effect should be selective and not affect the contractions of systemic arteries to the extent that severe hypotension occurs.[3] Previous experiments conducted by one of us (G.S.A.) in animals suggested that nimodipine might meet these requirements.[4-6] Nimodipine is a substituted 1,4-dihydropyridine that is lipid soluble and therefore should cross the blood–brain barrier. Its inhibition is selective because as a "calcium antagonist," it blocks the influx of extracellular calcium, the primary source of calcium for contraction of large cerebral arteries, whereas some systemic arteries use intracellular calcium for contraction.[7] Nimodipine was chosen for the present study because it was more potent in animals than its more commonly known analogue, nifedipine.

The objective of our prospective, randomized, double-blind, placebo-controlled trial of nimodipine was to test its effectiveness in preventing or altering the severity of ischemic neurologic deficits due to spasm. Only patients who were neurologically normal according to study criteria were entered, so that the development of a neurologic deficit could be accurately determined. A subarachnoid hemorrhage from an aneurysm had to have occurred within the 96 hours before treatment, so that all patients in the study were at risk for spasm. We found that nimodipine significantly reduced the occurrence of severe neurologic deficits from spasm. This report discusses the results at the end of the 21-day treatment period.

METHODS

Organization

Five university centers were responsible for recruiting, treating, and following patients between December 1979 and June 1982. Definitions of entry criteria, evaluation of patients during treatment, medical and surgical management, and outcome criteria were predetermined and specified in a protocol manual. A clinical-investigation committee at each institution approved the study protocol. Everyone involved in the study was blinded with respect to the allocation of placebo and nimodipine.

Study Population and Pre-entry Evaluation

Patients of both sexes and all races who met the following criteria were entered: age between 15 and 80 years; subarachnoid hemorrhage within 96 hours of the start of study medication; and normal results on a neurologic examination performed just before the start of medication, except for the following findings: a stiff neck, headache, fever or photophobia; drowsiness but with orientation at least to person, city, and year; or the presence of isolated cranial-nerve palsies. Pre-entry evaluation consisted of CAT scanning, documentation of a subarachnoid hemorrhage by either CAT scanning or cerebrospinal-fluid examination, and demonstration of an intracranial aneurysm by angiography.

From the Departments of Neurosurgery, Neurology, and Neuroradiology, Johns Hopkins Medical Institutions, Baltimore; and the Departments of Neurosurgery, University of Alberta (Alberta, Canada); Bowman-Gray School of Medicine (Winston-Salem, N.C.); University of North Carolina (Chapel Hill, N.C.); and University of Minnesota (Minneapolis). Address reprint requests to Dr. Allen at the Department of Neurosurgery, Meyer 5-181, Johns Hopkins Hospital, 600 N. Wolfe St., Baltimore, MD 21205.

Supported by a research grant from Miles Pharmaceuticals (West Haven, Conn.).

Effect of oral nimodipine on cerebral infarction and outcome after subarachnoid haemorrhage: British aneurysm nimodipine trial

J D Pickard, G D Murray, R Illingworth, M D M Shaw, G M Teasdale, P M Foy, P R D Humphrey, D A Lang, R Nelson, P Richards, J Sinar, S Bailey, A Skene

Wessex Neurological Centre, Southampton General Hospital, Southampton SO9 4XY
J D Pickard, MCHIR, *professor of clinical neurological sciences*
R Nelson, FRCS, *senior registrar in neurosurgery*
S Bailey, RGN, *Medical Research Council research sister*

Medical Statistics Unit, Department of Surgery, University of Glasgow, Glasgow G11 6NT
G D Murray, PHD, *senior lecturer in medical statistics*

Regional Neurosciences Centre, Charing Cross Hospital, London W6 8RF
R Illingworth, FRCS, *consultant neurosurgeon*
P Richards, FRCS, *consultant neurosurgeon*

Mersey Regional Department of Medical and Surgical Neurology, Walton Hospital, Liverpool L9 1AE
M D M Shaw, FRCS, *consultant neurosurgeon*
P M Foy, FRCS, *consultant neurosurgeon*
P R D Humphrey, MRCP, *consultant neurologist*

Institute of Neurological Sciences, Southern General Hospital, Glasgow G51 4TF
G M Teasdale, FRCS, *professor of neurosurgery*
D A Lang, FRCS, *registrar in neurosurgery*
J Sinar, FRCS, *registrar in neurosurgery*

Abstract

Objective—To determine the efficacy of oral nimodipine in reducing cerebral infarction and poor outcomes (death and severe disability) after subarachnoid haemorrhage.

Design—Double blind, placebo controlled, randomised trial with three months of follow up and intention to treat analysis. To have an 80% chance with a significance level of 0·05 of detecting a 50% reduction in an incidence of cerebral infarction of 15% a minimum of 540 patients was required.

Setting—Four regional neurosurgical units in the United Kingdom.

Patients—In all 554 patients were recruited between June 1985 and September 1987 out of a population of 1115 patients admitted with subarachnoid haemorrhage proved by the results of lumbar puncture or computed tomography, or both. The main exclusion criterion was admission to the neurosurgical units more than 96 hours after subarachnoid haemorrhage. There were four breaks of code and no exclusions after entry. One patient was withdrawn and in 130 treatment was discontinued early. All patients were followed up for three months and were included in the analysis, except the patient who had been withdrawn.

Interventions—Placebo or nimodipine 60 mg was given orally every four hours for 21 days to 276 and 278 patients, respectively. Treatment was started within 96 hours after subarachnoid haemorrhage.

End points—Incidence of cerebral infarction and ischaemic neurological deficits and outcome three months after entry.

Measurements—Demographic and clinical data, including age, sex, history of hypertension and subarachnoid haemorrhage, severity of haemorrhage according to an adaptation of the Glasgow coma scale, number and site of aneurysms on angiography, and initial findings on computed tomography were measured at entry. Deterioration, defined as development of a focal sign or fall of more than one point on the Glasgow coma scale for more than six hours, was investigated by using clinical criteria and by computed tomography, by lumbar puncture, or at necropsy when appropriate. All episodes of deterioration and all patients with a three month outcome other than a good recovery were assessed by a review committee.

Conclusions—Oral nimodipine 60 mg four hourly is well tolerated and reduces cerebral infarction and improves outcome after subarachnoid haemorrhage.

Introduction

Despite advances that have reduced considerably the risks of operation to secure a ruptured cerebral aneurysm the overall mortality and morbidity during the management of patients with subarachnoid haemorrhage who have survived and not been devastated by the initial ictus has not fallen dramatically. This is mainly because such patients rebleed and have delayed cerebral ischaemia. The management dilemma remains the need to weigh the risk of precipitating cerebral ischaemia by operation against that of rebleeding while awaiting surgery.

Subarachnoid haemorrhage provides the clearest clinical opportunity for pretreating ischaemia, but, although the calcium antagonist nimodipine has been reported to reduce the incidence of delayed cerebral ischaemia after subarachnoid haemorrhage,[1,2] definitive evidence is lacking. Previous trials were small and relied on selecting a subgroup of patients with cerebral ischaemia presumed to be due to cerebral vasospasm. Ischaemia may be the result of several factors[3-5] and cannot be attributed simply to an exaggerated contraction of cerebral arteries (vasospasm); thus defining such a subgroup is difficult and ignores any potential benefit of treatment in other causes of ischaemia.

Nimodipine has various effects on the cerebral circulation, not all of which may be beneficial. Cerebrovascular smooth muscle is more sensitive than systemic arterial smooth muscle to changes in extracellular calcium concentration and to calcium antagonists such as nimodipine.[6-8] In addition to being a moderate cerebral vasodilator, however, nimodipine impairs cerebrovascular reactivity.[9-11] Nimodipine does not reduce the incidence or severity of cerebral vasospasm detected by angiography in humans or primates,[12-17] but it reduces the size of cerebral infarcts in rats when given before but not after occlusion of a cerebral artery.[18]

We therefore conducted a prospective trial to establish the effect of nimodipine on the incidence of both ischaemic events and proved cerebral infarction and on outcome after subarachnoid haemorrhage.

Fig. 6.14 Title page

difference between nimodipine-treated patients and placebo-treated patients. Nimodipine also may reduce the severity of infarction by reducing size and by increasing fibrinolytic activity decreasing microthrombi [127]. Currently, there is interest in using nimodipine intra-arterially because of its potent vasodilatory effect [65, 167]. Moreover, intra-arterial nimodipine did show improvement on CT perfusion scans. Selective intra-arterial nimodipine has resulted in marked improvement in patients with refractory cerebral vasospasm without a sudden decrease in blood pressure.

In 1988, Flamm and coworkers published a dose-escalation trial using nicardipine infusions particularly because the drug was more often used for cerebral vasospasm in Japan and because oral drugs were more difficult to use in critically ill comatose patients [48]. Nicardipine is highly protein-bound in plasma and rapidly penetrates the brain. This led to a large placebo-controlled study by Clarke Haley [61, 62]. A marked reduction in angiographic vasospasm was found (51% vs. 33%), and a follow-up trial comparing a high dose with a low dose in 365 patients found less side effects in the low dose 0.075 mg/kg/h group but no difference in 3-month outcome [63]. A Cochrane analysis of seven clinical trials found that nimodipine reduces poor outcome (approximately 50%) given orally, but again there is no evidence that IV administration impacts on outcome [123].

There are very few candidate drugs that could potentially reverse the spasm in vasospasm. Our understanding of this complication after aneurysmal subarachnoid hemorrhage may move beyond the mechanistic explanation of smooth muscle contraction, and other mechanism (e.g., cortical spreading depression [91]) may play a role that could lead to new approaches. Moreover, management of these patients constantly changes and likely is now different from when these studies were performed.

Short Historical Note 48

ANTIFIBRINOLYTIC TREATMENT IN SUBARACHNOID HEMORRHAGE

The Title of the Paper

Vermeulen M, Lindsay KW, Murray GD, et al. Antifibrinolytic treatment in subarachnoid hemorrhage. N Engl J Med. 1984;311:432–7.

The Paper and the Times

A considerably better understanding of the management of aneurysmal subarachnoid hemorrhage (SAH) emerged in the early 1980s. The availability of computed tomography (CT) scanning—the first CT scanning in the United States was performed in 1973—dramatically improved recognition with first reports of CT patterns in SAH appearing in 1976 [83]. Complications of surgery, rebleeding, cerebral vasospasm, and acute hydrocephalus were well known to neurosurgeons and neurologists. Patients were categorized into a specific grade, and several systems were available (e.g., Botterell, Hunt and Hess) that not only identified patients eligible for surgery but also indicated prognosis. In the Hunt and Hess—system of five levels, a grade V indicated deep coma, decerebrate rigidity, and poor prognosis.

The potential harm of early surgical repair of the aneurysm during this time epoch was a major topic of debate, and most neurosurgeons opted for operating late. There was a sense that early surgery (in the first days after the ictus) resulted in higher operative mortality and morbidity. Typically, patients were admitted to intermediate or intensive care units (ICUs), and surgery was planned 2 weeks after the ictus. Such an approach warranted medical intervention of complications and prevention of rebleeding in particular.

Neurosurgeon Gibbs from Brook General Hospital in London published a case–control series in 1967 of 32 patients treated with an oral dose of ε-aminocaproic acid. The underlying premise of using antifibrinolytic treatment was summarized as follows: "the primary sealing of the hole in an aneurysm wall by a platelet plug, at first permeable to red cells, may be assumed responsible for the initial stemming of the leak within, say 4 min. Cells infiltrate the plug and the complex process of building a clot commences."

Rebleeding remained a poorly understood process, but Gibbs speculated that platelet adhesiveness, blood viscosity, and local fibrinogen could play a role. "It seems certain, however, that there is both continual building up and absorption of clot going on simultaneously—the laying down of fibrin and formed elements on the one hand, and fibrinolysis with digestion on the other. Perhaps, one of these ceases too soon or another too late [55]." His study did not show improved outcome, but he suggested that whole blood clot lysis time could be manipulated. Before 1984, 14 clinical trials had been published on antifibrinolytic drugs, but all had—by new strict statistical standards—methodological problems [155].

The Details of the Paper

A multicenter clinical trial was conducted from 1977 to 1982 (Fig. 6.15). A total of 479 patients with a SAH—seen within 72 hours after onset—were eligible for randomization into placebo or tranexamic acid. Patients were treated for 28 days with 6 g daily in the first week and 4 g/day in the remaining weeks. Treatment was continued until surgical clipping, but discontinued if the cerebral angiogram was normal. In contrast to prior studies, this clinical trial operated with strict CT scan or autopsy definitions of SAH, rebleeding, and delayed cerebral ischemia. Outcome was assessed with the Glasgow Outcome Scale.

The study found that the rate of rebleeding was reduced by more than 60% (24% in control group vs. 9% in the treated group). Cerebral infarction increased significantly from 27% in the placebo group to 45% in the tranexamic acid group, resulting in no overall improvement of outcome. The incidence of cerebral infarction started to diverge on day 6 of the treatment, suggesting a negative effect of the drug in the "vasospasm period." It was speculated that antifibrinolytic therapy could lend to thrombi formation in vasospastic arteries. The study concluded that "until some method can be found to minimize ischemic complications, tranexamic

ANTIFIBRINOLYTIC TREATMENT IN SUBARACHNOID HEMORRHAGE

M. Vermeulen, K. W. Lindsay, G. D. Murray, F. Cheah, A. Hijdra, J. P. Muizelaar, M. Schannong, G. M. Teasdale, H. van Crevel, and J. van Gijn

Abstract We enrolled 479 patients with subarachnoid hemorrhage in a multicenter, randomized, double-blind, placebo-controlled trial to determine whether treatment with the antifibrinolytic agent tranexamic acid improves outcome by preventing rebleeding. At three months there was no statistical difference between the outcomes in the tranexamic acid group and the control group. Of the 173 patients who died, 84 had received tranexamic acid and 89 placebo (95 per cent confidence interval for the difference in mortality rate, −6 to 11 per cent). Similarly, when analysis was restricted to patients with an angiographically demonstrated aneurysm, there was no significant difference between the groups. This absence of effect was not due to a lack of antifibrinolytic action, since the rate of rebleeding was reduced from 24 per cent in the control group to 9 per cent in the tranexamic acid-treated group (chi-square = 18.07, $P<0.001$), but resulted from a concurrent increase in the incidence of ischemic complications (15 per cent in the control group and 24 per cent in the tranexamic acid group; chi-square = 8.07, $P<0.01$). We conclude that until some method can be found to minimize ischemic complications, tranexamic acid is of no benefit in patients with subarachnoid hemorrhage. (N Engl J Med 1984; 311:432-7.)

PATIENTS who survive subarachnoid hemorrhage from a ruptured intracranial aneurysm have high mortality and morbidity from associated complications in the following weeks. Of these complications, rebleeding and cerebral ischemia are the most important.[1,2] Rebleeding has been attributed to fibrinolysis of the blood clot around the fundus of the aneurysm.[3] Antifibrinolytic agents have been used since 1967 to inhibit this dissolution,[4,5] but the varying attitudes toward the value of this treatment reflect the lack of convincing evidence from clinical studies so far.[6-8]

We studied the effect of the antifibrinolytic drug tranexamic acid in a randomized, double-blind trial. The design and conduct of this trial took account of the contrasts between "pragmatic" and "explanatory" studies[9] and of the need to study sufficient numbers of patients to detect or exclude a clinically important effect.[10] We aimed to determine whether, in practical, clinical circumstances, antifibrinolytic treatment led to improved functional outcome.

Methods

The trial began in November 1977 in Rotterdam, in October 1979 in Amsterdam, in October 1980 in Glasgow, and in January 1982 in London, and ended in all four centers on December 31, 1982.

Criteria for Eligibility

Patients eligible for this study were admitted to one of the centers, with symptoms and signs of subarachnoid hemorrhage and with confirmatory evidence on the initial CT scan or in the cerebrospinal fluid. If the CT scan was negative and therefore doubt existed about whether an aneurysm had ruptured,[11] angiography was carried out before randomization. Reasons for exclusion were a lapse of 72 hours since the presenting hemorrhage; the presence of deep-vein thrombosis, coagulation disorders, renal insufficiency, or pregnancy; previous treatment with antifibrinolytic agents; CT-scan evidence of a cause other than aneurysm; or negative angiography carried out before randomization (see above). If death appeared imminent, entry was delayed.

Randomization

Using random-number tables,[10] the pharmaceutical manufacturer supplied each center with boxes containing phials or tablets for a complete four-week course of either tranexamic acid or placebo. Each batch of six boxes was balanced with respect to the two treatments. The boxes were numbered consecutively, and their contents were administered to eligible patients in that order. For each patient the trial period commenced on opening the treatment box. The phials or tablets were marked only with the trial number. The trial code was broken in May 1983, after all events and outcomes had been recorded.

Treatment

Treatment was always started within 72 hours after the hemorrhage. The maximum duration of treatment was four weeks. In Rotterdam and Amsterdam the drugs were administered by intra-

From the Department of Neurology, University Hospital, Rotterdam; the Department of Neurosurgery, Royal Free Hospital, London; the Department of Statistics, University of Glasgow, and the Department of Neurosurgery, Institute of Neurological Sciences, The Southern General Hospital, Glasgow; the Research Department, Kabi AB, Stockholm; and the Departments of Neurology and Neurosurgery, Academisch Medisch Centrum, Amsterdam. Address reprint requests to Dr. Vermeulen at the Department of Neurology, University Hospital Dijkzigt, 40 Dr. Molewaterplein, 3015 GD Rotterdam, The Netherlands.

Supported by the Dutch Heart Foundation.

Fig. 6.15 Title page

acid is of no benefit in patients with subarachnoid hemorrhage."

The study investigators also commented on other factors. First, the lack of calcium channel antagonist administration (the beneficial effect of nimodipine was published just after completion of this study. Second, the need for more aggressive fluid management in prevention of delayed cerebral ischemia rather than fluid restriction and third, the use of antihypertensives, which might have resulted in a less than adequate cerebral perfusion pressure.

The Message and Acceptance

Long-term antifibrinolytic therapy in aneurysmal SAH worked well but to no avail. The drug—with its thrombotic characteristics—was administered during the critical vasospasm period usually starting after 3–4 days. Therefore, this clinical trial was followed—logically so—with a pilot study using a shorter course (4 days) of antifibrinolytic treatment. The results of this series of 119 patients treated between 1986 and 1987 were compared with the patient's outcomes from the previous randomized trial. Disappointedly, with this short treatment of tranexamic acid, the rate of rebleeding increased and approached the placebo rate in the double-blind controlled long-term treatment trial. The incidence of cerebral infarction did not decrease [165].

A Cochrane review in 2003 concluded that nine clinical trials (involving more than 1,000 patients) were conducted, with eight trials using either IV tranexamic acid (4–9 g daily) or oral ε-aminocaproic acid (24 g/day), but showing no impact on outcome despite reduction in rebleeding rate [128]. These trials have been considered problematic because patients were treated as late as 4 days after the hemorrhage excluding many patients who could additionally benefit from early treatment. Several studies and a more recent review of all clinical trials suggested that a short, ultra-early treatment in combination with early repair of the aneurysm—within 2 days of presentation—could reduce rebleeding rate and without negatively impacting on other complications [66, 68, 138].

Early endovascular treatment of intracranial aneurysms has changed the overall picture [113]. Delayed cerebral ischemia has been markedly reduced in good grade patients treated with endovascular coil embolization, and in this patient population the benefit of reduction of rebleeding might be greatest. It is questionable whether a new clinical trial will be performed, and many neurosurgical practices administer several doses of antifibrinolytic agents while planning for virtually immediate surgery or coiling. The pendulum has shifted again to favor its use, although this time, its administration is very short.

Short Historical Note 49

INTRA-ARTERIAL THROMBOLYSIS IN STROKE

The Title of the Paper

del Zoppo GJ, Ferbert A, Otis S, et al. Local intra-arterial fibrinolytic therapy in acute carotid territory stroke. Stroke. 1988;19:307–13.

Hacke W, Zeumer H, Ferbert A, Bruckmann H, del Zoppo GJ. Intra-arterial thrombolytic therapy improves outcome in patients with acute vertebrobasilar occlusive disease. Stroke. 1988;19:1216–22.

The Paper and the Times

Before thrombolysis became available in acute ischemic stroke [1], their efficacy was proven in acute coronary syndromes. Although thrombolytic drugs due to its potent clot dissolving effect could lead to unwanted hemorrhages—in the brain and elsewhere—an overall benefit was sought for patients with a potentially devastating stroke [38, 39]. Using certain thrombolytics using intravenous (IV) or intra-arterial (IA) routes might help some and hopefully not worsen too many patients. Previous attempts to surgically open an acute carotid or basilar artery occlusion were unsuccessful and commonly nothing but catastrophic.

The initial trials with IV thrombolytic agents (urokinase and streptokinase) in acute stroke were disappointing. However, after a tissue plasminogen activator (tPA) study showed favorable outcome in 30–50% of treated patients with IV treatment 3 h after onset—compared with 20–38% of patients treated with placebo—the FDA approved its use in 1996 [145]. These results were confirmed by the European Cooperative Acute Stroke Study (ECAS) I and II trials [59].

Patients with major strokes (e.g., National Institutes of Health Stroke Scale [NIHSS] scores of ≥22 or higher) had less benefit from IV tPA, and many patients "missed the window", therefore researchers sought to establish whether systemic administration could have a more dramatic effect. In these nonresponders and non-eligible patients, other more aggressive options were considered. Studies exploring the IA and IV routes, however, developed virtually parallel with each other.

The IA administration of thrombolytics surfaced as an option when endovascular techniques improved. With more skilled interventional neuroradiologists, the question came up whether IA administration could not be tried in the more severely affected patients. Improvement in delivery systems was also needed to guarantee local infusion right into the clot. Earlier studies involved fairly simple catheters with multiple openings for more efficient drug administration. Concerns about transforming bland cerebral infarcts into swollen hemorrhagic masses from acute reperfusion dominated the clinical research at the time, and there was little, if any, enthusiasm.

The Details of the Paper

Two papers described the use of IA thrombolysis in a substantial number of patients (Fig. 6.16). The studies were a collaboration between the Rheinische–Westfalische Technische Hochshule in Aachen Germany and the Scripps Clinic and Research Foundation. Both papers published in 1988 described encouraging results after IA infusion with urokinase or streptokinase. In 3 years, 20 patients with acute "carotid territory ischemia" were subjected to cerebral angiography within 8 h of presentation. Occlusions were documented in the internal carotid artery siphon ($n=2$) carotid artery T segment ($n=3$), internal carotid and middle cerebral artery ($n=3$), middle cerebral artery stem or branch ($n=11$), and posterior cerebral artery ($n=1$). Complete recanalization occurred in all internal carotid siphons, all carotid T segments, and in the majority of other locations. Fifteen patients demonstrated complete recanalization, but 10 of these 15 patients improved "partially to near completely" at discharge.

In four patients, intracerebral hemorrhage occurred, but with no evidence of clinical deterioration. None of the five patients with failed recanalization improved. Three patients died from swelling (with one patient after complete recanalization).

In Hacke's study, (Fig. 6.17) 43 patients with vertebrobasilar disease received intra-arterial

Local Intra-arterial Fibrinolytic Therapy in Acute Carotid Territory Stroke

A Pilot Study

Gregory J. del Zoppo, MD, Andreas Ferbert, MD, Shirley Otis, MD, Hartmut Brückmann, MD, Werner Hacke, MD, Jack Zyroff, MD, Laurence A. Harker, MD, and Hermann Zeumer, MD

The possibility that intra-arterial local infusion of fibrinolytic agents may achieve recanalization of previously occluded carotid territory arteries in acute stroke was tested in a prospective angiography-based open pilot study at two centers. Fifteen of 20 patients with acute symptoms (mean treatment–onset interval 7.6 hours) demonstrated complete recanalization; 10 of the 15 patients exhibited clinical improvement of varying degree by the time of hospital discharge. Four of the 20 patients suffered hemorrhagic transformation of the infarcted territory without clinical deterioration or demise. Because of the study format and the limited number of patients, dose responses for recanalization and risk relations were not established. We conclude that local intra-arterial fibrinolytic therapy may lead to cerebral arterial recanalization in acute carotid territory thrombotic stroke. The particular implications and limitations of this approach are discussed. (*Stroke* 1988;19:307–313)

Fig. 6.16 Title page

Intra-arterial Thrombolytic Therapy Improves Outcome in Patients With Acute Vertebrobasilar Occlusive Disease

Werner Hacke, MD, Hermann Zeumer, MD, Andreas Ferbert, MD, Hartmut Brückmann, MD, and Gregory J. del Zoppo, MD

In this retrospective analysis we report our treatment experience in 65 consecutive patients with clinical signs of severe brainstem ischemia with angiographically demonstrated thrombotic vertebrobasilar artery occlusions who received either local intra-arterial thrombolytic therapy (urokinase or streptokinase) (43 patients) or conventional therapy (antiplatelet agents or anticoagulants) (22 patients). We analyzed the data with respect to cerebral artery occlusion patterns, posttreatment arterial recanalization, and the clinical categories of favorable/unfavorable outcome and survival/death. In subgroup analyses, recanalization in patients who received thrombolytic therapy correlated significantly with clinical outcome; in 19 of 43 patients, recanalization was demonstrated angiographically, while in 24 patients the occlusion persisted. All patients without recanalization died, but 14 of the 19 patients displaying recanalization survived ($p = 0.000007$), 10 with a favorable clinical outcome. Only three of the 22 patients who received conventional therapy survived, all with a moderate clinical deficit. When we compared the treatment groups, highly significant differences in both outcome quality ($p = 0.017$) and survival ($p = 0.0005$) were found to depend on establishing recanalization. Our data support the concept that technically successful thrombolysis of vertebrobasilar artery occlusions is associated with beneficial clinical outcome. (*Stroke* 1988;19:1216–1222)

Fig. 6.17 Title page

thrombolysis. These patients, treated between 1985 and 1986, received urokinase or streptokinase at 100,000 units for up to a 4-h infusion, but with some patients with lower infusion rates for 48 h.

The occlusion patterns were top of the basilar ($n=9$), mid-basilar ($n=15$), caudal vertebrobasilar occlusion ($n=11$), and mixed occlusion patterns ($n=8$) Recanalization occurred in 6 of 9 patients, 5 of 15 patients, 5 of 11 patients, and 3 of 8 patients, respectively. Three patients died of a pontine hemorrhage. Two patients without recanalization developed a hemorrhage. Comatose patients with "tetraparesis" had a poor outcome despite recanalization.

The Message and Acceptance

These studies are landmarks not only because they documented recanalization of acutely occluded large cerebral arteries but also the result showed that an aggressive invasive approach to acute stroke could benefit certain patients [51].

Several clinical trials followed. The Prolyse in Acute Cerebral Thromboembolism II trial enrolled 180 patients (from 12,323 screened patients and 474 with cerebral angiograms) who had a median NIHSS score of 17 and M_1 or M_2 middle cerebral artery occlusion. Nine milligrams of recombinant prourokinase and heparin was compared with heparin alone within 6 h of ictus. At 3 months, 40% of the patients who received thrombolysis had a slight or no neurologic disability compared with 25% in the control group. The frequency of intracranial hematoma was 10% in the treated group and 2% in the control group. Recanalization occurred in 66% of the patients receiving the combination of prourokinase and heparin, but in only 19% of the controls [53].

The treatment of acute occlusion of the intracranial internal carotid artery at the level of its bifurcation (T-type occlusion) has been disappointing. It has led some experts to consider exclusion from thrombolysis, but success in some cases has been reported [146]. These large emboli are considered of aged thrombotic material that could be less responsive to thrombolytic agents.

IA thrombolysis is now a very feasible endovascular treatment of acute stroke [22, 56, 77, 146, 161, 166, 170]. tPA replaced urokinase and streptokinase, and prospective trials found similar benefit. In the following decades, neurointervention of acute ischemic stroke would see the emergence of mechanical fragmentation devices and expandable and retrievable stents. IA thrombolysis almost has become a second choice, and most neurointerventionalists will try mechanical disruption first after IV tPA has been administered. Now with several options available, the treatment choices are evolving, operator dependent, and may become guided in the first place by CT perfusion scan or magnetic resonance perfusion imaging. These imaging modalities may demonstrate whether there is salvageable tissue or not. Estimation of the penumbra and infarct core is useful because it may select patients who could benefit from escalating treatment with an endovascular procedure [98].

Short Historical Note 50

CORTICOSTEROIDS IN SPINAL CORD INJURY

The Title of the Paper

Bracken MB, Collings WF, Freeman DF. Efficacy of methylprednisolone in acute spinal cord injury. JAMA. 1984;251:45–52.

Bracken MB, Shepard MJ, Collings WF, et al. A randomized, controlled trial of methylprednisolone or naloxone in the treatment of acute spinal-cord injury. Results of the Second National Acute Spinal Cord Injury Study. N Engl J Med. 1990;322:1405–11.

Bracken MB, Shepard MJ, Holford TR, et al. Administration of methylprednisolone for 24 or 48 h or tirilazad mesylate for 48 h in the treatment of acute spinal cord injury. Results of the Third National Acute Spinal Cord Injury Randomized Controlled Trial. National Acute Spinal Cord Injury Study. JAMA. 1997;277:1597–604.

The Paper and the Times

The care of spinal cord injury has a long history of trial and error but also substantial progress. Corticosteroids were widely used for the treatment of acute spinal cord injury that affects approximately 40 million people each year in the United States. Animal experiments found improvement in spinal cord injury outcome after corticosteroid treatment and also reported histological confirmation that showed white matter sparing. One of the possible explanations for a positive effect of corticosteroids on injured cord was that corticosteroids could suppress the neuronal breakdown by inhibiting lipid peroxidation and hydrolysis. Earlier studies also showed that this breakdown occurred within 8 h after injury, leaving open a window of therapeutic intervention [8, 17]. However, in some studies there was a discrepancy between histological improvement and clinical outcome [15, 24, 25, 37, 44]. Depending on species tested, some investigators could not confirm a change in outcome after corticosteroid use [168].

In 1975, the National Acute Spinal Cord Injury Study (NASCIS) group was established with a mandate to evaluate pharmacologic therapies in the first hours after spinal cord injury. The study group completed three trials known as NASCIS I, NASCIS II, and NASCIS III.

The Details of the Paper

All three studies were multicenter, blinded prospective, randomized controlled trials (Fig. 6.18–Fig. 6.20). NASCIS I compared different doses of methylprednisolone in 330 patients after acute spinal cord injury. NASCIS I used a low-dose regimen with a loading dose of methylprednisolone 100 mg followed by 25 mg every 6 h for 10 days, and this was compared with a moderate-dose regimen of 1,000 mg bolus followed by 250 mg every 6 h for 10 days. NASCIS I found no difference between these two regimens, but there was a trend toward better outcome for moderate dose methylprednisolone if it was administered within 8 h. Wound infections of both trauma and operative sites were more common. The authors speculated that high dose methylprednisolone did not reach therapeutic levels. Additionally, they found that although there were significantly increased wound infection and skin ulcers in high dose corticosteroids steroid patients, there also was 78% increased risk for pulmonary embolism among patients treated with the higher dose.

NASCIS II investigated three groups. Methylprednisolone was given as a bolus of 30 mg/kg body weight followed by 5.4 mg/kg for 23 h and compared with naloxone used as a bolus of 5.4 mg/kg followed by an infusion of 4 mg/kg for 23 h and a group with placebo only. NASCIS II concluded that patients who received methylprednisolone within 8 h of injury had a statistically significant improvement in motor and sensory function, but there was no beneficiary effect of naloxone. This study could demonstrate that a large proportion of patients had improved motor function, pinprick sensation, and sensation of touch. All these differences were still present 6 months later.

Finally, NASCIS III compared methylprednisolone bolus and maintenance infusion similar to the NASCIS II trial except this time the drug was continued for another 23 or 47 h. This trial showed no statistical significant additional benefit for continuing methylprednisolone treatment for 48 h or any statistical significant benefit for ultra-early administration of methylprednisolone.

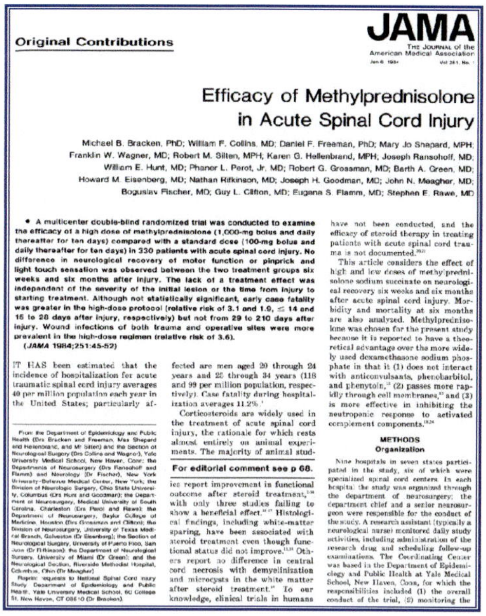

Original Contributions

JAMA

The Journal of the American Medical Association

Jan 6, 1984 Vol 251, No. 1

Efficacy of Methylprednisolone in Acute Spinal Cord Injury

Michael B. Bracken, PhD; William F. Collins, MD; Daniel F. Freeman, PhD; Mary Jo Shepard, MPH; Franklin W. Wagner, MD; Robert M. Silten, MPH; Karen G. Hellenbrand, MPH; Joseph Ransohoff, MD; William E. Hunt, MD; Phanor L. Perot, Jr, MD; Robert G. Grossman, MD; Barth A. Green, MD; Howard M. Eisenberg, MD; Nathan Rifkinson, MD; Joseph H. Goodman, MD; John N. Meagher, MD; Boguslav Fischer, MD; Guy L. Clifton, MD; Eugene S. Flamm, MD; Stephen E. Rawe, MD

• A multicenter double-blind randomized trial was conducted to examine the efficacy of a high dose of methylprednisolone (1,000-mg bolus and daily thereafter for ten days) compared with a standard dose (100-mg bolus and daily thereafter for ten days) in 330 patients with acute spinal cord injury. No difference in neurological recovery of motor function or pinprick and light touch sensation was observed between the two treatment groups six weeks and six months after injury. The lack of a treatment effect was independent of the severity of the initial lesion or the time from injury to starting treatment. Although not statistically significant, early case fatality was greater in the high-dose protocol (relative risk of 3.1 and 1.9, ≤ 14 and 15 to 28 days after injury, respectively) but not from 29 to 210 days after injury. Wound infections of both trauma and operative sites were more prevalent in the high-dose regimen (relative risk of 3.6).

(*JAMA* 1984;251:45-52)

IT HAS been estimated that the incidence of hospitalization for acute traumatic spinal cord injury averages 40 per million population each year in the United States; particularly affected are men aged 20 through 24 years and 25 through 34 years (118 and 99 per million population, respectively). Case fatality during hospitalization averages 11.2%.[1]

Corticosteroids are widely used in the treatment of acute spinal cord injury, the rationale for which rests almost entirely on animal experiments. The majority of animal studies report improvement in functional outcome after steroid treatment,[2-10] with only three studies failing to show a beneficial effect.[11-13] Histological findings, including white-matter sparing, have been associated with steroid treatment even though functional status did not improve.[11,14] Others report no difference in central cord necrosis with demyelinization and microcysts in the white matter after steroid treatment.[15] To our knowledge, clinical trials in humans have not been conducted, and the efficacy of steroid therapy in treating patients with acute spinal cord trauma is not documented.[20,21]

This article considers the effect of high and low doses of methylprednisolone sodium succinate on neurological recovery six weeks and six months after acute spinal cord injury. Morbidity and mortality at six months are also analyzed. Methylprednisolone was chosen for the present study because it is reported to have a theoretical advantage over the more widely used dexamethasone sodium phosphate in that it (1) does not interact with anticonvulsants, phenobarbitol, and phenytoin,[22] (2) passes more rapidly through cell membranes,[23] and (3) is more effective in inhibiting the neutropenic response to activated complement components.[18,24]

For editorial comment see p 68.

METHODS

Organization

Nine hospitals in seven states participated in the study, six of which were specialized spinal cord centers. In each hospital the study was organized through the department of neurosurgery; the department chief and a senior neurosurgeon were responsible for the conduct of the study. A research assistant (typically a neurological nurse) monitored daily study activities, including administration of the research drug and scheduling follow-up examinations. The Coordinating Center was based in the Department of Epidemiology and Public Health at Yale Medical School, New Haven, Conn, for which the responsibilities included (1) the overall conduct of the trial, (2) monitoring the

From the Department of Epidemiology and Public Health (Drs Bracken and Freeman, Mss Shepard and Hellenbrand, and Mr Silten) and the Section of Neurological Surgery (Drs Collins and Wagner), Yale University Medical School, New Haven, Conn; the Departments of Neurosurgery (Drs Ransohoff and Flamm) and Neurology (Dr Fischer), New York University-Bellevue Medical Center, New York; the Division of Neurologic Surgery, Ohio State University, Columbus (Drs Hunt and Goodman); the Department of Neurosurgery, Medical University of South Carolina, Charleston (Drs Perot and Rawe); the Department of Neurosurgery, Baylor College of Medicine, Houston (Drs Grossman and Clifton); the Division of Neurosurgery, University of Texas Medical Branch, Galveston (Dr Eisenberg); the Section of Neurological Surgery, University of Puerto Rico, San Juan (Dr Rifkinson); the Department of Neurological Surgery, University of Miami (Dr Green); and the Neurological Section, Riverside Methodist Hospital, Columbus, Ohio (Dr Meagher).

Reprint requests to National Spinal Cord Injury Study, Department of Epidemiology and Public Health, Yale University Medical School, 60 College St, New Haven, CT 06510 (Dr Bracken).

Fig. 6.18 Title page

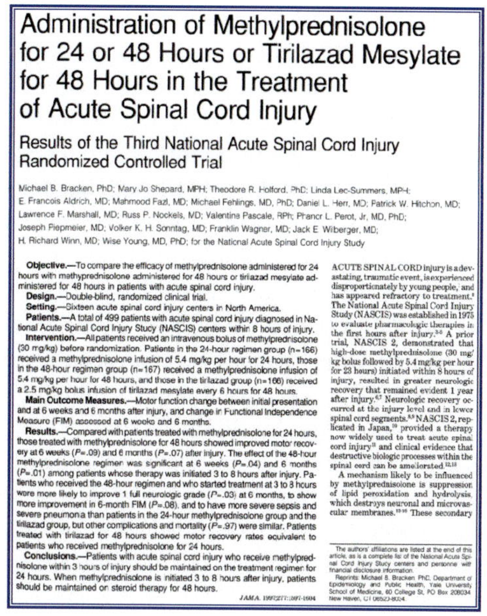

Administration of Methylprednisolone for 24 or 48 Hours or Tirilazad Mesylate for 48 Hours in the Treatment of Acute Spinal Cord Injury

Results of the Third National Acute Spinal Cord Injury Randomized Controlled Trial

Michael B. Bracken, PhD; Mary Jo Shepard, MPH; Theodore R. Holford, PhD; Linda Leo-Summers, MPH; E. Francois Aldrich, MD; Mahmood Fazl, MD; Michael Fehlings, MD, PhD; Daniel L. Herr, MD; Patrick W. Hitchon, MD; Lawrence F. Marshall, MD; Russ P. Nockels, MD; Valentina Pascale, RPh; Phanor L. Perot, Jr, MD, PhD; Joseph Piepmeier, MD; Volker K. H. Sonntag, MD; Franklin Wagner, MD; Jack E. Wilberger, MD; H. Richard Winn, MD; Wise Young, MD, PhD; for the National Acute Spinal Cord Injury Study

Objective.—To compare the efficacy of methylprednisolone administered for 24 hours with methyprednisolone administered for 48 hours or tirilazad mesylate administered for 48 hours in patients with acute spinal cord injury.

Design.—Double-blind, randomized clinical trial.

Setting.—Sixteen acute spinal cord injury centers in North America.

Patients.—A total of 499 patients with acute spinal cord injury diagnosed in National Acute Spinal Cord Injury Study (NASCIS) centers within 8 hours of injury.

Intervention.—All patients received an intravenous bolus of methylprednisolone (30 mg/kg) before randomization. Patients in the 24-hour regimen group (n=166) received a methylprednisolone infusion of 5.4 mg/kg per hour for 24 hours, those in the 48-hour regimen group (n=167) received a methylprednisolone infusion of 5.4 mg/kg per hour for 48 hours, and those in the tirilazad group (n=166) received a 2.5 mg/kg bolus infusion of tirilazad mesylate every 6 hours for 48 hours.

Main Outcome Measures.—Motor function change between initial presentation and at 6 weeks and 6 months after injury, and change in Functional Independence Measure (FIM) assessed at 6 weeks and 6 months.

Results.—Compared with patients treated with methylprednisolone for 24 hours, those treated with methylprednisolone for 48 hours showed improved motor recovery at 6 weeks (P=.09) and 6 months (P=.07) after injury. The effect of the 48-hour methylprednisolone regimen was significant at 6 weeks (P=.04) and 6 months (P=.01) among patients whose therapy was initiated 3 to 8 hours after injury. Patients who received the 48-hour regimen and who started treatment at 3 to 8 hours were more likely to improve 1 full neurologic grade (P=.03) at 6 months, to show more improvement in 6-month FIM (P=.08), and to have more severe sepsis and severe pneumonia than patients in the 24-hour methylprednisolone group and the tirilazad group, but other complications and mortality (P=.97) were similar. Patients treated with tirilazad for 48 hours showed motor recovery rates equivalent to patients who received methylprednisolone for 24 hours.

Conclusions.—Patients with acute spinal cord injury who receive methylprednisolone within 3 hours of injury should be maintained on the treatment regimen for 24 hours. When methylprednisolone is initiated 3 to 8 hours after injury, patients should be maintained on steroid therapy for 48 hours.

JAMA. 1997;277:1597-1604

ACUTE SPINAL CORD injury is a devastating, traumatic event, is experienced disproportionately by young people,[1] and has appeared refractory to treatment.[2] The National Acute Spinal Cord Injury Study (NASCIS) was established in 1975 to evaluate pharmacologic therapies in the first hours after injury.[3-5] A prior trial, NASCIS 2, demonstrated that high-dose methylprednisolone (30 mg/kg bolus followed by 5.4 mg/kg per hour for 23 hours) initiated within 8 hours of injury, resulted in greater neurologic recovery that remained evident 1 year after injury.[6,7] Neurologic recovery occurred at the injury level and in lower spinal cord segments.[8,9] NASCIS 2, replicated in Japan,[10] provided a therapy now widely used to treat acute spinal cord injury[11] and clinical evidence that destructive biologic processes within the spinal cord can be ameliorated.[12,13]

A mechanism likely to be influenced by methylprednisolone is suppression of lipid peroxidation and hydrolysis, which destroys neuronal and microvascular membranes.[13-16] These secondary

The authors' affiliations are listed at the end of this article, as is a complete list of the National Acute Spinal Cord Injury Study centers and personnel with financial disclosure information.

Reprints: Michael B. Bracken, PhD, Department of Epidemiology and Public Health, Yale University School of Medicine, 60 College St, PO Box 208034, New Haven, CT 06520-8034.

Fig. 6.20 Title page

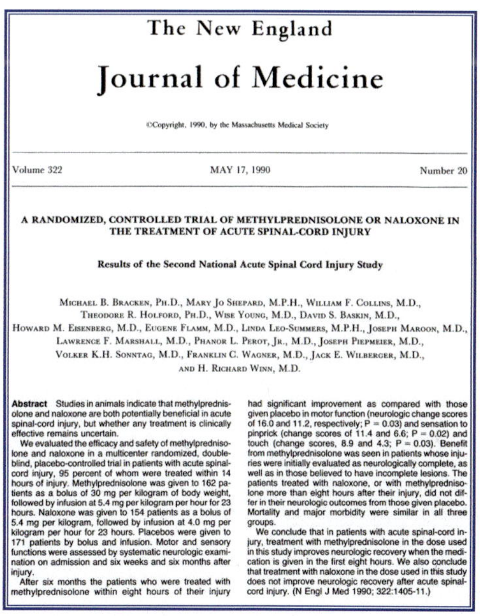

The New England

Journal of Medicine

©Copyright, 1990, by the Massachusetts Medical Society

Volume 322 MAY 17, 1990 Number 20

A RANDOMIZED, CONTROLLED TRIAL OF METHYLPREDNISOLONE OR NALOXONE IN THE TREATMENT OF ACUTE SPINAL-CORD INJURY

Results of the Second National Acute Spinal Cord Injury Study

Michael B. Bracken, Ph.D., Mary Jo Shepard, M.P.H., William F. Collins, M.D., Theodore R. Holford, Ph.D., Wise Young, M.D., David S. Baskin, M.D., Howard M. Eisenberg, M.D., Eugene Flamm, M.D., Linda Leo-Summers, M.P.H., Joseph Maroon, M.D., Lawrence F. Marshall, M.D., Phanor L. Perot, Jr., M.D., Joseph Piepmeier, M.D., Volker K.H. Sonntag, M.D., Franklin C. Wagner, M.D., Jack E. Wilberger, M.D., and H. Richard Winn, M.D.

Abstract Studies in animals indicate that methylprednisolone and naloxone are both potentially beneficial in acute spinal-cord injury, but whether any treatment is clinically effective remains uncertain.

We evaluated the efficacy and safety of methylprednisolone and naloxone in a multicenter randomized, double-blind, placebo-controlled trial in patients with acute spinal-cord injury, 95 percent of whom were treated within 14 hours of injury. Methylprednisolone was given to 162 patients as a bolus of 30 mg per kilogram of body weight, followed by infusion at 5.4 mg per kilogram per hour for 23 hours. Naloxone was given to 154 patients as a bolus of 5.4 mg per kilogram, followed by infusion at 4.0 mg per kilogram per hour for 23 hours. Placebos were given to 171 patients by bolus and infusion. Motor and sensory functions were assessed by systematic neurologic examination on admission and six weeks and six months after injury.

After six months the patients who were treated with methylprednisolone within eight hours of their injury had significant improvement as compared with those given placebo in motor function (neurologic change scores of 16.0 and 11.2, respectively; P = 0.03) and sensation to pinprick (change scores of 11.4 and 6.6; P = 0.02) and touch (change scores, 8.9 and 4.3; P = 0.03). Benefit from methylprednisolone was seen in patients whose injuries were initially evaluated as neurologically complete, as well as in those believed to have incomplete lesions. The patients treated with naloxone, or with methylprednisolone more than eight hours after their injury, did not differ in their neurologic outcomes from those given placebo. Mortality and major morbidity were similar in all three groups.

We conclude that in patients with acute spinal-cord injury, treatment with methylprednisolone in the dose used in this study improves neurologic recovery when the medication is given in the first eight hours. We also conclude that treatment with naloxone in the dose used in this study does not improve neurologic recovery after acute spinal-cord injury. (N Engl J Med 1990; 322:1405-11.)

Fig. 6.19 Title page

The Message and Acceptance

The treatment of acute spinal cord injury with methylprednisolone—despite three major trials—has remained controversial. Significant criticisms of all three trials followed, and most objections pertained to the alleged degree of improvement. There was a concern that the motor score recovery improvement did not correlate with functional improvement [33, 54, 108]. In the post hoc analysis of NASCIS III, sensory and motor changes were not seen among the treatment group at 6 weeks, 6 months, or 1 year follow-up. NASCIS III also showed higher incidences of severe sepsis and pneumonia that were not found in the NASCIS II study. Other concerns were identified that included certain statistical comparisons, simplification of subgroup analysis, and post hoc analysis of study data including only 127 patients treated with 8 h of injury rather than the entire population.

An interesting study from Canada documented a shifted practice away from corticosteroid use in acute spinal cord injury over the past 5 years [75].

Eventually, the American Association of Neurologic Surgeons/Congress of Neurologic Surgeons (WANS/CNS) Joint Section on Disorders of the Spine and Peripheral Nerve stated the following:

> Treatment with methylprednisolone for either 24 or 48 h is recommended as an option in the treatment of patients with acute spinal cord injuries that should be undertaken only with the knowledge that the evidence suggesting harmful side effects is more consistent than any suggestion of clinical benefit.

The true practice in the United States is not known and likely varies.

Short Historical Note 51

PLASMAPHERESIS AND IMMUNOGLOBULIN IN GUILLAIN-BARRÉ SYNDROME

The Title of the Paper

Plasmapheresis and acute Guillain-Barré syndrome. The Guillain-Barré syndrome Study Group. Neurology. 1985;35:1096–104.

van der Meché FG, Schmitz PI, and the Dutch Guillain-Barré Study Group. A randomized trial comparing intravenous immune globulin and plasma exchange in Guillain-Barré syndrome. N Engl J Med. 1992;326: 1123–9.

The Paper and the Times

Since its first description, the treatment of Guillain-Barré syndrome (GBS) was largely supportive [74]. Many patients received corticosteroids, although its effect was highly questionable and possibly with undesirable side effects. One of the first studies that suggested an effect of plasma exchange (PLEX) was by Brettle et al. from Hammersmith Hospital who described a single case of a patient with GBS who after a second PLEX noted dramatic and sustained improvement of proximal limb power. After four exchanges, the patient was able to sit and stand unaided [18]. Other observations were made by Ropper et al., also showing improvement in four patients with GBS by PLEX. These initial encouraging responses in a few cases prompted the development of a prospective study comparing PLEX with supportive "conventional" therapy. The study of 245 patients was organized by Guy McKhann from Johns Hopkins University School of Medicine. The trial was notable for specific inclusion criteria, strict definition of the disease, and outcome assessment using a previously tested grading scale [73].

PLEX became the standard of treatment, but 3 years after this trial, IV immunoglobulin (IVIG) was introduced as an alternative treatment for GBS. IVIG became a consideration after a patient with chronic inflammatory polyneuropathy (CIDP) fortuitously was treated with plasma infusion rather than PLEX and, to the surprise of all, improved [154]. This led to consideration of IVIG as the possible active component.

IVIG—using pooled large quantities of human IgG—has been rarely used in neurologic disorders and mostly in autoimmune thrombocytopenia. The reasoning was simple: If IVIG could work in other autoimmune disorders, it could work in autoimmune CIDP. In subsequent studies, patients with a CIPD and a successful response to plasma infusion had similar results with IVIG [156].

The first experience with IVIG in GBS was reported in 1988 in six patients with rapid deteriorating GBS. (In another two patients, IVIG was combined with fresh frozen plasma infusion after worsening with PLEX.) In four of six patients, a significant improvement in motor function was observed, and again after a repeat IVIG infusion in a patient with an early relapse [84].

The ease of use IVIG was the major incentive to study it prospectively. Although in the early days of GBS treatment concerns were raised about the potential of virus transmission and risk for anaphylaxis in IgA-deficient patients, of IVIG has been found to be safe, comparable in expense with PLEX, and to cause few side effects [19, 46, 71, 72, 76].

The Details of the Paper

In the PLEX study, patients were randomized into PLEX or a conventional therapy group and basically analyzed for time on the respirator and outcome (Fig. 6.21). The study concluded PLEX had an important effect on recovery. Medical benefit was most apparent when time on the ventilator was taken into consideration. Median time for patients to reach grade 2 (to be able to walk unassisted) declined from 85 to 53 days, and similar benefit was found in patients who were on the ventilator. Outcome at 6 months was similar for all patients.

The study was criticized because of lack of a sham plasmapheresis. The observers knew which patients were treated, and this could have influenced time on the ventilator and earlier weaning. Of note is that the earlier and more rapid recovery of the PLEX was not observed in this study, and

Fig. 6.21 Title page

Article abstract—We compared plasmapheresis with conventional therapy in 245 patients with the Guillain-Barré syndrome of recent onset. Statistically significant differences, favoring the plasmapheresis group, were found in terms of improvement at 4 weeks, time to improve one clinical grade, time to independent walking, and outcome at 6 months. Plasmapheresis was not effective for all patients, but was particularly effective for patients who received this treatment within 7 days of onset and for patients who required mechanical ventilation after entry into the study. Plasmapheresis appears to be of benefit in patients with Guillain-Barré syndrome of recent onset.

NEUROLOGY 1985;35:1096-1104

Plasmapheresis and acute Guillain-Barré syndrome

The Guillain-Barré Syndrome Study Group*

The present study was designed to determine whether plasmapheresis has a beneficial effect on the course and outcome of the acute Guillain-Barré syndrome (GBS). This paper presents the results of a randomized trial of plasmapheresis versus conventional care on 245 patients severely ill with acute GBS. This syndrome is an inflammatory demyelinating disease of peripheral nerves that annually affects at least 1.7 per 100,000 population.[1] Since the marked decline in the incidence of poliomyelitis in the United States, GBS has become the major cause of rapid flaccid paralysis in healthy persons. Although most patients with GBS recover spontaneously, 10 to 23% require mechanical ventilation, 7 to 22% are left with some disability, 3 to 10% relapse, and 2 to 5% die.[2-4] The likelihood of permanent disability increases with severity and duration of disease, and patients may require prolonged stays in the hospital.[4] Among 159 cases at the Massachusetts General Hospital between 1962 and 1979, the average hospital stay was 61 days, and 30% of the patients required mechanical ventilation for an average of 49 days (Drs. Brad Truax and Allan Ropper, unpublished). At present, there is no effective therapy other than supportive care. Corticosteroids have been recommended, but one cooperative trial showed no benefit.[5] Clearly, treatment that shortened the duration of acute and chronic morbidity would be desirable.

The present study of plasmapheresis was initiated in 1980 for several reasons: (1) anecdotal reports that some patients with the acute GBS responded to plasmapheresis[6-8]; (2) the response of some patients with chronic relapsing polyneuropathy to plasmapheresis[9-12]; and (3) reports of circulating factors in the serum of GBS patients that impede peripheral nerve function in experimental situations.[13-17]

While this study was in progress, two other lines of investigation underscored the need for a large-scale randomized study of the efficacy of plasmapheresis. First, Koski et al[18] observed that patients with acute GBS had circulating antibodies to human peripheral nerve myelin that decreased as the patient improved. Second, several reports, with many fewer patients, cited conflicting results about the efficacy of plasmapheresis.[19,20]

In the present randomized trial, we compared patients receiving plasmapheresis with a similar group who received conventional care in terms of complications and mortality, and possible beneficial effects of plasmapheresis. Among other secondary questions, we were interested in whether the timing of plasmapheresis affected the course of the disease. To evaluate efficacy, we used two general approaches: evaluation of outcome at predetermined times (4 weeks and 6 months) and evaluation of predetermined degrees of improvement as a continuous function of time (improvement of one clinical grade and ability to walk unaided). The methods to attain and assess these outcomes were specified in advance of patient entry and were adhered to strictly in the subsequent analysis. The study showed a significant beneficial effect of plasmapheresis.

Methods. The design was based on several considerations. The number of patients included, the methods of data collection, and the statistical techniques were preplanned so that the results would provide definitive data.

The study was initiated in the fall of 1980, and the last patient was enrolled in April 1984. The patients were randomized into two groups:

A RANDOMIZED TRIAL COMPARING INTRAVENOUS IMMUNE GLOBULIN AND PLASMA EXCHANGE IN GUILLAIN–BARRÉ SYNDROME

F.G.A. van der Meché, M.D., Ph.D., P.I.M. Schmitz, Ph.D.,
and the Dutch Guillain–Barré Study Group*

Abstract *Background.* The subacute demyelinating polyneuropathy known as Guillain–Barré syndrome improves more rapidly with plasma exchange than with supportive care alone. We conducted a multicenter trial to determine whether intravenous immune globulin is as effective as the more complicated treatment with plasma exchange.

Methods. To enter the study, patients had to have had Guillain–Barré syndrome for less than two weeks and had to be unable to walk independently. They were randomly assigned to receive either five plasma exchanges (each of 200 to 250 ml per kilogram of body weight) or five doses of a preparation of intravenous immune globulin (0.4 g per kilogram per day). The predefined outcome measure was improvement at four weeks by at least one grade on a seven-point scale of motor function.

Results. After 150 patients had been treated, strength had improved by one grade or more in 34 percent of those treated with plasma exchange, as compared with 53 percent of those treated with immune globulin (difference, 19 percent; 95 percent confidence interval, 3 percent to 34 percent; P = 0.024). The median time to improvement by one grade was 41 days with plasma exchange and 27 days with immune globulin therapy (P = 0.05). The immune globulin group had significantly fewer complications and less need for artificial ventilation.

Conclusions. In the acute Guillain–Barré syndrome, treatment with intravenous immune globulin is at least as effective as plasma exchange and may be superior. (N Engl J Med 1992;326:1123-9.)

Fig. 6.22 Title page of IVIG study

differences became apparent after many weeks of observation. Very few of the investigators expected a positive effect of PLEX on the course of GBS when they were asked to speculate before release of the results.

The IVIG study was limited to patients with severe GBS—unable to stand unassisted—and patients were randomized into two groups: patients treated with PLEX and patients treated with IVIG but again outcome assessment was not blinded (Fig. 6.22). Patients were treated with IVIG 0.4 g/day for 5 days compared with PLEX 200–250 mL/kg body weight in five sessions within 7–14 days. The trial was prematurely discontinued after a difference of 19% in favor of IVIG was found. Most noticeable in this trial was that there was less improvement by one functional grade in the IVIG group at 4 weeks. In the North American trial, 52% of the patients improved one grade as opposed to 34% in the IVIG study. The study also found that in a considerable proportion of patients (16%), one or more sessions of PLEX had to be discontinued because of hypotension or other side effects.

The Message and Acceptance

The PLEX study was followed by a study that compared PLEX in combination with IVIG. No difference was found between IVIG and PLEX, and combining both therapies—PLEX followed by IVIG—did not result in better outcome [58].

IVIG has also been compared with corticosteroids, and again, no additional benefit was found [153].

PLEX has remained an important treatment modality in a patient with GBS [50, 52], although IVIG has become the preferred first line approach [70–73, 152].

The most interesting observation in the past 10 years is that IgG levels in GBS after IVIG vary, and that in some patients little change of IgG levels after IVIG treatment was noted, and that it related to poor outcome. This observation calls for dose ranging studies [89].

Possible disadvantages of IVIG have accumulated over the years and initially tempered enthusiasm. The adverse effects, all rare, were aseptic meningitis, acute renal failure, ischemic stroke, and anaphylactic shock. Early anecdotal series have suggested a high relapse rate in patients receiving IVIG [27, 76]. But a large comparative trial has not confirmed a higher relapse rate [58].

There is still insufficient understanding of how IVIG works in inflammatory disorders [23]. There are many potential pathways, and they include inhibition of autoantibody mediated injury. IVIG also may counteract the interaction of T cells with antigen presenting cells. IVIG reduces interleukin 1 and tumor necrosis factor and increases transforming growth factor production. IVIG also prevents binding and complement activation of autoantibodies to their antigen by anti-idiotypic antibodies. Each of these mechanisms may be operative.

What happened with IVIG in CIDP? The ICE (immunoglobulin CIDP efficacy) trial in 117 patients showed that continued IVIG infusion 1 g/kg every 3 weeks protected patients from relapse. Most notable side effects were seen in 34% of the patients and involved headache, hypertension, and fever [69].

References

1. Adams Jr HP, del Zoppo G, Alberts MJ, et al. Guidelines for the early management of adults with ischemic stroke. A guideline from the American Heart Association/American Stroke Association Stroke Council, Clinical Cardiology Council, Cardiovascular Radiology, and Intervention Council and the Atherosclerotic peripheral vascular disease and quality of care outcomes in research interdisciplinary working groups. Circulation. 2007;115:e478–534.
2. Al-Khotani A, Parrent A, Jenkins ME, et al. Decompressive craniectomy in stroke. Can J Neurol Sci. 2010;37:868–9.
3. Allen GS, Ahn HS, Preziosi TJ, et al. Cerebral arterial spasm – a controlled trial of nimodipine in patients with subarachnoid hemorrhage. N Engl J Med. 1983;308:619–24.
4. Allen GS, Ahn HS, Preziosi TJ, et al. Cerebral arterial spasm – a controlled trial of nimodipine in patients with subarachnoid hemorrhage. N Engl J Med. 1983; 308:619–24.
5. Allen GS, Bahr AL. Cerebral arterial spasm. 10. Reversal of acute and chronic spasm in dogs with orally administered nifedipine. Neurosurgery. 1979;4: 43–7.
6. Allen GS, Banghart SB. Cerebral arterial spasm. 9. In vitro effects of nifedipine on serotonin-, phenylephrine-, and potassium-induced contractions of canine basilar and femoral arteries. Neurosurgery. 1979;4: 37–42.
7. American Heart Association guidelines for cardiopulmonary resuscitation and emergency cardiovascular care. Circulation. 2005;112:IV1–211.
8. Anderson DK, Saunders RD, Demediuk P, et al. Lipid hydrolysis and peroxidation in injured spinal cord: partial protection with methylprednisolone or vitamin E and selenium. Cent Nerv Syst Trauma. 1985;2: 257–67.
9. Arrich J, Holzer M, Herkner H, et al. Cochrane corner: hypothermia for neuroprotection in adults after cardiopulmonary resuscitation. Anesth Analg. 2010;110:1239.
10. Auer LM. Pial arterial and venous reaction to intravenous infusion of nimodipine in cats. J Neurosurg Sci. 1982;26:213–8.
11. Auer LM, Ito Z, Suzuki A, et al. Prevention of symptomatic vasospasm by topically applied nimodipine. Acta Neurochir (Wien). 1982;63:297–302.
12. Batjer HH, Reisch JS, Allen BC, et al. Failure of surgery to improve outcome in hypertensive putaminal hemorrhage. A prospective randomized trial. Arch Neurol. 1990;47:1103–6.
13. Bauer RB, Tellez H. Dexamethasone as treatment in cerebrovascular disease. 2. A controlled study in acute cerebral infarction. Stroke. 1973;4:547–55.
14. Bernard S. Hypothermia after cardiac arrest: expanding the therapeutic scope. Crit Care Med. 2009;37: S227–33.
15. Black P, Markowitz RS. Experimental spinal cord injury in monkeys: comparison of steroids and local hypothermia. Surg Forum. 1971;22:409–11.
16. Bladin PF. Status epilepticus, the grim reaper of the mental health system in early Victoria. J Clin Neurosci. 2003;10:655–60.
17. Braughler JM, Hall ED. Correlation of methylprednisolone levels in eat spinal cord with its effects on (Na^+ + K^+)-ATPase, lipid peroxidation, and alpha motor neuron function. J Neurosurg. 1983;56:838–44.
18. Brettle RP, Gross M, Legg NJ, et al. Treatment of acute polyneuropathy by plasma exchange. Lancet. 1978;18:1100.
19. Bril V, Ilse WK, Pearce R, et al. Pilot trial of immunoglobulin versus plasma exchange in patients with Guillain-Barré syndrome. Neurology. 1996;46:100–3.
20. Broderick J, Brott T, Duldner JE, et al. Volume of intracerebral hemorrhage: a powerful and easy way to use prediction of 30 year mortality. Stroke. 1993;24:987–93.
21. Brott T, Broderick J, Kothari R, et al. Early hemorrhage growth in patients with intracerebral hemorrhage. Stroke. 1990;28:1–5.
22. Bruckmann H, Ferbert A, del Zoppo GJ, et al. Acute vertebral basilar thrombosis: angiologic-clinical comparison and therapeutic implications. Acta Radiol. 1987;369:38–42.
23. Buchwald B, Ahangari R, Weishaupt A, et al. Intravenous immunoglobulins neutralize blocking antibodies in Guillain-Barré syndrome. Ann Neurol. 2002;51:673–80.
24. Campbell JB, DeCrescito V, Tomasula JJ, et al. Experimental treatment of spinal cord contusions in the cat. Surg Neurol. 1973;1:102–6.
25. Campbell JB, DeCrescito V, Tomasula JJ, et al. Effects of antifibrinolytic and steroid therapy on the contused spinal cord cats. J Neurosurg. 1974;40:726–33.
26. Carter CH. Use of parenteral diphenylhydantoin (Dilantin) sodium in control of status epilepticus. AMA Arch Neurol Psychiatry. 1958;79:136–7.
27. Castro LH, Ropper AH. Human immune globulin infusion in Guillain-Barré syndrome: worsening during and after treatment. Neurology. 1993;43:1034–6.
28. Chen JW, Waterlain CG. Status epilepticus: pathophysiology and management in adults. Lancet Neurol. 2006;5:246–56.
29. Claassen J, Hirsch LJ, Emerson RG, et al. Treatment of refractory status epilepticus with pentobarbital, propofol, or midazolam: a systematic review. Epilepsia. 2002;43:146–53.
30. Clark K, Nash TM, Hutchison GC. The failure of circumferential craniotomy in acute traumatic cerebral swelling. J Neurosurg. 1968;29:367–71.
31. Clark LP, Prout TP. Status epilepticus: a clinical and pathological study in epilepsy. Am J Insanity. 1904;61: 1081–3.
32. Cohen RJ, Allen GS. Cerebral arterial spasm: the role of calcium in in vitro and in vivo analysis of treatment with nifedipine and nimodipine. In: Wilkins RH, editor. Cerebral arterial spasm. Baltimore: Williams & Wilkins; 1980. p. 527–32.

33. Coleman WP, Benzel D, Cahill DW, et al. A critical appraisal of the reporting of the national acute spinal cord injury studies (II and III) of methylprednisolone in acute spinal cord injury. J Spinal Disord. 2000;13: 185–99.
34. Collier GK. The intravenous use of paraldehyde. NY State J Med. 1914;14
35. Cooper DJ, Rosenfeld JV, Murray L, et al. Decompressive craniectomy in diffuse traumatic brain injury. N Engl J Med. 2011;364:1493–502.
36. Cushing H. The establishment of cerebral hernia as a decompressive measure for inaccessible brain tumors; with the description of intermuscular methods of making the bone defect in temporal and occipital regions. Surg Gynecol Obstet. 1905;1: 297–314.
37. De la Torre JC, Johnson CM, Goode DJ, et al. Pharmacologic treatment and evaluation of permanent experimental spinal cord trauma. Neurology. 1975;25: 508–14.
38. Del Zoppo GJ. tPA and scuPA: new concepts in the treatment of acute ischemic stroke. In: Poeck K, Ringelstein EB, Hacke W, editors. New trends in diagnosis and management of stroke. Berlin: Springer; 1987. p. 115–27.
39. del Zoppo GJ, Zeumer H, Harker LA. Thrombolytic therapy in acute stroke: possibilities and hazards. Stroke. 1986;17:595–607.
40. Demchuk AM, Dowlatshahi D, Rodriguez-Luna D et al. Prediction of hematoma growth and outcome in patients with intracerebral hemorrhage using the CT-angiography spot sign (PREDICT): A prospective observational study. Lancet Neurol. 2012;11:307–14.
41. Desai P, Prasad K. Dexamethasone is not necessarily unsafe in primary supratentorial intracerebral hemorrhage. J Neurol Neurosurg Psychiatry. 1998;65: 799–800.
42. Diringer MN, Skolnick BE, Mayer SA, et al. Thromboembolic events with recombinant activated factor VII in spontaneous intracerebral hemorrhage: results from the Factor Seven for Acute Hemorrhagic Stroke (FAST) trial. Stroke. 2010;41:48–53.
43. Dreler JP, Windmuller O, Petzold G, et al. Ischemia triggered by red blood cell products in the subarachnoid space is inhibited by nimodipine administration or moderate volume expansion/hemodilution in rats. Neurosurgery. 2002;51:1457–65.
44. Ducker TB, Hamit HF. Experimental treatments of acute spinal cord injury. J Neurosurg. 1969;30: 693–7.
45. Dumas F, Grimaldi D, Zuber B, et al. Is hypothermia after cardiac arrest effective in both shockable and nonshockable patients? Insights from a large registry. Circulation. 2011;123:877–86.
46. Feasby T, Banwell B, Benstead T, et al. Guidelines on the use of intravenous immune globulin for neurologic conditions. Transfus Med Rev. 2007;21: S57–107.
47. Feigin VL, Anderson N, Rinkel GJ, et al. Corticosteroids for aneurysmal subarachnoid hemorrhage and primary intracerebral hemorrhage. Cochrane Database Syst Rev. 2005;(3):CD004583.
48. Flamm ES, Adams Jr HP, Beck DW, et al. Dose-escalation study of intravenous nicardipine in patients with aneurysmal subarachnoid hemorrhage. J Neurosurg. 1988;68:393–400.
49. Freeman WD, Brott TG, Barrett KM, et al. Recombinant factor VIIa for rapid reversal of warfarin anticoagulation in acute intracranial hemorrhage. Mayo Clin Proc. 2004;79:1495–500.
50. French Cooperative Group on plasma exchange in Guillain-Barré syndrome. Appropriate number of plasma exchanges in Guillain-Barré syndrome. Ann Neurol. 1997;41:298–306.
51. Furlan AJ. Acute stroke therapy: Beyond IV tPA. Cleve Clin J Med. 2002;69:730–34.
52. French Cooperative Group on plasma exchange in Guillain-Barré syndrome: efficiency of plasma exchange in Guillain-Barré syndrome: role of replacement fluids. Ann Neurol. 1987;22:753–61.
53. Furlan A, Higashida R, Wechsler L, et al. Intra-arterial prourokinase for acute ischemic stroke. The PROACT II study: a randomized controlled trial. Prolyse in acute cerebral thromboembolism. JAMA. 1999;282: 2003–11.
54. Galandiuk S, Raque G, Appel S, et al. The two-edged sword of large-dose steroids for spinal cord trauma. Ann Surg. 1993;218:419–25.
55. Gibbs JR, O'Gorman P. Fibrinolysis in subarachnoid hemorrhage. Postgrad Med J. 1967;43:779–84.
56. Gonner F, Remonda L, Mattle H, et al. Local intra-arterial thrombolysis in acute ischemic stroke. Stroke. 1998;29:1894–900.
57. Gowers WRG. Epilepsy and other chronic convulsive diseases. 2nd ed. London: JA Churchill; 1901.
58. Guillain-Barré Syndrome Steroid Trial Group. Double-blind trial of intravenous methylprednisolone in Guillain-Barré syndrome. Lancet 1993;341: 586–90.
59. Hacke W, del Zoppo GJ, Harker LA. Thrombosis and cerebrovascular disease. In: Poeck K, Ringelstein EB, Hacke W, editors. New trends in diagnosis and management of stroke. Berlin: Springer; 1987. p. 59–74.
60. Hacke W, Schwab S, Horn M, et al. "Malignant" middle cerebral artery territory infarction: clinical course and prognostic signs. Arch Neurol. 1996;53:309–15.
61. Haley Jr EC, Kassell NF, Torner J. A randomized controlled trial of high-dose intravenous nicardipine in aneurysmal subarachnoid hemorrhage. A report of the Cooperative Aneurysm Study. J Neurosurg. 1993;78: 537–47.
62. Haley Jr EC, Kassell NF, Torner JC. A randomized trial of nicardipine in subarachnoid hemorrhage: angiographic and transcranial Doppler ultrasound results. A report of the Cooperative Aneurysm Study. J Neurosurg. 1993;78:548–53.
63. Haley Jr EC, Kassell NF, Torner JC, et al. A randomized trial of two doses of nicardipine in aneurysmal subarachnoid hemorrhage. A report of the Cooperative Aneurysm Study. J Neurosurg. 1994;80:788–96.

64. Han DH, Lee S. Effect of nimodipine treatment on outcome in surgical cases of aneurysmal SAH. J Neurosurg. 1993;78:346A.
65. Hanggi D, Turowski B, Beseoglu K, et al. Steiger HJ. Intraarterial nimodipine for severe cerebral vasospasm after aneurysmal subarachnoid hemorrhage: influence on clinical course and cerebral perfusion. AJNR Am J Neuroradiol. 2008;29:1053–60.
66. Harrigan MR, Rajneesh KF, Ardelt AA, Fisher 3rd WS. Short-term antifibrinolytic therapy before early aneurysm treatment in subarachnoid hemorrhage: effects on rehemorrhage, cerebral ischemia, and hydrocephalus. Neurosurgery. 2010;67:935–9.
67. Heros RC, Zervas NT, Varsos V. Cerebral vasospasm after subarachnoid hemorrhage: an update. Ann Neurol. 1983;14:599–608.
68. Hillman J, Fridriksson S, Nilsson O, et al. Saveland H, Jakobsson KE. Immediate administration of tranexamic acid and reduced incidence of early rebleeding after aneurysmal subarachnoid hemorrhage: a prospective randomized study. J Neurosurg. 2002;97:771–8.
69. Hughes RA, Donofrio P, Bril V, et al. ICE Study Group. Intravenous immune globulin (10% caprylate-chromatography purified) for the treatment of chronic inflammatory demyelinating polyradiculoneuropathy (ICE study): a randomized placebo-controlled trial. Lancet Neurol. 2008;7:136–44.
70. Hughes RA, Raphael JC, Swan AV, et al. Intravenous immunoglobulin for Guillain-Barré syndrome. Cochrane Database Syst Rev. 2006;(1):CD002063.
71. Hughes RA, Swan AV, Raphael JC, et al. Immunotherapy for Guillain-Barré syndrome; a systematic review. Brain. 2007;130:2245–57.
72. Hughes RA, Swan AV, van Doorn PA. Intravenous immunoglobulin for Guillain-Barré syndrome. Cochrane Data base Syst Rev. 2010;(6):CD002063.
73. Hughes RA, Wijdicks EFM, Barohn R, et al. Quality Standards Subcommittee of the American Academy of Neurology. Immunotherapy in Guillain-Barré syndrome. American Academy of Neurology practice parameter. Neurology. 2003;61:736–40.
74. Hughes RA, Wijdicks EFM, Benson E, et al. Supportive care for patients with Guillain-Barré syndrome. Arch Neurol. 2005;62:1194–8.
75. Hurlbert RJ, Hamilton MG. Methylprednisolone for acute spinal cord injury: 5-year practice reversal. Can J Neurol Sci. 2008;3:541–5.
76. Irani DN, Cornblath DR, Chaudhry V, et al. Relapse in Guillain-Barré syndrome after treatment with human immune globulin. Neurology. 1993;43:872–5.
77. Jahan R, Duckwiler GR, Kidwell CS, et al. Intraarterial thrombolysis for treatment of acute stroke: experience in 26 patients with long-term follow-up. AJNR Am J Neuroradiol. 1999;20:1291–9.
78. Joseph M, Ziadi S, Nates J, et al. Increases in cardiac output can reverse flow deficits from vasospasm independent of blood pressure: a study using xenon computed tomographic measurement of cerebral blood flow. Neurosurgery. 2003;53:1044–51.
79. Juvela S, Heiskanen O, Poranen A, et al. The treatment of spontaneous intracerebral hemorrhage. A prospective randomized trial of surgical and conservative treatment. J Neurosurg. 1989;70:755–8.
80. Kassel NF, Peerless SJ, Durward QJ, et al. Treatment of ischemic deficits from vasospasm with intravascular volume expansion and induced arterial hypertension. Neurosurgery. 1982;11:337–43.
81. Kastrau F, Wolter M, Huber W, et al. Recovery from aphasia after hemicraniectomy for infarction of the speech-dominant hemisphere. Stroke. 2005;36:825–9.
82. Kelley RE, Berger JR, Schienberg P, et al. Active bleeding in hypertensive intracerebral hemorrhage: computed tomography. Neurology. 1982;32:852–6.
83. Kendal BE, Lee BCB, Claveria E. Computed tomography and angiography in subarachnoid hemorrhage. Br J Radiol. 1976;49:483–501.
84. Kleyweg RP, van der Meche FG, Meulstee J. Treatment of Guillain-Barré syndrome with high-dose gammaglobulin. Neurology. 1988;38:1639–41.
85. Kocher T. Die Therapie des Hirndruckes. In: Hölder A, editor. Hirnerschütterung, Hirndruck und chirurgische Eingriffe bei Hirnkrankheiten. Vienna: A Hölder; 1901. p. 262–6.
86. Korenkov AI, Pahnke J, Frei K, et al. Treatment with nimodipine or mannitol reduces programmed cell death and infarct size following focal cerebral ischemia. Neurosurg Rev. 2000;23:145–50.
87. Krieger DW, Demchuk AM, Kasner SE, et al. Early clinical and radiological predictors of fatal brain swelling in ischemic stroke. Stroke. 1999;30:287–92.
88. Kuboyama K, Safar P, Radovsky A, et al. Delay in cooling negates the beneficial effect of mild resuscitative cerebral hypothermia after cardiac arrest in dogs: a prospective, randomized study. Crit Care Med. 1993;21:1348–58.
89. Kuitwaard K, de Gelder J, Tio-Gillen AP, Hop WC, van Gelder T, van Toorenenbergen AW, et al. Pharmacokinetics of intravenous immunoglobulin and outcome in Guillain-Barré syndrome. Ann Neurol. 2009;66:597–603.
90. Lee KH, Lukovits T, Friedman JA. "Triple-H" therapy for cerebral vasospasm following subarachnoid hemorrhage. Neurocrit Care. 2006;4:68–76.
91. Leng LZ, Fink ME, Iadecola C. Spreading depolarization: a possible new culprit in the delayed cerebral ischemia of subarachnoid hemorrhage. Arch Neurol. 2011;68:31–6.
92. Lennihan L, Mayer SA, Fink ME, et al. Effect of hypervolemic therapy on cerebral blood flow after subarachnoid hemorrhage: a randomized controlled trial. Stroke. 2000;31:383–91.
93. Lin J, Hanigan WC, Tarantino M, et al. The use of recombinant activated factor VII to reverse warfarin-induced anticoagulation in patients with hemorrhages in the central nervous system: preliminary findings. J Neurosurg. 2003;98:737–40.
94. Maramattom BV, Bahn MM, Wijdicks EFM. Which patient fares worse after early deterioration due to swelling from hemispheric stroke? Neurology. 2004;63:2142–5.

95. Mayer SA, Solomon RA, Fink ME, et al. Effect of 5% albumin solution on sodium balance and blood volume after subarachnoid hemorrhage. Neurosurgery. 1998;42:759–67.
96. McKissock W, Richardson A, Taylor J. Primary intracerebral hematoma: a controlled trial of surgical and conservative treatment in 180 unselected cases. Lancet. 1961;2:221–6.
97. Meldrum B. Status epilepticus: the past and the future. Epilepsia. 2007;48:33–4.
98. Meyers PM, Schumacher HC, Connolly Jr ES, et al. Current status of endovascular stroke treatment. Circulation. 2011;123:2591–601.
99. Moody RA, Ruamsuke S, Mullan S. An evaluation of decompression in experimental head injury. J Neurosurg. 1968;29:586–90.
100. Morgenstern LB, Frankowski RF, Shedden P, Pasteur W, Grotta JC. Surgical treatment for intracerebral hemorrhage (STICH). A single-center, randomized clinical trial. Neurology. 1998;51:1359–63.
101. Neligan A, Shorvon SD. History of epilepsy 1909–2009: the ILAE Century. The history of status epilepticus and its treatment. Epilepsia. 2009;50:56–68.
102. Neligan A, Shorvon SD. The frequency and prognosis of convulsive status epilepticus of different causes: a systematic review. Arch Neurol. 2010;67: 931–40.
103. Nielsen N, Friberg H, Gluud C, et al. Hypothermia after cardiac arrest should be further evaluated – a systematic review of randomised trials with meta-analysis and trial sequential analysis. Int J Cardiol. 2011;151:333–41.
104. Nielsen N, Hovdenes J, Nilsson S, et al. Outcome, timing and adverse events in therapeutic hypothermia after out-of-hospital cardiac arrest – a report from the Hypothermia Network Registry. Acta Anaesthesiol Scand. 2009;53:926–34.
105. Nolan JP, Morley PT, Hoek TL, Hickey RW, Advancement Life Support Task Force of the International Liaison Committee on Resuscitation. Therapeutic hypothermia after cardiac arrest: an advisory statement by the Advancement Life Support Task Force of the International Liaison Committee on Resuscitation. Resuscitation. 2003;57:231–5.
106. Nolan JP, Neumar RW, Adrie C, et al. Post-cardiac arrest syndrome: epidemiology, pathophysiology, treatment, and prognostication: a scientific statement from the International Liaison Committee on Resuscitation; the American Heart Association Emergency Cardiovascular Care Committee; the Council on Cardiovascular Surgery and Anesthesia; the Council on Cardiopulmonary, Perioperative, and Critical Care; the Council on Clinical Cardiology; the Council on Stroke. Resuscitation. 2008;79: 350–79.
107. Norris JW, Hachinski VC. High dose steroid treatment in cerebral infarction. BMJ. 1986;292:21–3.
108. Pandya KA, Weant KA, Cook AM. High-dose methylprednisolone in acute spinal cord injuries: proceed with caution. Orthopedics. 2010;33:327–31.
109. Patterson HA, Le Damon GA, Levi P. A comparative study of various methods of the administration of luminal in epilepsy. J Nerv Ment Dis. 1926;63:275.
110. Peroutka SJ, Allen GS. Calcium channel antagonist binding sites labeled by ^{3}H-nimodipine in human brain. J Neurosurg. 1983;59:933–7.
111. Pfeifer R, Jung C, Purle P, et al. Survival does not improve when therapeutic hypothermia is added to post-cardiac arrest care. Resuscitation. 2011;82: 1168–73.
112. Piriyawat P, Morgenstern LB, Yawn DH, et al. Grotta JC. Treatment of acute intracerebral hemorrhage with epsilon-aminocaproic acid: a pilot study. Neurocrit Care. 2004;1:47–51.
113. Plowman RS, Clarke A, Clarke M, et al. Sixteen-year single-surgeon experience with coil embolization for ruptured intracranial aneurysms: recurrence rate and incidence of late rebleeding. J Neurosurg. 2011;114:863–74.
114. Prasad K, Mendelow AD, Gregson B. Surgery for primary supratentorial intracerebral hemorrhage. Cochrane Database Syst Rev. 2008;(4):CD000200.
115. Pratt CH. The treatment of epilepsy. Can Med Assoc J. 1928;19:303–12.
116. Pritz MB, Giannotta SL, Kindt GW, et al. Treatment of patients with neurological deficits associated with cerebral vasospasm by intravascular volume expansion. Neurosurgery. 1978;3:364–8.
117. Rabinstein AA, Atkinson JL, Wijdicks EFM. Emergency craniotomy in patients worsening due to expanded cerebral hematoma: to what purpose? Neurology. 2002;58:1367–72.
118. Rabinstein AA, Mueller-Kronast N, Maramattom BV, et al. Factors predicting prognosis after decompressive hemicraniectomy for hemispheric infarction. Neurology. 2006;67:891–3.
119. Rabinstein AA, Wijdicks EFM. Surgery for intracerebral hematoma: the search for the elusive right candidate. Rev Neurol Dis. 2006;3:163–72.
120. Rabinstein AA, Wijdicks EFM, Nichols DA. Complete recovery after early intra-arterial recombinant tissue plasminogen activator thrombolysis of carotid T occlusion. AJNR Am J Neuroradiol. 2002;23:1596–9.
121. Radberg JA, Olson JE, Radberg CT. Prognostic parameters in spontaneous intracerebral hematomas with special reference to anticoagulant treatment. Stroke. 1991;22:571–6.
122. Ransohof J, Benjamin V, Gage L, et al. Hemicraniectomy in the management of acute subdural hematoma. J Neurosurg. 1971;34:70–6.
123. Rinkel GJ, Feigin VL, Algra A, et al. Calcium antagonists for aneurysmal subarachnoid hemorrhage. Cochrane Database Syst Rev. 2005;(3):CD000277.
124. Robertson EG. Cerebral lesions due to intracranial aneurysms. Brain. 1949;72:150–85.
125. Robinson MT, Rabinstein AA, Meschia JF, et al. Safety of recombinant activated factor VII in patients with warfarin-associated hemorrhages of the central nervous system. Stroke. 2010;41:1459–63.

126. Roine RO, Kaste M, Kinnunen A, et al. Nimodipine after resuscitation from out-of-hospital ventricular fibrillation. A placebo-controlled, double-blind, randomized trial. JAMA. 1990;264:3171–7.
127. Roos YB, Levi M, Carroll TA, et al. Nimodipine increases fibrinolytic activity in patients with aneurysmal subarachnoid hemorrhage. Stroke. 2001;32:1860–2.
128. Roos YB, Rinkel G, Vermeulen M, et al. Antifibrinolytic therapy for aneurysmal subarachnoid hemorrhage. Cochrane Database Syst Rev. 2003;(2):CD001245.
129. Rosenwasser RH, Jallo JI, Getch CC, et al. Complications of Swan-Ganz catheterization for hemodynamic monitoring in patients with subarachnoid hemorrhage. Neurosurgery. 1995;37:872–5.
130. Russek HI, Zohman BL, Russek AS. Cortisone in immediate therapy of apoplectic stroke. J Am Geriatr Soc. 1954;2:216–22.
131. Scarcella G. Encephalomalacia simulating the clinical and radiological aspects of brain tumor; a report of 6 cases. J Neurosurg. 1956;13:278–92.
132. Shanahan WT. Report of the meeting of the American association for the study and the care and treatment of epileptics. Baltimore, Maryland 25th, 1914: II. Treatment of status epilepticus. Epilepsia. 1915;5: 283–91.
133. Shorvon S. Status epilepticus: its clinical features and treatment in children and adults. Cambridge: Cambridge University Press; 1994.
134. Silbergleit R, Durkalski V, Lowenstein D et al. Intramuscular versus intravenous therapy for prehospital status epilepticus. N Engl J. Med. 2012:366: 591–600.
135. Solomon RA, Fink ME, Lennihan L. Early aneurysm surgery and prophylactic hypervolemic hypertensive therapy for the treatment of aneurysmal subarachnoid hemorrhage. Neurosurgery. 1988;23:699–704.
136. Solomon RA, Fink ME, Lennihan L. Prophylactic volume expansion therapy for the prevention of delayed cerebral ischemia after early aneurysm surgery. Results of a preliminary trial. Arch Neurol. 1988;45:325–32.
137. Spiller WG, Franzier CH. Cerebral decompression. Palliative operations in the treatment of tumors of the brain, based on the observation of fourteen cases. JAMA. 1906;47:679–83.
138. Starke RM, Connolly ES. Rebleeding after aneurysmal subarachnoid hemorrhage. Neurocrit Care. 2011;15:241–7.
139. Starke RM, Kim GH, Fernandez A, et al. Impact of a policy of early antifibrinolytic therapy for the prevention of acute rebleeding after aneurysmal subarachnoid hemorrhage. Stroke. 2008;39:2617–21.
140. Stertz F, Safar P, Tisherman SA, et al. Mild hypothermic cardiopulmonary resuscitation improves outcome after cardiac arrest in dogs. Crit Care Med. 1991;19:379–89.
141. Sutherland CS, Hill MD, Kaufmann AM, et al. Recombinant factor VIIa plus surgery for intracerebral hemorrhage. Can J Neurol Sci. 2008;35: 567–72.
142. Teernstra OPM, Evers SMAA, Lodder J, et al. Stereotactic treatment of intracerebral hematoma by means of a plasminogen activator: a multicenter randomized controlled trial (SICHPA). Stroke. 2003;34:968–74.
143. Tellez H, Bauer RB. Dexamethasone as treatment in acute cerebrovascular disease. I. A controlled study in intracerebral hemorrhage. Stroke. 1973;4:541–6.
144. The Guillain-Barré Syndrome Study Group. Plasmapheresis and acute Guillain-Barré syndrome. Neurology. 1985;35:1096–104.
145. The National Institute of Neurological Disorders and Stroke rt-PA Stroke Study Group. Tissue plasminogen activator for acute ischemic stroke. N Engl J Med. 1995;333:1581–7.
146. Theron J, Courtheoux P, Casasco A, et al. Local intraarterial fibrinolysis in the carotid territory. AJNR Am J Neuroradiol. 1989;10:753–65.
147. Treatment of convulsive status epilepticus. Recommendations of the Epilepsy Foundation of America's Working Group on Status Epilepticus. JAMA. 1993;270:854–9.
148. Treiman DM, Meyers PD, Walton NY, et al. A comparison of four treatments for generalized convulsive status epilepticus. Veterans Affairs Status Epilepticus Cooperative Study Group. N Engl J Med. 1998;339:792–8.
149. Tuhrim S. Intracerebral hemorrhage – improving outcome by reducing volume? N Engl J Med. 2008;358:2174–6.
150. Vahedi K, Hofmeijer J, Juettler E, et al. Early decompressive surgery in malignant infarction of the middle cerebral artery: a pooled analysis of three randomized controlled trials. Lancet Neurol. 2007;6:215–22.
151. van Doorn PA, Kuitwaard K, Walgaard C, et al. IVIG treatment and prognosis in Guillain-Barré syndrome. J Clin Immunol. 2010;30:S74–8.
152. van Doorn PA, Ruts L, Jacobs BC. Clinical features, pathogenesis, and treatment of Guillain-Barré syndrome. Lancet Neurol. 2008;7:939–50.
153. van Koningsveld R, Schmitz PI, Meché FG, et al. Effect of methylprednisolone when added to standard treatment with intravenous immunoglobulin for Guillain-Barré syndrome: randomized trial. Lancet. 2004;363:192–6.
154. Vermeulen M. A patient that changed my practice: the first chronic inflammatory demyelinating polyneuropathy patient to be treated with intravenous immunoglobulin. Pract Neurol. 2002;2:354–7.
155. Vermeulen M, Muizelaar JP. Do antifibrinolytic agents prevent rebleeding after rupture of a cerebral aneurysm? A review. Clin Neurol Neurosurg. 1980; 82:25–30.
156. Vermeulen M, van der Meché FGA, Speelman JD, et al. Busch HFM. Plasma and gamma-globulin infusion in chronic inflammatory polyneuropathy. J Neurol Sci. 1985;70:317–26.
157. Wada R, Aviv RI, Fox AJ, et al. CT angiography "spot sign" predicts hematoma expansion in acute intracerebral hemorrhage. Stroke. 2007;38:1257–62.

158. Walker MC, Smith SJ, Shorvon SD. The intensive care treatment of convulsive status epilepticus in the UK. Results of a national survey and recommendations. Anaesthesia. 1995;50:130–5.
159. Wallis W, Kutt H, McDowell F. Intravenous diphenyl hydantoin in the treatment of acute repetitive seizures. Neurology. 1968;18:513–25.
160. Wasterlain CG, Treiman DM. Status epilepticus. Mechanism and management. Boston: The MIT Press; 2006.
161. Wechsler LR, Jungreis CA. Intra-arterial thrombolysis for carotid circulation ischemia. Crit Care Clin. 1999;15:701–18.
162. Weinrauch V, Safar P, Tisherman S, et al. Cerebral benefit of mild or moderate hypothermia and cardiac risk of deep resuscitative hypothermia after cardiac arrest in dogs. Stroke. 1992;23:1454–62.
163. Wijdicks EFM, Diringer MN. Middle cerebral artery territory infarction and early brain swelling: progression and effect of age on outcome. Mayo Clin Proc. 1998;73:829–36.
164. Wijdicks EFM, Fugate J. Anoxic-ischemic encephalopathy. In: Bradley WG, Darroff RB, Fenichel GM, Jankovic J, Mazziotta J (Eds) Bradley's Neurology in Clinical Practice. 6th ed. Philadelphia: Elsevier; 2012.
165. Wijdicks EFM, Hasan D, Lindsay KW, et al. Short-term tranexamic acid treatment in aneurysmal subarachnoid hemorrhage. Stroke. 1989;20:1674–9.
166. Wijdicks EFM, Nichols DA, Thielen KR, et al. Intra-arterial thrombolysis in acute basilar artery thromboembolism: the initial Mayo Clinic experience. Mayo Clin Proc. 1997;72:1005–13.
167. Wolf S, Martin H, Landscheidt JF, et al. Continuous selective intraarterial infusion of nimodipine for therapy of refractory cerebral vasospasm. Neurocrit Care. 2010;12:346–51.
168. Yeo JD, Stabback S, McKenzie B. Central necrosis following contusion to the sheep's spinal cord. Paraplegia. 1977;14:276–85.
169. Zaganas I, Halpin AP, Oleinik A, et al. A comparison of acute hemorrhagic stroke outcomes in 2 populations: the Crete-Boston Study. Stroke. 2011;42:3640–2.
170. Zeumer H, Hundgen R, Ferbert A, et al. Local intra-arterial fibrinolytic therapy in inaccessible internal carotid occlusion. Neuroradiology. 1984;26:315–7.
171. Zuccarello M, Brott T, Derex L, et al. Early surgical treatment for intracerebral hemorrhage. A randomized feasibility study. Stroke. 1999;30:1833–9.

7 First Studies on Outcome

E.F.M. Wijdicks, *Famous First Papers for the Neurointensivist*,
DOI 10.1007/978-1-4614-3182-4_7, © Springer Science+Business Media New York 2013

Short Historical Note 52

THE GLASGOW COMA SCALE AND GLASGOW OUTCOME SCALE

The Title of the Paper

Teasdale G, Jennett B. Assessment of coma and impaired consciousness. A practical scale. Lancet. 1974;2: 81–4.

Jennett B, Bond M. Assessment of outcome after severe brain damage. Lancet. 1975;1:480–4.

The Paper and the Times

It is in the nature of things that prolonged coma from a major structural injury to the brain may lead to poor outcome. However, the assessment of comatose patients is complex because it requires a detailed neurologic evaluation that includes a reliable history, neurologic examination, and also interpretation of laboratory tests, neuroimaging, and sometimes electrophysiologic studies [23].

The key findings of the neurologic examination can be encapsulated into practical scales that allow physicians to communicate with each other and with other health care workers more effectively. Ideally, a coma scale would include the bare minimum of the unconscious state, and grading a patient over time must indicate changes in clinical condition. The scale or score may also indicate prognosis, but any coma study necessarily would include a heterogeneous group of patients with structural brain injury, and thus likely only those with very low scores may do poorly no matter what the cause. Prognosis of coma from nonstructural injury is far more difficult to predict.

Coma scales originated in neurosurgical intensive care units. Charting neurologic status and physiologic functions at the bedside was common practice. The need for a clinical bedside tool was universal. Ommaya, a neurosurgeon at the National Institute of Neurological Diseases and Blindness in Bethesda, Maryland, developed one of the earliest systems in 1966—a comprehensive scoring system called a "vital sign card". It later became briefly known at the Ommaya Coma Scale [48].

Before the publication of the Glasgow Coma Scale (GCS), (Fig. 7.1) coma scales were not systematically used and—in day-to-day practice—descriptions of coma were likely much less detailed. Neurologists or neurosurgeons would communicate a full neurologic examination, but other specialists would probably commonly use ambiguous terms such as unresponsiveness or somnolence.

Prognosis could be determined early on but more accurately after the patient had been resuscitated and had entered a relative stable clinical state. Furthermore, classification of disability had always been a problematic assessment with easy pitfalls and limitations. Before Jennett and Bond devised a practical scale that later became known as the Glasgow Outcome Scale (GOS) (Fig. 7.2) several scales had been devised in Europe that pertained to outcome in head injury survivors. Outcomes that had been described previously included categories such as "permanent invalid," "slight sequelae," "partially reintegrated," "mental restitution," and were all poor interpretations of a patient's functional well-being or handicap. When traumatic brain injury databases became well organized, there was a demand for tools that could evaluate outcome and also could predict futility.

The Details of the Paper

In 1974, Teasdale and Jennett published "Assessment of Coma and Impaired Consciousness: A Practical Scale," which was a "spin-off" of the National Institutes of Health-sponsored international studies on coma and prognosis of severe brain injury [37]. The first version of this scale was known initially as the "Coma Index" but soon became known as the Glasgow Coma Scale. The GCS was constructed mainly to improve communication between physicians and nurses when describing different states of impaired consciousness.

To provide a tool for repeated measurements that could be charted hourly at the bedside and to "restrict routine observations to the minimum," Teasdale and Jennett excluded certain tests from the scale (e.g., brainstem reflexes) that they believed would be difficult for "inexperienced

ASSESSMENT OF COMA AND IMPAIRED CONSCIOUSNESS

A Practical Scale

Graham Teasdale Bryan Jennett

University Department of Neurosurgery, Institute of Neurological Sciences, Glasgow G51 4TF

Summary A clinical scale has been evolved for assessing the depth and duration of impaired consciousness and coma. Three aspects of behaviour are independently measured—motor responsiveness, verbal performance, and eye opening. These can be evaluated consistently by doctors and nurses and recorded on a simple chart which has proved practical both in a neurosurgical unit and in a general hospital. The scale facilitates consultations between general and special units in cases of recent brain damage, and is useful also in defining the duration of prolonged coma.

Introduction

A WIDE range of conditions may be associated with coma or impaired consciousness. Apart from acute brain damage due to traumatic, vascular, or infective lesions, there are metabolic disorders such as hepatic or renal failure, hypoglycæmia or diabetic ketosis, and also drug overdose. In gauging deterioration or improvement in the acute stage of such conditions, as well as in predicting the ultimate outcome, the degree and duration of altered consciousness usually overshadow all other clinical features in importance. It is therefore vital to be able to assess and to record changing states of altered consciousness reliably.

Need for a Clinical Scale

Impaired consciousness is an expression of dysfunction in the brain as a whole. This may be due to agents acting diffusely, such as drugs or metabolic imbalance; or to the combination of remote and local effects produced by brain damage which was initially focal. Such focal brain damage may affect some of the responses which are used to assess the level of consciousness, and any scale devised for general use must allow for this possibility. A simpler scale might suffice for metabolic or drug coma, when the likelihood of structural brain damage is small, but in an emergency there may be insufficient information to assign patients confidently to a particular diagnostic category. Moreover, coma of mixed origin is not uncommon, as when head injury is suspected of being associated with ingestion of drugs or alcohol, or with a vascular accident. These seem good reasons for devising a generally applicable scheme of assessment.

Fig. 7.1 Title page

ASSESSMENT OF OUTCOME AFTER SEVERE BRAIN DAMAGE

A Practical Scale

Bryan Jennett Michael Bond

Institute of Neurological Sciences, and Departments of Neurosurgery and Psychological Medicine, University of Glasgow

Summary Persisting disability after brain damage usually comprises both mental and physical handicap. The mental component is often the more important in contributing to overall social disability. Lack of an objective scale leads to vague and over-optimistic estimates of outcome, which obscure the ultimate results of early management. A five-point scale is described—death, persistent vegetative state, severe disability, moderate disability, and good recovery. Duration as well as intensity of disability should be included in an index of ill-health; this applies particularly after head injury, because many disabled survivors are young.

Introduction

MANY patients now survive illnesses which would previously have proved fatal, especially those associated with acute failure in one bodily system or another. In most systems survival is followed by good recovery, and, even if functional reserve is subsequently diminished, the patient can usually accommodate to this. But when the brain is the organ affected, the persisting disability usually comprises both mental and physical handicaps which can seriously impair the quality of life. This makes the assessment of outcome after brain damage a matter of some complexity, calling for the exercise of considerable effort and skill. In practice the state of health of survivors is often described in vague terms which make it difficult to judge what degree of recovery has really occurred.

Need for a Scale

The outcome of serious illness concerns not only the patient and his family but therapeutic teams and the whole community. As medicine becomes more expensive, and major illness increasingly the corporate concern of society rather than a private contract between patient and physician, there is growing awareness of the need to assess the results of different types of management. In cases of brain damage, not only is the initial treatment dependent on the use of scarce resources, but the outcome may be permanent disablement which requires continuing social support. If measures of the efficacy of health services are to take account of humanitarian benefits, as well as economic costs and benefits, then some attempt must be made to measure the quality of life. The Institute of Social

Fig. 7.2 Title page

junior doctors or nurses" to perform or interpret. The GCS, therefore, assessed only eye motor, and verbal responses. Teasdale and Jennett's reasoning for the use of these three components was as follows:

> Motor responses: "The case with which motor responses can be elicited in the limbs, together with the wide range of different patterns which can occur, makes motor activity a suitable guide to the functioning state of the central nervous system."
> Verbal responses: "Probably the commonest definition of the end of coma, or the recovery of consciousness, is the patient's first understandable utterance."
> Eye responses: "Spontaneous eye opening, with sleep/wake rhythms, is most highly scored on this part of the scale, and it indicates that the arousal mechanisms in the brainstem are active."

The GCS was initially an unnumbered system. The practice of assigning a number to the responses (using "1" for the lowest score rather than "0") was introduced in a later article that also expanded the motor responses, adding abnormal flexion [70].

Meanwhile, the new computer database on traumatic head injury in Glasgow would need a standardized outcome assessment. Jennett and Bond's paper on what became known as the *Glasgow Outcome Scale* was basically was a description of the nature of disability in survivors of brain damage. The GOS divided outcome into death or survival and in surviving patients whether there was a persistent vegetative state, severe disability, moderate disability, or good recovery. The GOS was used in their intensive care unit for some years, and they found "a good measure of agreement between different assessors." No formal studies were presented in this paper, but its publication was a landmark development because it pointed out limitations of existing systems, summarized the difficulty in judging disability, and proposed a solution. The authors clearly emphasized that, when assessing disability, there is a patient component and a physician component. In other words, the patient may feel he is markedly handicapped while the physician feels that the patient is doing quite well considering the severity of his injury. The authors also acknowledged that the disability might be underestimated and a routine encounter with the patient may not reveal the extent of the cognitive deficit. Death requires no further description, but the authors were careful in determining that death could be ascribable to primary brain damage or, for example to severe pneumonia or sepsis. However, there was no clear distinction in the GOS between brain death, death from systemic complications or withdrawal of support in a patient with a major complication. The more difficult categories to assess were severe and moderate disability. Severe disability indicated that patients were dependent on daily care. Patients with moderate disability were independent and could travel alone, although a major handicap might be present. The good recovery category usually was seen as "resumption of normal life," with minor neurologic or psychological deficits. The authors also had the fortitude to describe that return to work was a poor index of recovery. Moreover, the distinction of whether the patient will be institutionalized or home often had more to do with the support of the family rather than the disability.

The Message and Acceptance

Although users of the GCS began creating sum scores for the three components (giving a total range of 3–15 points), this method was never the intention of the originators of the scale: "…while we do not favor its use in day-to-day clinical practice, we find no reason to doubt that it will continue to be used widely in the analysis and reporting of a series of patients with head injury or other forms of acute brain damage." GCS sum scores such as 3, 8, and 15 have immediate familiarity and use of the sum scores even led to the slogan, "Glasgow 8, intubate."

There have been criticisms over the years [28, 61]. First, GCS is skewed toward the motor part (six items vs. four for eyes and five for verbal). Second, the verbal component of the GCS is unusable in intubated patients. Several techniques and mathematical models have been devised to circumvent this problem. One technique is pseudoscoring, adding the average value of the motor and eye score to the sum in place of the missing verbal score. Another study using linear regression model found that the predicted verbal response correlated well with the actual verbal score, but the model is limited to patients with high GCS sum scores and nonintubated patients [59].

In clinical practice, most institutions substitute T (for "tube") in the verbal component, but it is not clear how sum scores are calculated using this substitution. These attempts over the years to modify or simplify the GCS may be indicative of dissatisfaction with its use in patients with severe brain injury. Several other alternative coma scales have been proposed [65, 66, 68, 83]. None of the new coma scales have yet proven to be able to stand the test of time.

Additionally, when GCS is tested, physicians' knowledge of the GCS is marginal. On average, when asked to name the individual scale components, physicians could identify three of the four possible eye responses, three of the six motor responses, and two of the five verbal responses. Approximately half of the neurologists and internists did not accurately name the verbal response [55].

The outcome scale became known as the GOS. (In a follow-up article, it was briefly called the Glasgow Global Outcome Scale [11].) The GOS was less easily accepted than the GCS, and many other scales have been developed. Nonetheless, the contribution was quite significant with dividing disability into being dependent (assistance with personal needs) and independent (able to look after oneself). It also included persistent vegetative state as a condition that should be separately recognized.

The GCS and GOS became adopted by most European countries and, through the ambassadorial work of neurosurgeon Langfitt, became a frequently used scale in the United States [58]. The scales would become universal metrics for severely brain injured patients. In his paper in 1978, Langfitt forcefully stated:

> The author believes that the Glasgow Coma Scale and the Glasgow outcome measures should be adopted by neurosurgical units throughout the world to evaluate their patients with head injuries. Since other coma scales have merit, and changes such as the recent addition of a 15th point undoubtedly will be made in the Glasgow Coma Scale, there should be agreement to adopt the Coma Scale for a specified period of time, perhaps a 5-year period from 1978 to 1982. During that time, the applicability of the Coma Scale can be thoroughly tested and suggested changes catalogued in a central location [58].

The GOS has remained a preferred outcome system in assessing patients with traumatic head injury, particularly in Europe and the United Kingdom. Two decades later, Teasdale et al. published an extended GOS (8-point version) [71].

Nevertheless, the original GOS is still used in the two major traumatic brain injury data banks (The IMPACT and CRASH). The Cerebral Performance Category (CPC) and Rankin Scale also are used although they are basically modifications of the GOS. The CPC most often is used in studies of anoxic-ischemic encephalopathy. The Rankin Scale is most often used in studies on stroke. Albeit appropriately validated, the instruments that assess clinical outcomes vary considerably among studies and even vary in studies with the same patient populations.

Short Historical Note 53

OUTCOME AFTER NONTRAUMATIC COMA

The Title of the Paper

Levy DE, Bates D, Caronna JJ, et al. Prognosis in nontraumatic coma. Ann Intern Med. 1981;94:293–301.

The Paper and the Times

In the early 1960s, intensive care units (ICUs) were mushrooming in the United States and throughout the rest of the world. As a result, a discussion on medical costs and, in particular, high ICU costs, prompted a review of care in patients with hopeless neurologic conditions. Often, these discussions focused on the pressing issue of how to approach the long-term care of persistently comatose patients. Prognosis of acute neurologic conditions was nothing more than an educated empirical guess. Usually, a combination of persistent coma, abnormal pupil reflexes, and reflexive motor responses in a demonstrable severe brain injury would indicate a poor outcome, but guidelines had not been developed. Cohorts of comatose patients after traumatic brain injury had been published, but prognostic information about "nontraumatic" coma was not available. In these times, it was fashionable to longitudinally study a large number of patients with repeated neurologic examinations and then trying retrospectively to obtain useful predictors of outcome [19, 20]. The early studies mostly involved comatose patients following cardiopulmonary resuscitation (CPR) [47, 64, 88]. This study would involve all patients in nontraumatic coma. The study was a UK–US collaboration and a result of deliberations between neurosurgeon Bryan Jennett and neurologist Fred Plum [87].

The Details of the Paper

The study is an extension of the Bates paper that originally included 310 patients [7]. Levy's paper has been better referenced due to its inclusion of useful algorithms. The study followed 500 patients in nontraumatic coma seen in New York Hospital—Cornell Medical Center, The Royal Victoria Infirmary (New Castle upon Tyne) and San Francisco General Hospital. Patients were identified by the investigators retrospectively while attending neurology rounds, visiting intensive care units and emergency departments, and daily for 3.5 years (Fig. 7.3). Patients in coma could be enrolled if coma lasted at least 6 h. Patients were followed daily to 1 month. The patient population was a mix of disorders such as subarachnoid hemorrhage ($n=38$), cerebrovascular disease ($n=143$), hypoxic-ischemic encephalopathy ($n=210$), hepatic encephalopathy ($n=51$), and a variety of other disorders (e.g., metabolic disturbances, infectious mass lesions). Outcome was determined by the Glasgow Outcome Scale.

The authors were able to determine outcome in certain subsets of patients. As expected, there was worse outcome in structural brain injury and best outcome in metabolic derangements causing abnormal level of consciousness.

The study found that the absence of pupillary light responses, corneal reflexes, and oculovestibular responses were each associated with a very low probability (<5%) of independent outcome (Fig. 7.4). But, no single sign predicted good outcome.

Clinical signs were then grouped in those seen at days 1, 3, and 7 and analyzed. On the first day, absent pupillary light responses or corneal reflexes predicted a poor outcome. Patients who would speak, opened eyes to noise, fixated on the examiner or were orienting—not unexpectedly—would do well.

At day 3, no patient recovered with absent pupil responses to light, no corneal reflexes, or no motor responses. At day 7, any absent brainstem reflex would indicate poor outcome. The data were then summarized in algorithms shown in Fig. 7.5.

The paper also reported some other interesting findings. The data also showed a major difference between UK and US patients with 71% and 46% of patients, respectively, dying within the first 3 days. The study found that 24 patients with a (retrospectively determined) poor prognosis still survived more than 200 hospital days, indicating a reluctance of physicians and families to withdraw support.

ANNALS
of Internal Medicine
MARCH 1981 • VOLUME 94 • NUMBER 3
Published Monthly by the American College of Physicians

Prognosis in Nontraumatic Coma

DAVID E. LEVY, M.D.; DAVID BATES, M.B.; JOHN J. CARONNA, M.D.; NIALL E. F. CARTLIDGE, M.B.; ROBIN P. KNILL-JONES, M.B.; ROBERT H. LAPINSKI, Ph.D.; BURTON H. SINGER, Ph.D.; DAVID A. SHAW, M.B.; and FRED PLUM, M.D.; New York, New York; San Francisco, California; Newcastle-upon-Tyne, England; and Glasgow, Scotland

We conducted serial neurologic examinations on 500 patients in nontraumatic coma to identify factors predicting recovery. Overall, 81 patients (16%) led an independent life at some point within the first year; the remainder either died without recovery from coma (61%), never improved beyond the vegetative state (12%), or regained consciousness but remained dependent on others for daily activities (11%). Functional recovery did not depend on age but was to some degree related to the cause of coma (subarachnoid hemorrhage and other cerebrovascular disease having the worst recovery; hypoxia-ischemia, intermediate; and hepatic and miscellaneous causes, best) and especially to early clinical signs of brain dysfunction. Even within hours of the onset of coma, only one of 120 patients lacking two of corneal, pupillary, and oculovestibular responses ever regained independent function. The study identifies clinical features of comatose patients that appear within the first week and that are important for predicting recovery and designing future therapeutic trials.

and expensive technological resources when dealing with coma.

A preliminary report by our group (1) based on 310 patients in coma studied prospectively from onset suggested that some early clinical signs might correlate with prognosis. That analysis proved the power of the clinical method, but its applicability was limited by the fact that it gave outcomes from coma in a small number of patients and only on a 1-month basis. We have now extended the analysis to 500 patients in coma from nontraumatic causes and lengthened the follow-up to 1 year.

Fig. 7.3 Title page

Table 5. Moderate Disability or Good Recovery Within 1 Year Related to Absent Neurologic Responses at Admission and Cause of Coma

Absent Neurologic Response	Patients Achieving Independent Function with Coma Caused by:*									
	HI		SAH		CVD		HEP		Misc.	
	%	*n*	%	*n*	%	*n*	%	*n*	%	*n*
Verbal	13	(82)	13	(30)	7	(103)	27	(30)	32	(25)
Eye opening	11	(185)	9	(33)	8	(111)	35	(31)	27	(37)
Pupillary reaction	0	(52)	6	(17)	4	(55)	0	(2)	0	(8)
Corneal	4	(71)	0	(12)	4	(48)	0	(5)	12	(8)
Spontaneous eye movements	6	(140)	8	(24)	5	(55)	45	(11)	17	(23)
Oculocephalic	7	(83)	6	(18)	2	(51)	50	(2)	0	(12)
Oculovestibular	5	(56)	0	(17)	2	(41)	0	(2)	0	(6)
Motor	4	(102)	0	(9)	6	(32)	20	(5)	29	(14)
Deep tendon reflexes	3	(63)	0	(10)	10	(21)	14	(7)	20	(15)
Skeletal muscle tone	9	(124)	12	(16)	5	(39)	20	(10)	14	(21)

* The numbers in parentheses are the number of patients lacking the specific neurologic response. The percentage indicates how many of these patients were to achieve a best 1-year functional state of moderate disability or good recovery. HI = hypoxia-ischemia; SAH = subarachnoid hemorrhage; CVD = other cerebrovascular disease; HEP = hepatic encephalopthy; and Misc. = miscellaneous.

Fig. 7.4 Data on subcategories

The Message and Acceptance

Despite lack of computed tomography scan data, lack of details on level of care, lack of details in specific disease groups (i.e., cerebrovascular categories), and very wide confidence intervals of the reported percentages (due to small groups of patients in each prognosis category), the algorithms became a popular tool for neurologists. How they have influenced practice is not known, but pupil, corneal, and oculocephalic responses now were part of the clinical tools to assess the degree of coma and outcome probability. The study, however, eloquently found that assessment of injury to the brainstem was crucial in order to prognosticate accurately.

With better description of the structural injury and subclassification, the prognostic rules changed and became more refined. Therefore, an absent corneal reflex is more important in a massive hemispheric hemorrhage than in a cerebellar hematoma. The rules of prognostication may also be different in patients who are aggressively resuscitated or become neurosurgical candidates.

Very few studies have addressed outcome after nontraumatic coma, and most have concentrated on prognostication of coma after CPR. Recently, a study group performed an evidence-based comprehensive review on prognostication in comatose survivors after cardiac arrest and that resulted in new guidelines endorsed by the American Academy of Neurology. It became quickly clear by the authors writing this guideline that studies on prognostication had flaws and after careful selection criteria only 22 papers were selected. The definitions of coma and outcome were Glasgow Coma Scale score sum score 8 or less, "persistent unresponsiveness," and "not regaining consciousness." Poor outcome was defined as death or persisting unconsciousness after 1 month or death, persisting unconsciousness, or severe disability requiring full nursing care after 6 months.

Only a few reliable prognosticators of poor outcome after cardiopulmonary resuscitation were identified; if they were present, severe disability, persistent vegetative state, or death was very likely (defined as a false-positive rate approaching zero) [85].

The current practice has evolved over the years, but neurologists use the following basic principles of prognostication in comatose patients after CPR:

Exclusion of confounders such as prior use of sedatives or neuromuscular blocking agents, hypothermia, and presence of organ failure (including shock).

Identification of possible loss of all brain function and consideration of brain death.

Identification of key poor prognostic signs such as myoclonus status epilepticus, absent pupil or corneal reflex after 72 h from resumption of circulation, or a motor response not better than extensor responses.

Identification of abnormal laboratory tests such as increased neuron-specific enolase (NSE) or absent cortical potentials on somatosensory evoked potential studies.

These indicators of poor prognosis in comatose survivors are derived from studies in patients not treated with therapeutic hypothermia. Assessment of clinical markers—particularly motor responses—is more difficult due to possible prolonged effects of sedation after hypothermia [25]. Moreover, the prognostic value of a single sample of serum NSE is very uncertain. Serial measurements showing an increase may have more value but this remains to be proven [24]. Failure to awaken several days after CPR may prompt magnetic resonance imaging (MRI), but its value as an independent predictor is not yet established. Finding quantitative MRI evidence of diffuse laminar cortical necrosis in an unchanged comatose patient obviously predicts a poor outcome but MRI may remain nearly normal initially in patients bound for longterm nursing care.

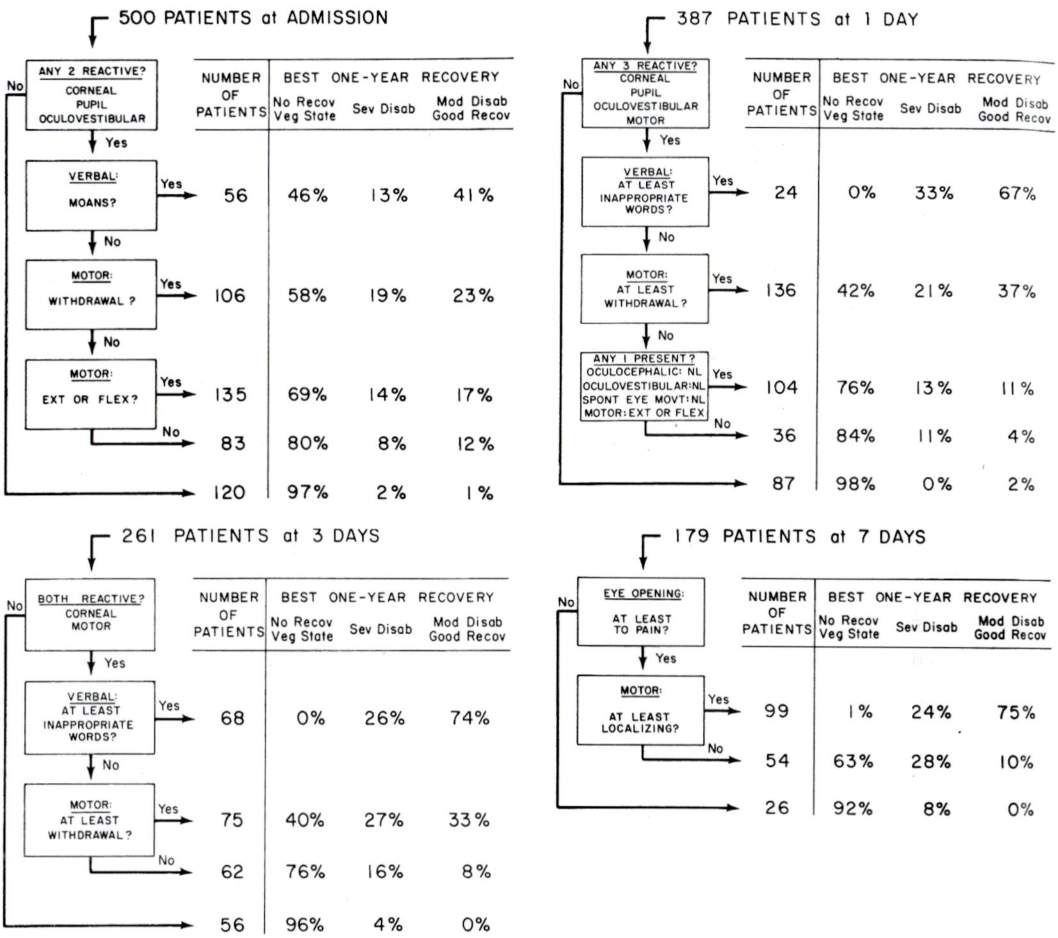

Figure 2. Estimating prognosis in nontraumatic coma. All patients surviving various early intervals after onset of coma are categorized on the basis of sequential criteria relating to their clinical examinations. Best levels of recovery within 1 year are given for each of the prognostic groups. No Recov=no recovery; Veg State=vegetative state; Sev Disab=severe disability; Mod Disab=moderate disability; Good Recov=good recovery; Mot=motor responses; Ext=extensor; Flex=flexor; Spont Eye Movt=spontaneous eye movements; Nl=normal. Nonreactive motor responses means the absence of any motor response to pain.

Fig. 7.5 The outcome algorithms

Short Historical Note 54

OUTCOME AFTER TRAUMATIC BRAIN INJURY

Title of the Paper

Jennett B, Teasdale G, Braakman R, Minderhoud J, Knill-Jones R. Predicting outcome in individual patients after severe head injury. Lancet. 1976;1:1031–4.

The Paper and the Times

The agony of a family suddenly confronted with severe traumatic brain injury (TBI) starts early. Family members often enter an ambivalent period of waiting and hoping. Some comatose patients are stable, but many require aggressive management of increased intracranial pressure (ICP) and that may include decompressive craniectomy. Even in the most aggressively treated patient, the outlook is uncertain, perhaps acceptable, hopefully not too grim, but rarely detailed enough to make radical decisions on level of care early on.

As early as the 1970s, articles from Scandinavian countries claimed to have identified clinical features that would portend poor outcome [15, 49]. Prediction of good outcome has always been tentative because certain major complications (i.e., pulmonary embolus, sepsis) could not be predicted. The Scandinavian studies focused on patients awakening from coma and the probability of them being able to return to work or care for themselves. No systematic studies on detailed neurologic findings linked to outcome categories in large population were known until Bryan Jennett's effort to study severe TBI in Glasgow (Scotland), Rotterdam and Groningen (The Netherlands) (Fig. 7.6).

The Details of the Paper

A database of 600 prospectively collected patients was used to calculate predictions of outcome. Outcome was defined at 6 months and with clinical observations on days 1–7. The clinical examination included pupil responses, eye movements, and motor responses. The outcome categories included death, persistent vegetative state (PVS), severely disabled, moderately disabled, and good recovery as defined in the Glasgow Outcome Scale.

The study importantly stated that "no individual predictions have been made in a prospective fashion while the patient was still under treatment." Additionally, the authors stated that "the patients in each of the centers were treated by a considerable number of neurosurgeons and neurologists who were not involved in the investigation and who were not asked to modify their practice."

The authors considered it a "preliminary report." The outcomes were distributed similarly during the 8 years of the study, making it less likely that patient care was influenced by the study. Bayesian probability statistics were used. A confident prediction was considered with a probability of 0.97 or more. The authors selected 200 existing patients at random, and outcome was predicted after comparison with the remainder 400 cases in the series. The study results found that confident predictions were made in 44% of patients seen within 24 h and this increased to 52–61% with data obtained after 3 days.

The study identified several factors associated with outcome. These were age over 20 years with increasing mortality beyond this cutoff age and even more likelihood of morbidity after 60 years. No differences were found between the decades. A major correlation was found between outcome and eye movement abnormalities (95% of patients with absent eye movements died or remained in PVS), pupil responses (95% of patients with absent pupil reflexes died or remained in PVS), and motor responses (83% of patients with extensor responses died or remained in PVS). The presence of an intracranial hematoma—whether left or right—was associated with a worse outcome.

The authors also identified "optimistic errors" as a result of "unexpected complications" in three patients. These were patients predicted to have a good recovery, but died or were left disabled.

The Message and Acceptance

The foresight of neurosurgeon Bryan Jennett to foster an international head injury databank and carry it through to a large data set remains

PREDICTING OUTCOME IN INDIVIDUAL PATIENTS AFTER SEVERE HEAD INJURY

B. JENNETT G. TEASDALE

University Department of Neurosurgery, Institute of Neurological Sciences, Glasgow

R. BRAAKMAN

Department of Neurosurgery, Academic Hospital, Rotterdam, The Netherlands

J. MINDERHOUD

Department of Neurology, Academic Hospital, Groningen, The Netherlands

R. KNILL-JONES

Hospital Health Services Research Unit, University Department of Medicine, Western Infirmary, Glasgow

Summary Clinical data available in the first few days after severe head injury have been collected prospectively on 600 patients from Glasgow and the Netherlands and stored on computer; the patients in the two countries were similar in initial severity and in their outcome on a defined scale at 6 months. Calculated predictions of outcome were made in 200 randomly selected cases, using Bayesian statistics to compare the data from each patient with those from the 400 remaining cases whose outcome was known. Confident predictions (>0·97 probability) were made in 44% of cases within the first 24 hours of coma, and in 52–61% when data up to 3 days were available. The higher confidence-rate occurred when prediction was limited to two outcomes (death or survival). Comparison of predicted with actual outcomes showed that 96–98% of confident predictions were correct. More logical clinical decisions should be possible when these predictions are available.

Fig. 7.6 Title page

a seminal moment in the understanding of TBI. The paper was the first to use mathematical calculations for predicting outcome. The authors were quick to point out that these predictions could only assist physicians and noted that hospital administrators should not use the data to guide the use of resources. The study's main message, however, was that severe TBI often resulted in a poor outcome.

The study spawned a major increase in TBI databanks throughout the world [13, 41, 42, 44, 67]. Gradually, the number of clinical predictors increased, and computed tomographic (CT) data were added—largely unavailable in Jennett's series [44, 46]. Systemic variables (hypotension, anemia) also became recognized as possible predictors.

Any predictive model recognizes pitfalls. Percentages can be "read" both positively and negatively, but these models are definitively better than clinical judgment based on experience. No physician can claim to have sufficient clinical acumen as to be absolutely certain. Poor outcome is more difficult to predict in younger patients [39, 40].

The most important factors with high predictive power are coma after adequate resuscitation, age of 65 years, abnormal pupils or abnormal pupils for at least one observation, shock on admission, persistently increased ICP, hypoxemia on admission, and CT scan abnormalities representing multiple contusions.

Currently, multiple prediction models in head injury exist. One of the largest databases of TBI (IMPACT; International Mission for Prognosis and Analysis of Clinical trials in Traumatic brain injury) uses admission characteristics to calculate a prognosis estimate. These are age, motor response, pupil responses, presence of hypoxia and hypotension, CT categorization into severity of lesions and presence of a mass lesion, presence of traumatic subarachnoid hemorrhage, epidural mass, and also serum glucose and hemoglobin values (calculator at www.tbi-impact.org) [44]. Another database is the CRASH prognostic model (calculator at www.crash.lshtm.ac.uk) [46].

CT categorization now plays an important part in calculation of risk for poor outcome [78]. Shear lesions frequently are found on CT scans in patients with diffuse closed head injury. They commonly are located in the frontal cortex and white matter interface, basal ganglia, thalamus, and internal capsule. Shearing abnormalities of the corpus callosum often are associated with small lesions in the thalamus, splenium, or septum pellucidum, consistent with a fronto-occipital direction of acceleration.

The Marshall CT classification introduces CT features that may be important cutoff points. In this classification, a high- or mixed-density mass lesion implies contusion or hemorrhage. The extent of the lesion is determined by its volume, the cutoff being 25 cc. The higher risk for raised ICP is determined by present, absent, or compressed basal cisterns and the degree of midline shift—the cutoff point being 5 mm. These pathologies fall into the classes based on the severity:

Grade 1: No visible intracranial pathology.

Grade 2: Cisterns present with midline shift 0–5 mm; no high- or mixed-density lesion >25 mL.

Grade 3: Cisterns compressed or absent with midline shift 0–5 mm.

Grade 4: Midline shift >5 mm or surgically evacuated lesion and nonevacuated high- or mixed-density lesion >25 mL.

Grade 5: Any lesion surgically removed.

Grade 6: High- or mixed-density lesion >25 mL not surgically removed.

The main aim of the Marshall classification was to identify those TBI patients who are at higher risk for deterioration or death [43].

Prognostic features on magnetic resonance imaging scans have not been systematically studied in large groups of patients, but one study claimed a very poor outcome when corpus callosum lesions appeared in conjunction with brainstem lesions [42].

Short Historical Note 55

OUTCOME AFTER CEREBRAL HEMORRHAGE

The Title of the Paper

Tuhrim S, Dambrosia JM, Price TR, et al. Prediction of intracerebral hemorrhage survival. Ann Neurol. 1988;24:258–63.

The Paper and the Times

Stroke (called cerebrovascular accident in the 1950s) is mostly understood as ischemic injury caused by occlusion of a large cerebral artery or as a intracerebral hemorrhage (ICH). Early studies were hampered by lack of angiographic verification, lack of computed tomography (CT) scans, reliance on autopsy confirmation, as well as other imperfections such as a careful neurologic examination over time.

In the 1980s, studies on outcome started to appear, mostly to obtain a better sense of the natural history [22, 29, 50]. These studies could then be a benchmark toward the evaluation of medical or surgical treatments. For example, better insight in prognostic factors could address the potential benefits of surgical evacuation of a cerebral hematoma. Furthermore, outcome studies could identify causes of worsening that could lead to its better recognition. It was also recognized early on that the natural history of acute stroke also may be biased by referral patterns and in some hospital series including the more severely affected patients. This prompted the development of studies of patients from a defined geographic location ("population-based studies").

Medical complications only recently received attention. Modern intensive care unit care undoubtedly impacted on outcome, and a better outcome became apparent when patients with cerebral hemorrhage were transferred to more secure settings, rather than being simply observed on the ward.

The complex interaction of many factors could make studying the natural history an almost futile undertaking. Most studies of patients with a recent cerebral hemorrhage identified that the neurologic examination of the patient and initial clot size (more than 50 mL) was a potent predictor of outcome. The initial studies undoubtedly used heterogeneous groups; later studies were far more location specific, in particular when CT scans became available in the early 1970s. Limited deficits in a patient with a presumed ischemic stroke could now be linked to a hemorrhagic stroke, and the epidemiology of stroke changed as a result of that. The study cited here was an important first attempt to sort out the melee of factors that could contribute to outcome in cerebral hemorrhage (Fig. 7.7).

The Details of the Paper

The data were obtained through the pilot phase of the stroke databank, a cooperative effort of four hospitals and the National Institute of Neurological Disorders and Stroke [76]. The 30-day survival status of 82 patients with cerebral hemorrhage was the basis of this study. Tuhrim et al. identified multiple variables that were possibly related to ICH outcome. He included medical history (21 variables), demographics (11 variables), stroke course (8 variables), physical examination (4 variables), neurologic examination (20 variables), and laboratory values (7 variables) [75]. All variables that were statistically significant were entered into a multiple logistic regression model.

Factors associated with outcome were Glasgow Coma Scale (GCS) score, systolic blood pressure, vertical gaze palsy, severity of weakness, presence of brainstem–cerebellar deficits, and clinical course and size of parenchymal hemorrhage. The major prognostic factors included GCS (≤8), size of hemorrhage (large, more than one lobe; small, less than half lobe), and pulse pressure (≤40, 41–65, or more than 65) (Fig. 7.8).

The Message and Acceptance

Application of Tuhrim's model resulted in 90% correct prediction. The worst prognosis was seen in a patient with a GCS less than 8, hemorrhage involving more than one lobe, and a pulse pressure greater than 65 mmHg. The prognostic value of

Prediction of Intracerebral Hemorrhage Survival

Stanley Tuhrim, MD,* James M. Dambrosia, PhD,† Thomas R. Price, MD,‡ Jay P. Mohr, MD,§
Philip A. Wolf, MD,‖ Albert Heyman, MD,# and Carlos S. Kase, MD‖

The Pilot Stroke Data Bank obtained information on 94 patients with intracerebral hemorrhage. These data were used to identify factors predictive of 30-day outcome from among 85 demographic, historical, clinical, and laboratory variables generally available to clinicians on the day of admission. The 9 univariate factors statistically associated with outcome were Glasgow Coma Scale score, systolic blood pressure, pulse pressure, horizontal and vertical gaze palsies, severity of weakness, presence of brainstem-cerebellar deficits, interval stroke course, and parenchymal hemorrhage size. Beginning with these factors, a step-down variable selection procedure was used to derive a logistic regression model, containing only Glasgow Coma Scale score, pulse pressure, and hemorrhage size, that could be used to categorize correctly 92% of the patients as alive or dead at 30 days after onset.

Tuhrim S, Dambrosia JM, Price TR, Mohr JP, Wolf PA, Heyman A, Kase CS. Prediction of intracerebral hemorrhage survival. Ann Neurol 1988;24:258–263

Fig. 7.7 Title page

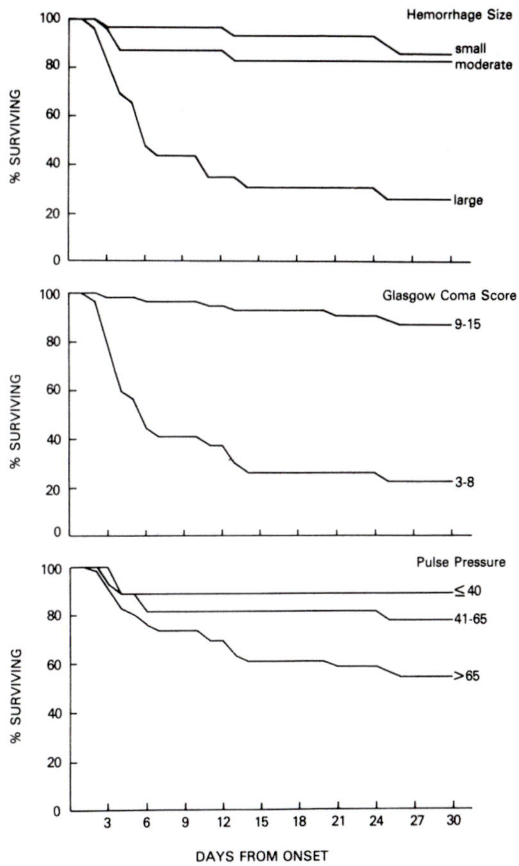

Fig 1. Survival curves for patients in each category of the 3 variables in the logistic regression model.

Fig. 7.8 Outcomes per variable

the pulse pressure was novel. (Pulse pressure is a surrogate of increased intracranial pressure). The model was later validated, now including hyperglycemia and intraventricular hemorrhage (IVH) extension as additional variables [50]. This time, IVH contributed significantly [77, 90].

Current ICH models have included GCS score, National Institutes of Health Stroke Scale, ICH volume, location (supra- or infratentorial), age, and presence of comorbidity. However, no universal scale has emerged and there remains a lack of a standard [16, 26, 30–32, 35, 57].

Further differentiation by specific lesion site was helpful in determining prognosis. Studies found that extension of the hemorrhage mattered greatly. For example, extension of a putaminal hemorrhage into the posterior limb of the capsule would markedly reduce chance of motor recovery [45]. Further classification would include lesions involving anterior limb of capsule and thalamus. Moreover, the significance of IVH depended on the location, with poor outcome in putaminal hemorrhage, but much higher chance of recovery in caudate hemorrhage. Presence of acute hydrocephalus (often a result of shift and compression by a large hematoma) also became recognized as a poor prognosticator in ganglionic hemorrhage with little improvement after placement of a ventriculostomy. Keeping the ventriculostomy open with thrombolytics-allowing clearance of intraventricular hemorrhage-may change the odds of a poor outcome.

In the early 1980s, anticoagulation-associated hemorrhage received more attention, and immediate reversal of warfarin became a major part of management. The impact of rapid normalisation of INR on outcome remains unknown.

Outcome prediction in patients presenting early with cerebral hemorrhage likely relates best to clinical assessment of brainstem injury. With it, the outcome is poor; without it, the degree of midline shift is a reflection of size and predicts morbidity.

Short Historical Note 56

OUTCOME AFTER ANEURYSMAL SUBARACHNOID HEMORRHAGE

The Title of the Paper

Kassell NF, Torner JC, Haley EC Jr, Jane JA, Adams HP, Kongable GL. The international cooperative study on the timing of aneurysm surgery. Part 1: overall management results. J Neurosurg. 1990;73:18–36.
Kassell NF, Torner JC, Jane JA, Haley EC Jr, Adams HP. The international cooperative study on the timing of aneurysm surgery. Part 2: surgical results. J Neurosurg. 1990;73:37–47.

The Paper and the Times

Outcome after aneurysmal subarachnoid hemorrhage (SAH) has been difficult to predict. At presentation, patients seem to do well, but the neurologic condition often changes for the worse, and in these patients the overall outcome of aneurysmal SAH—despite revolutionary changes in aneurysmal repair and better intensive care—remains quite poor. It has been long known that about 10% of patients become deeply comatose and die (mostly become brain dead) within 24–28 h and very little can be done to prevent this outcome [56]. Still, there is a considerable proportion of patients who are less affected by SAH, have their aneurysm coiled or clipped, and are left with only a scar of the craniotomy or ventriculostomy site and are able to return to work without major adjustments in responsibilities.

Prognostication of aneurysmal SAH also was biased by surgical selection (no surgery because of advanced age, poor condition, major early medical complication such as cardiopulmonary injury) or referral patterns (patients in poor condition do not reach tertiary centers that typically report on these patients in the medical literature) [80]. In addition, the quality of neurorehabilitation may play a role [72].

A landmark moment came after the publication of the prospective clinical trial, The International Cooperative Study. The main aim was to collect detailed information about the natural history and results of various interventions from several centers, as well as to define the relationship between timing of surgery and outcome. Initial data for 249 patients were published during the period from 1974 to 1977 and concluded that the mortality and morbidity remained high despite antifibrinolytic drugs to reduce rebleeding; therefore, the authors suggested earlier repair of the aneurysm [1].

In the late 1970s and 1980s, most US and UK neurosurgeons operated "late" (several days later mostly after 10 days). The main reason was "soft swollen brains" or the belief that "early operation could precipitate or exacerbate cerebral vasospasm." In contrast, Japanese neurosurgeons would operate early allowing aggressive management of cerebral vasospasm that normally would not result in an increased risk of rebleeding. According to Kassell, there was only a "small (nonvocal) minority" that felt there was no difference in outcome between early and delayed surgery. In reality, timing of surgery likely was an expression of arbitrary and personal choice.

The Details of the Paper

The study was a prospective, observational epidemiologic study. A randomized controlled trial was considered, but the assumption was that few neurosurgeons would be willing to randomize patients, and there were anticipated difficulties obtaining consent (Figs. 7.9 and 7.10).

Participants included 68 neurosurgical centers in 14 countries (US, 24; Japan, 12; Italy, 8; and UK, 5), and they entered 3,521 patients. The patients were stratified by age, gender, hypertension, and site and size of aneurysm. Assessments were performed by neurologists unaware of the timing of surgery. The data forms included demographic data, neurologic assessments on admission (≤3 days from first SAH), results from CT scan and cerebral angiogram, neurologic and medical complications, operative condition, and surgical techniques. The Glasgow Outcome Scale was used to obtain a 6 months follow-up assessment.

The paper identified several important factors associated with poor outcome. Leading cause of poor outcome was cerebral vasospasm resulting in death or disability in 14% of patients. Rebleeding was the second most common cause of poor outcome in 8%. Other contributing factors were operative complications, intracerebral hematoma, and hydrocephalus. Other major

The International Cooperative Study on the Timing of Aneurysm Surgery

Part 1: Overall management results

Neal F. Kassell, M.D., James C. Torner, Ph.D., E. Clarke Haley, Jr., M.D., John A. Jane, M.D., Ph.D., Harold P. Adams, M.D., Gail L. Kongable, B.S.N., and Participants

Department of Neurological Surgery, University of Virginia Health Sciences Center, Charlottesville, Virginia, and Department of Neurology, University of Iowa, Iowa City, Iowa

✓ The International Cooperative Study on the Timing of Aneurysm Surgery evaluated the results of surgical and medical management in 3521 patients between December, 1980, and July, 1983. At admission, 75% of patients were in good neurological condition and surgery was performed in 83%. At the 6-month evaluation, 26% of the patients had died and 58% exhibited a complete recovery. Vasospasm and rebleeding were the leading causes of morbidity and mortality in addition to the initial bleed. Predictors for mortality included the patient's decreased level of consciousness and increased age, thickness of the subarachnoid hemorrhage clot on computerized tomography, elevated blood pressure, preexisting medical illnesses, and basilar aneurysms. The results presented here document the status of management in the 1980's.

Key Words • **aneurysm** • **multicenter management study** **subarachnoid hemorrhage** • **Cooperative Aneurysm Study**

Fig. 7.9 Title page

The International Cooperative Study on the Timing of Aneurysm Surgery

Part 2: Surgical results

Neal F. Kassell, M.D., James C. Torner, Ph.D., John A. Jane, M.D., Ph.D., E. Clarke Haley, Jr., M.D., Harold P. Adams, M.D., and Participants

Department of Neurological Surgery, University of Virginia Health Sciences Center, Charlottesville, Virginia, and Department of Neurology, University of Iowa, Iowa City, Iowa

✓ A prospective, observational clinical trial was conducted by the International Cooperative Study on the Timing of Aneurysm Surgery to determine the best time in relation to the hemorrhage for surgical treatment of ruptured intracranial aneurysms. Sixty-eight centers contributed 3521 patients in a $2\frac{1}{2}$-year period beginning in December, 1980. Analysis by a prespecified "planned" surgery interval demonstrated that there was no difference in early (0 to 3 days after the bleed) or late surgery (11 to 14 days). Outcome was worse if surgery was performed in the 7 to 10-day post-bleed interval. Surgical results were better for patients operated on after 10 days. Patients alert on admission fared best; however, alert patients had a mortality rate of 10% to 12% when undergoing surgery prior to Day 11 compared with 3% to 5% when surgery was performed after Day 10. Patients drowsy on admission had a 21% to 25% mortality rate when operated on up to Day 11 and 7% to 10% with surgery thereafter. Overall, early surgery was neither more hazardous nor beneficial than delayed surgery. The postoperative risk following early surgery is equivalent to the risk of rebleeding and vasospasm in patients waiting for delayed surgery.

Fig. 7.10 Title page

findings included better outcome in patients who were alert on presentation, and were younger. Good outcome was still observed in more than one in four patients older than 70 years.

Better outcome also was related to size of the aneurysm (<12 mm) and location (patients with an anterior circulation aneurysms had better outcome than those whose aneurysm was located on the posterior circulation). The study also identified other less well known indicators for good outcome and included lower admission blood pressure, thin clot on CT, absent comorbidity, absence of cerebral vasospasm, better motor response, and good orientation on admission. At 6 months, 75% of the patients had a favorable outcome with a good recovery in 58%, but there was still a 25% mortality rate. The authors stated in the second part of the manuscript on surgical results

> The risk of waiting 2 weeks for surgery is accompanied by a 12% risk for rebleeding and 30% risk of focal ischemic deficits. … Early surgery is feasible from a technical perspective and reduces the risk of rebleeding; however, in this study, it did not appear to have a major influence on the incidence of mortality or morbidity from vasospasm.

The investigators were "somewhat surprised" that clipping of the aneurysm did not appear to be more difficult when done early and the risk for premature leak or rupture was not dependent on timing of surgery.

The Message and Acceptance

The message of the International Cooperative Study was that 75% of patients in a good condition and seen within 3 days may have a good recovery at 6 months.

The impact of the International Cooperative Study on care of patients was significant. It is likely it changed practice all over the world with more neurosurgeons now opting for surgical repair within 3 days of presentation. It also showed the problems with early aneurysmal clipping in elderly patients presenting in a poor grade and with associated comorbidity. However, contrary to this belief, several reports did later show that early aggressive management of poor grade patients could still lead to significant improvement in outcome in approximately 40–50% [6, 38].

Management of SAH also changed dramatically with the introduction of endovascular coil embolisation of aneurysms. In the early 2000s, studies reported 30–50% good outcome in poor-grade SAH patients [9, 79]. Coiling thus has been a particularly important development in good-grade SAH patients [53]. In some series, mortality was reduced by 50% [52, 56, 69]. Newer endovascular techniques for patients—otherwise bound to become disabled after surgical repair—also may change the equation. Flow diverters (pipeline endovascular stent) may have a role in treatment of complex giant aneurysms [18].

Treatment of aneurysmal SAH has remained highly individualized. There is insufficient data to unmistakably prove that care in the neurosciences ICU, aggressive cerebrospinal fluid diversion, and ultra-early use of antifibrinolytic agents change outcome. Every physician in this field understands very well that multiple factors impact on outcome [2]. However it is fair to say that high volume centers and years of expertise in caring for these very complex patients must yield better results.

Short Historical Note 57

OUTCOME OF CATASTROPHIC NEUROLOGIC INJURY: PERSISTENT VEGETATIVE STATE

The Title of the Paper

Multi-Society Task Force on PVS. Medical aspects of the persistent vegetative state: parts I and II. N Engl J Med. 1994;330:1499–508, 1572–9.

The Paper and the Times

Once the term *persistent vegetative state* (PVS) had been coined in 1972, it became an established neurologic condition [10, 84]. In the 1990s, position papers by major US and UK medical organizations moved toward the definitions of medical interventions in these patients [4, 14, 33, 51]. Both nasogastric and fluid administration through IV access were considered a "form of medical treatment" [17]. This would then imply that family or any other legal guardian could stop these interventions. Interruption of nutrition and hydration in children also was considered acceptable but more problematic [5].

PVS became an issue in legal proceedings where the "persistent" label of the condition was debated. A comprehensive review was deemed necessary, and a multisociety task force was formed in 1991 and included representatives of the American Academy of Neurology, Child Neurology Society, American Neurologic Association, American Association of Neurological Surgeons, and American Academy of Pediatrics [73, 74]. The task force was chaired by Stephan Ashwal, pediatric neurologist from Loma Linda University School of Medicine, in California, and Ronald Cranford from Hennepin County Medical Center, Minneapolis. Consultants to the task force included leading experts in traumatic head injury, anoxic brain injury, and bioethics.

Details of the Paper

Two comprehensive manuscripts dealt with definition and clinical aspects, related terms and conditions, causes and clinical course, and ancillary diagnostic studies (Figs. 7.11 and 7.12). The review would become quickly "famous" after introducing a new term: *permanent vegetative state*. Permanent would mean irreversibility; persistent could mean "a condition from the past and continuing disability with an uncertain future." The task force stated:

> A permanent vegetative state, on the other hand, means an irreversible state, which like all clinical diagnoses in medicine, is based on probabilities, no absolutes. A patient in a persistent vegetative state becomes permanently vegetative when the diagnostic of irreversibility can be established with a high degree of clinical certainty—that is, when the chance that the patient will regain consciousness is exceedingly small. We believe there are sufficient data on the prognosis for neurologic recovery to allow us to distinguish between persistent and permanent vegetative factors in an individual patient, can be used by a physician to determine when the persistent vegetative state becomes permanent—that is, when a physician can tell the patient's family or surrogate with a high degree of medical certainty that there is no further hope for recovery of consciousness or that, if consciousness were recovered, the patient would be left severely disabled.

The task force found that the prevalence of PVS was not known, mostly as a result of a lack of accepted criteria and the fact that the diagnosis was not in the International Classification of Diseases (ICD). The task force also concluded that neurodiagnostic testing could not predict recovery potential or even confirm the clinical diagnosis.

The second part of the document focused on recovery and outcome, pain and suffering, and treatment and determination of the level of treatment, including withdrawal of nutrition and hydration. Only five verified cases were found in the literature with late recovery, albeit still in a debilitated state.

The task force also focused on costs for caring for patients in a PVS and concluded in 1994 that the total annual costs for the care of adults and children in a PVS would amount to 1–7 billion dollars. The task force also finally concluded that recovery from a post-traumatic PVS is unlikely after 12 months. Recovery from a nontraumatic PVS was rare after 3 months. The task force noted a 70% mortality in 3 years and 84% in 5 years. Mortality from untreated infections or sepsis was high in the first 3 years. Prolonged survival could be achieved only with meticulous care and aggressive medical intervention with each complication.

MEDICAL ASPECTS OF THE PERSISTENT VEGETATIVE STATE

(First of Two Parts)

THE MULTI-SOCIETY TASK FORCE ON PVS*

Abstract This consensus statement of the Multi-Society Task Force summarizes current knowledge of the medical aspects of the persistent vegetative state in adults and children.

The vegetative state is a clinical condition of complete unawareness of the self and the environment, accompanied by sleep–wake cycles, with either complete or partial preservation of hypothalamic and brain-stem autonomic functions. In addition, patients in a vegetative state show no evidence of sustained, reproducible, purposeful, or voluntary behavioral responses to visual, auditory, tactile, or noxious stimuli; show no evidence of language comprehension or expression; have bowel and bladder incontinence; and have variably preserved cranial-nerve and spinal reflexes. We define persistent vegetative state as a vegetative state present one month after acute traumatic or nontraumatic brain injury or lasting for at least one month in patients with degenerative or metabolic disorders or developmental malformations.

The clinical course and outcome of a persistent vegetative state depend on its cause. Three categories of disorder can cause such a state: acute traumatic and nontraumatic brain injuries, degenerative and metabolic brain disorders, and severe congenital malformations of the nervous system.

Recovery of consciousness from a posttraumatic persistent vegetative state is unlikely after 12 months in adults and children. Recovery from a nontraumatic persistent vegetative state after three months is exceedingly rare in both adults and children. Patients with degenerative or metabolic disorders or congenital malformations who remain in a persistent vegetative state for several months are unlikely to recover consciousness. The life span of adults and children in such a state is substantially reduced. For most such patients, life expectancy ranges from 2 to 5 years; survival beyond 10 years is unusual. (N Engl J Med 1994;330:1499-508.)

THE term "persistent vegetative state" was coined by Jennett and Plum in 1972 to describe the condition of patients with severe brain damage in whom coma has progressed to a state of wakefulness without detectable awareness.[1] Such patients have sleep–wake cycles but no ascertainable cerebral cortical function. Jennett and Plum thought that patients in a persistent vegetative state could be distinguished clinically from those with other conditions associated with prolonged unconsciousness.

In 1983 the President's Commission for the Study of Ethical Problems in Medicine and Biomedical and Behavioral Research accepted the definition of persistent vegetative state proposed by Jennett and Plum and defined unconsciousness as the inability "to experience the environment." In the commission's judgment, a persistent vegetative state is only one form of permanent unconsciousness.[2] The others include coma after a traumatic or nontraumatic injury, with death occurring before the recovery of sufficient brain-stem function to allow a stable vegetative state; the end stages of degenerative neurologic conditions, such as Alzheimer's or Creutzfeldt–Jakob disease; coma from untreatable mass lesions such as neoplasms or vascular masses; and anencephaly in infants.

Because of the diagnostic, prognostic, and therapeutic uncertainties concerning the persistent vegetative state, several professional medical organizations began a comprehensive examination of their standards of medical care for patients with this condition.[3-7] In 1989, the American Academy of Neurology published a position paper that defined persistent vegetative state, classified artificial nutrition and hydration as forms of medical treatment, and stated that patients or their surrogates could decide to terminate treatment and that there were no medical or ethical distinctions between withholding and withdrawing treatment.[8] A 1990 survey by the American Neurological Association found that 88 percent of responding members agreed with this document.[9] In a 1991 survey by the Child Neurology Society, 92 percent of respondents agreed with the position paper as it related to adults, but only 72 percent thought that it was applicable to infants and children.[10] In addition, 75 percent of the respondents to this survey indicated that they would not withdraw nutrition and hydration from children in a persistent vegetative state.

In 1990, the Council on Scientific Affairs and the Council on Ethical and Judicial Affairs of the American Medical Association issued a report that provided

Address reprint requests to the Multi-Society Task Force on PVS, American Academy of Neurology, 2221 University Ave. S.E., Minneapolis, MN 55414.

This statement has been approved by the American Academy of Neurology, Child Neurology Society, American Neurological Association, American Association of Neurological Surgeons, and American Academy of Pediatrics. The results of the literature search, as well as correspondence and other documents generated by the task force, are available through the American Academy of Neurology in Minneapolis.

*The members of the task force are Stephen Ashwal, M.D., cochairman (Loma Linda University School of Medicine, Loma Linda, Calif.), Child Neurology Society; Ronald Cranford, M.D., cochairman (Hennepin County Medical Center, Minneapolis), American Academy of Neurology; James L. Bernat, M.D. (Dartmouth Medical School, Hanover, N.H.), American Academy of Neurology; Gastone Celesia, M.D. (Loyola University Stritch School of Medicine, Maywood, Ill.), American Neurological Association; David Coulter, M.D. (Boston University School of Medicine, Boston), Child Neurology Society; Howard Eisenberg, M.D. (Maryland Institute of Emergency Medical Services Systems, Baltimore), American Association of Neurological Surgeons; Edwin Myer, M.D. (Medical College of Virginia, Richmond), American Academy of Pediatrics; Fred Plum, M.D. (New York Hospital–Cornell University Medical College, New York), American Neurological Association; Marion Walker, M.D. (Primary Children's Hospital and Medical Center, Salt Lake City), American Academy of Pediatrics; Clark Watts, M.D. (University of Texas Health Sciences Center, San Antonio), American Association of Neurological Surgeons; and Teresa Rogstad, project administrator, American Academy of Neurology.

Fig. 7.11 Title page

The Message and Acceptance

Hope for a clinically meaningful recovery after the diagnosis is made is unrealistic, with recovery extremely rare and not better than a severely disabled fully dependent state of living. All "improved" patients remained in a severely disabled state, fully dependent on care, were bed or wheelchair bound and needed permanent gastrostomy and urinary catheter.

For some families, there may be incredulity seeing their loved one with wide-open eyes while no interaction is registered, and they may need time to accept the irreversibility of the condition [74]. Others may follow their guiding principles or moral values and wish to continue the maintenance of life in any circumstance. Long term survival (30–40 years) in PVS has been reported. For most of us, an irreversible prolonged condition, in which one is unconscious and permanently disconnected from outside stimuli is unacceptable.

The case of Terri Schiavo in Florida generated not only controversy about the need for prolonged care but also a major dispute about her neurologic condition. Unprecedented in this case was a major focus on distinguishing a persistent vegetative state from a minimally conscious state. Far more surprising, being in a minimally conscious state was considered by her family members and their supporters as a major opportunity for therapeutic intervention despite Schiavo's unchanged catastrophic neurologic state for 15 years. In US study of media coverage of PVS, 1,141 articles were found in four North American newspapers on the Schiavo case [54]. The most frequent headline themes featured the legal (31%), end-of-life (25%), and political (22%) aspects of the case. Medical information about diagnosis and treatment was found in only 9% of headlines and suggested that the message to the public was inadequate.

The outcome of PVS seems quite clear. However one recent study found six additional patients that recovered outside the task force brackets [21]. Improvement from anoxic injury was 22 months from onset. However, all six patients remained severely disabled.

Furthermore, treatments in PVS may evolve [60]. A recent study from Tokyo found that deep brain stimulation (DBS) implanted in the mesencephalic reticular formation and centro-parafasciculars nucleus complex resulted in obeying verbal commands (DBS was initiated 4–8 months after onset of coma) [36, 89]. The bedridden statuses of patients did not change, but some patients "could communicate with some speech or other responses." Most patients did not recover over a 10-year follow-up period. Whether DBS is feasible in PVS is highly doubtful and such interventions may create false hope.

The outcome of PVS may also be determined by level of care. Withdrawal of support or no aggressive care of complications in sick, elderly patients may be more common than in patients who are young and in essence healthy. These clinical decisions may impact on the utility of any prognostic model.

SPECIAL ARTICLE

MEDICAL ASPECTS OF THE PERSISTENT VEGETATIVE STATE

(Second of Two Parts)

THE MULTI-SOCIETY TASK FORCE ON PVS*

PROGNOSIS FOR RECOVERY

There are two dimensions of recovery from a persistent vegetative state: recovery of consciousness and recovery of function. Recovery of consciousness can be verified by reliable evidence of awareness of self and the environment, consistent voluntary behavioral responses to visual and auditory stimuli, and interaction with others. Recovery of function is characterized by communication, the ability to learn and to perform adaptive tasks, mobility, self-care, and participation in recreational or vocational activities. Recovery of consciousness may occur without functional recovery, but functional recovery cannot occur without recovery of consciousness. In some instances, during the early stages of recovery of consciousness, external manifestations may not be immediately apparent. Repeated examinations over time are necessary to ensure the consistency and accuracy of signs of recovery.

The prognosis for cognitive and functional recovery depends on the cause of the underlying brain disease. The Glasgow Outcome Scale classifies outcome in five categories: good recovery, moderate disability, severe disability, persistent vegetative state, and death.[108] Patients with a good recovery have the capacity to resume normal occupational and social activities, although there may be minor physical or mental deficits or symptoms. Patients with moderate disability are independent and can resume almost all activities of daily living. They are disabled to the extent that they can no longer participate in a variety of social and work activities. Patients with severe disability are no longer capable of engaging in most previous personal, social, and work activities. Such patients have limited communication skills and abnormal behavioral and emotional responses. They are partially or totally dependent on assistance from others in performing the activities of daily living.

Acute Traumatic and Nontraumatic Injuries

Recovery of consciousness after 12 months is unlikely in adults and children who have had traumatic injuries. Recovery of consciousness after three months is rare in adults and children with nontraumatic injuries (Fig. 1 and Tables 3 and 4).

Traumatic Injuries in Adults

For patients in a vegetative state as a result of traumatic brain injury, the prognosis for recovery remains unfavorable. Recovery of consciousness and function was determined by reviewing data from previously described series of patients rather than individual case reports. Data were available on 434 patients in a vegetative state one month after a severe head injury (Fig. 1 and Table 3)[47,49,50,106,109,110] (and Tillet JA: personal communication). Recovery of consciousness varied with time. Three months after injury, 33 percent of the patients had recovered consciousness; 67 percent had died or remained in a vegetative state. Recovery had occurred in 46 percent of the patients at 6 months and in 52 percent at 12 months. Recovery after 12 months was reported in only 7 of the 434 patients.[47,49] One patient recovered consciousness 30 months after injury and remained severely disabled.[47,111] The Traumatic Coma Data Bank study reported that 6 of 93 adult patients in a vegetative state recovered consciousness one to three years after injury.[49]

Fig. 7.12 Title page

Short Historical Note 58

OUTCOME OF CATASTROPHIC NEUROLOGIC INJURY: BRAIN DEATH

The Title of the Paper

National Institute of Neurological and Communicative Disorders and Stroke Monograph No. 24. The NINCDS Collaborative Study of Brain Death (NIH Pub. No. 81–2286) 1980 (Summary published in JAMA. 1977;237:982–6).

The Paper and the Times

Widespread catastrophic injury involving the hemispheres and brainstem can be irreversible, lead to apnea, hemodynamic collapse, and cardiac arrest. Even when comatose patients are maintained on a ventilator with vasopressors to maintain blood pressure, this condition has been recognized as the end of life. This clinical condition, appropriately named brain death, became better characterized in the late 1960s and allowed organ donation after appropriate consent. In most hospitals, physicians were now able to peruse the "Harvard Criteria" and use it as a point of reference [81]. In the medical community, there was little question about the meaning of brain death, that is, death of the person.

Still, at least in the United States, there was an inclination to study the evolution of brain death in neurologically injured patients in more detail and to test the validity of used criteria. In the United States, most early papers on brain death involved electroencephalographic (EEG) descriptions. One of the most influential was by Silverman and associates [62, 63]. The paper involved a questionnaire send to members of the American Academy of Neurology, American Electroencephalographic Society, and American Neurologic Association producing data on 2,650 isoelectric EEGs [63]. The survey found that most members considered that any EEG activity could mean a patient might survive. In this study, however, only three patients with a true isoelectric EEG recovered, all with an overdose of drugs.

The study also concluded that there was uncertainly on how long a depressed or isoelectric EEG should exist for it to become permanent. This became the impetus for the development of a pilot study. The study became known as the NINDS Collaborative Study on Brain Death or "The Collaborative Study" (Fig. 7.13). Patients simply would have to meet two criteria—unresponsive coma and apnea—and changes in neurologic examination, and EEG would be followed over time. The study would be a starting point for what later became the report of the medical consultants on the diagnosis of death to the President's Commission for the Study of Ethical Problems in Medicine and Biomedical and Behavioral Research [27]. These criteria would become the standard for more than a decade until publication of the American Academy of Neurology practice parameters [3].

The Details of the Paper

The study originated in early 1970, after the National Advisory Council for Neurologic Diseases and Stroke approved a grant to Daniel Silverman at the time chairman of the American EEG Society Ad hoc Committee [62].

The study involved nine centers throughout the United States but was coordinated from the University of New Mexico (Earl Walker, Neurosurgeon). The other main investigators were Drs. Gaetano Molinari and Julius Korein. The study was conducted between July 1971 and October 1972, with some centers enrolling for shorter periods of time.

The study was a "nonintervention" study. Pronouncement of death was always left to the responsible physicians. Residents and neurologic associates often were involved in gathering clinical data. Comatose patients were identified and no effort made by the patient to override the ventilator for at least 15 min was considered sufficient to diagnose apnea. (Apnea was not formally tested and "judged impractical.") Physicians could terminate artificial respiration if they felt doing so was warranted.

The study enrolled 503 cases all seen as early as 15 min after the ictus. The investigators were specifically asked to examine several brainstem reflexes, to obtain blood for toxic studies and an EEG. The study excluded 155 patients due to submission of nonuniform data.

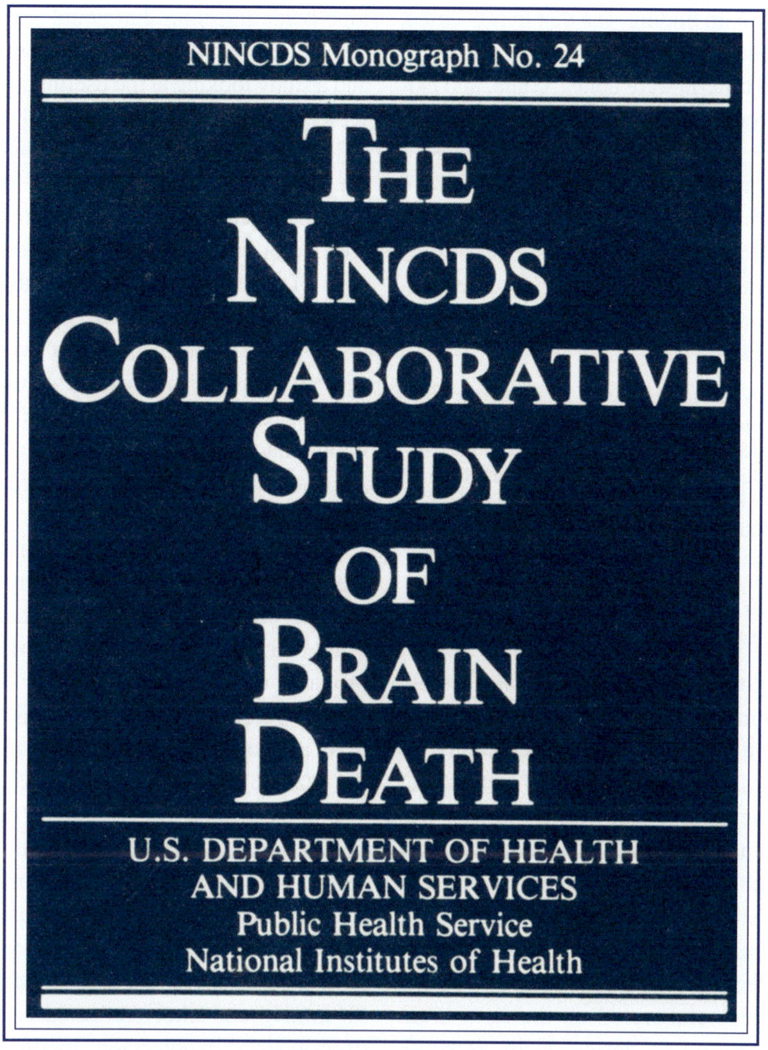
NINCDS Monograph No. 24

THE NINCDS COLLABORATIVE STUDY OF BRAIN DEATH

U.S. DEPARTMENT OF HEALTH
AND HUMAN SERVICES
Public Health Service
National Institutes of Health

Fig. 7.13 Title page

The study's main finding was that in 503 cases, 87% of patients died from cardiac standstill. However, if the criteria were apnea, coma, and isoelectric EEG, only patients with an intoxication improved. One of the other main conclusions of the study was that autopsy data could neither prove nor disprove the accuracy of clinical examination.

The study concluded that the 503 cases provided "an appraisal of the currently accepted criteria." The study also recommended use of a confirmatory test:

> A confirmatory test to demonstrate the absence of CBF is suggested when an early diagnosis of cerebral death is desired, particularly if one or more of the criterial factors are indefinite or cannot be tested. This would allow a diagnosis of a dead brain to be made in patients with small amounts of sedative drugs in the blood, in patients who are undergoing therapeutic procedures that make examination of one or more cranial nerves impossible, and in patients with small pupils.

The study found difficulties with assessment of brain death in the hospitals piloted. One of the most important findings was the difficulty of eliminating drug intoxication as a confounder mostly because levels were not obtained in a timely manner and in half of the patients were not performed at all. EEG was found to be additionally useful, and when all drug-induced cases of coma were eliminated, no patient recovered after a 30-min isoelectric EEG.

The study also elaborated on the term brain death and suggested to define death as death by cardiorespiratory criteria or by neurologic criteria rather than to use the terms cardiac death, cerebral death, or brain death. Later, Korein suggested that cerebral death was best defined by loss of function of the supratentorial part of the brain, placing less emphasis on the brainstem.

The Message and Acceptance

The study was a pilot study, but a later definitive study was never completed. Review of this period clearly suggests that the impetus of the study was a lack of consensus on the reliability of the EEG. The study investigators had a major interest in the neuropathology and electrophysiology of brain death.

The spin-off studies were substantial. The study produced an atlas of EEG in coma and cerebral death, the New York participants developed an isotope bolus injection that could detect absence of cerebral uptake and thus no cerebral blood flow, and a study looking at the usefulness of barbiturate screening in patients suspected of brain death [8, 12]. A considerable effort was made to examine the neuropathology of patients declared brain death. A separate study in 240 autopsies found that "respirator brain" was not a well-defined entity in 15% of cases and that recognizable light microscopic changes may require 24 h to develop. The investigators found a dusky and swollen brain with necrotic tonsillar herniation, cerebral lysis, and necrosis or even a mushy brain, but all without any inflammatory response or cellular glial response. A correlation between "respirator brain" and isoelectric EEG was clearly evident.

The study gained extreme prominence, and the US collaborative study is still often cited as the only US prospective study that looked into brain death, but only a fraction of those patients probably met the criteria.

The US collaborative study was far from definitive, and its problems have been recognized over the years [82]. When the EEG was isoelectric, the options were a do-not-resuscitate order or to treat until cardiac standstill. The patient population was notable for a considerable number of patients with anoxic-ischemic encephalopathy (20%) and intoxications (15%). More than one-third of the patients had systolic blood pressures less than 90 mmHg and likely reflected cardiac shock or drug-induced hypotension. In almost 20% of the patients, cough reflexes were not tested, and even oculovestibular reflexes were not tested in one of ten patients. Apnea was diagnosed when the patient was not overriding the ventilator and a formal CO_2 challenge was not performed. Careful analysis of the patient data shows a gradual increase in missing brainstem reflexes from mesencephalon to medulla oblongata.

Confounders were identified until after patient enrollment, and several confounders were not investigated (i.e., liver and kidney function or other metabolic derangements). Moreover, the toxicology screens were performed in only 313 of 503 patients.

Despite a detailed report published by the NINDS, the study data are difficult to sort out and interpret. The major critique has been that the investigators had more interest in pathology, flow studies, and neuropathology as a definitive test for brain death and did not specifically focus on clinical examination. This line of thinking unfortunately is still present with some physicians looking for a better test of brain death and accepting brain death only when there is demonstrable absent intracranial circulation or isoelectric EEG.

Similar prospective studies have not been performed in other countries. In the United Kingdom, however, Jennett et al. published an article in 1981 about 609 patients in three neurosurgical intensive care units in Cambridge, Glasgow, and Swansea. In 326 patients, ventilators were continued and the heart stopped within days (median 3.5–4.5 days). Jennett also validated brain death by looking at 1,003 surviving patients with traumatic head injury and found none with a combination of apnea, fixed pupils, absent eye movements, or other unresponsiveness [34].

Despite an overwhelming empirical evidence of irreversibility after loss of all brainstem function and rapid cardiovascular collapse requiring incremental doses of vasopressors in more than thousands of cases throughout the world, strictly speaking, a prospective study with repeat examinations over several days to weeks has not been performed [86]. Such a study would be impossible, effectively stop organ donation for the time of the study, and unnecessarily increase deaths on the transplant waiting list.

References

1. Adams Jr HP, Kassell NF, Torner JC, et al. Early management of aneurysmal subarachnoid hemorrhage. A report of the Cooperative Aneurysm Study. J Neurosurg. 1981;54:141–5.
2. Alleyne Jr CH. Aneurysmal subarachnoid hemorrhage: have outcomes really improved? Neurology. 2010;74:1486–7.
3. American Academy of Neurology practice parameters for determining brain death in adults (summary statement). Neurology 1995;45:1012–4.
4. Anonymous. An appraisal of the criteria of cerebral death. A summary statement. A collaborative study. JAMA 1977;237:982–6.
5. Ashwal S, Bale Jr JF, Coulter DL, et al. The persistent vegetative state in children: report of the Child Neurology Society Ethics Committee. Ann Neurol. 1992;32:570–6.
6. Bailes JE, Spetzler RF, Hadley MN, et al. Management morbidity and mortality of poor grade aneurysm patients. J Neurosurg. 1990;72:559–66.
7. Bates D, Caronna JJ, Cartlidge NEF, et al. A prospective study of nontraumatic coma: methods and results in 310 patients. Ann Neurol. 1977;2:211–20.
8. Bennett DR, Hughes JR, Korein J, et al. Atlas of electroencephalography in coma and cerebral death. New York: Raven Press; 1976.
9. Bergui M, Bradac GB. Acute endovascular treatment of ruptured aneurysms in poor grade patients. Neuroradiology. 2004;46:161–4.
10. Bernat JL. The natural history of chronic disorders of consciousness. Neurology. 2010;75:206.
11. Bond MR, Jennett WB, Brooks DN, et al. The nature of physical, mental and social deficits contributing to the categories of good recovery, moderate and severe disability in the Glasgow global outcome scale. Acta Neurochir Suppl. 1979;28:126–7.
12. Braunstein P, Korein J, Kircheff I. Bedside assessment of cerebral circulation. Lancet. 1972;I:1291–2.
13. Butcher I, McHugh GS, Lu J, et al. The prognostic value of cause of injury in traumatic brain injury: results from the IMPACT study. J Neurotrauma. 2007; 24:281–6.
14. Cantor NL. The permanently unconscious patient, nonfeeding and euthanasia. Am J Law Med. 1989;15: 381–437.
15. Carlsson C-A, von Essen C, Lofgren J. Factors affecting the clinical course of patients with severe head injuries. 1. Influence of biological factors. 2. Significance of posttraumatic coma. J Neurosurg. 1968;29:242–51.
16. Cheung RT, Zou LY. Use of the original, modified, or new intracerebral hemorrhage score to predict mortality and morbidity after intracerebral hemorrhage. Stroke. 2003;34:1717–22.
17. Council on Scientific Affairs and Council on Ethical and Judicial Affairs. Persistent vegetative state and the decision to withdraw or withhold life support. JAMA. 1990;263:426–30.
18. D'Urso PI, Lanzino G, Cloft HJ, et al. Flow diversion for intracranial aneurysms: a review. Stroke. 2011;42: 2363–8.
19. Earnest MP, Breckinridge JC, Yarnell PR, et al. Quality survival after out-of-hospital cardiac arrest: predictive value of early neurologic evaluation. Neurology. 1979;29:56–60.
20. Edgren E, Hedstrand U, Nordin M, et al. Ronquist G. Prediction of outcome after cardiac arrest. Crit Care Med. 1987;15:820–5.
21. Etraneo A, Moretta P, Loreto V, et al. Late recovery after traumatic, anoxic, or hemorrhagic long-lasting vegetative state. Neurology. 2010;75:239–45.
22. Fieschi C, Carolei A, Fiorelli M, et al. Changing prognosis of primary intracerebral hemorrhage: results of a clinical and computed tomographic follow-up study of 104 patients. Stroke. 1988;19:192–5.
23. Fischer J, Mathieson C. The history of the Glasgow Coma Scale: implications for practice. Crit Care Nurs Q. 2001;23:52–8.

24. Fugate JE, Wijdicks EFM, Mandrekar J, et al. Predictors of neurologic outcome in hypothermia after cardiac arrest. Ann Neurol. 2010;68:907–14.
25. Fugate JE, Wijdicks EFM, White RD, et al. Does therapeutic hypothermia affect time to awakening in cardiac arrest survivors? Neurology. 2011;77:399–401.
26. Godoy DA, Pinero G, Di Napoli M. Predicting mortality in spontaneous intracerebral hemorrhage: can modification to original score improve the prediction? Stroke. 2006;37:1038–44.
27. Guidelines for the determination of death: report of the medical consultants on the diagnosis of death to the President's Commission for the Study of Ethical Problems in Medicine and Biomedical and Behavioral Research. JAMA 1981; 246: 2184–6.
28. Healey C, Osler TM, Rogers FB, et al. Improving the Glasgow Coma Scale score: motor score alone is a better predictor. J Trauma. 2003;54:671–8.
29. Helweg-Larson S, Sommer W, Strange P, et al. Prognosis for patients treated conservatively for spontaneous intracerebral hematomas. Stroke. 1984;15:1045–8.
30. Hemphill 3rd JC, Bonovich DC, Besmertis L, et al. The ICH score: a simple, reliable grading scale for intracerebral hemorrhage. Stroke. 2001;32:891–7.
31. Hemphill 3rd JC, Farrant M, Neill Jr TA. Prospective validation of the ICH score for 12-month functional outcome. Neurology. 2009;73:1088–94.
32. Hwang BY, Appelboom G, Kellner CP, et al. Clinical grading scales in intracerebral hemorrhage. Neurocrit Care. 2010;13:141–51.
33. Jennett B, Dyer C. Persistent vegetative state and the right to die: the United States and Britain. BMJ. 1991;302:1256–8.
34. Jennett B, Gleave J, Wilson P. Brain death in three neurosurgical units. Br Med J. 1981;282:533–9.
35. Juvela S. Risk factors for impaired outcome after spontaneous intracerebral hemorrhage. Arch Neurol. 1995;52:1193–200.
36. Katayama Y, Tsubokawa T, Yamamoto T, et al. Characterization and modification of brain activity with deep brain stimulation in a persistent vegetative state. Pacing Clin Electrophysiol. 1991;14:116–21.
37. Langfitt TW. Measuring the outcome from head injuries. J Neurosurg. 1978;48:673–8.
38. Le Roux PD, Elliot JP, Newell DW, et al. Predicting outcome in poor-grade patients with subarachnoid hemorrhage: a retrospective review of 159 aggressively managed cases. J Neurosurg. 1996;85: 39–49.
39. Lingsma HF, Roozenbeek B, Steyerberg EW, et al. Maas AIR. Early prognosis in traumatic brain injury: from prophecies to predictions. Lancet Neurol. 2010; 9:543–54.
40. Maas AIR, Marmarou A, Murray GD, et al. Prognosis and clinical trial design in traumatic brain injury: the IMPACT study. J Neurotrauma. 2007;24:232–8.
41. Maas AIR, Stocchetti N, Bullock R. Moderate and severe traumatic brain injury in adults. Lancet Neurol. 2008;7:728–41.
42. Marquez de la Plata C, Ardelean A, Koovakkattu D, et al. Magnetic resonance imaging of diffuse axonal injury: quantitative assessment of white matter lesion volume. J Neurotrauma. 2007;24:591–8.
43. Marshall LF, Marshall SB, Klauber MR, et al. A new classification of head injury based on computerized tomography. J Neurosurg. 1991;75(Suppl): S14–20.
44. McHugh GS, Engel DC, Butcher I, et al. Prognostic value of secondary insults in traumatic brain injury: results from the IMPACT study. J Neurotrauma. 2007;24:287–93.
45. Mizukami M, Nishijima M, Kin H. Computed tomographic findings of good prognosis for hemiplegia in hypertensive putaminal hemorrhage. Stroke. 1981;12:648–52.
46. MRC CRASH Trial Collaborators. Predicting outcome after traumatic brain injury: practical prognostic models based on large cohort of international patients. BMJ. 2008;336:425–9.
47. Mullie A, Verstringe P, Buylaert W, et al. Predictive value of Glasgow coma score for awakening after out-of-hospital cardiac arrest. Cerebral resuscitation 6. Study Group of the Belgian Society for Intensive Care. Lancet. 1988;1:137–40.
48. Ommaya AK. Trauma to the nervous system. Ann R Coll Surg Engl. 1966;39:317–47.
49. Overgaard J, Hvid-Hansen O, Land A-M, et al. Prognosis after head injury based on early clinical examination. Lancet. 1973;2:631–5.
50. Portenoy RK, Lipton RB, Berger AR, et al. Intracerebral haemorrhage: a model for the prediction of outcome. J Neurol Neurosurg Psychiatry. 1987;50:976–9.
51. President's Commission for the Study of Ethical Problems in Medicine and Biomedical and Behavioral Research. Deciding to forego life-sustaining treatment: a report on the ethical, medical, and legal issues in treatment decisions. Washington, D.C.: Government Printing Office; 1983. p. 171–92.
52. Rabinstein AA, Lanzino G, Wijdicks EFM. Multidisciplinary management and emerging therapeutic strategies in aneurysmal subarachnoid haemorrhage. Lancet Neurol. 2010;9:504–19.
53. Rabinstein AA, Pichelmann MA, Friedman JA, et al. Symptomatic vasospasm and outcomes following aneurysmal subarachnoid hemorrhage: a comparison between surgical repair and endovascular coil occlusion. J Neurosurg. 2003;98:319–25.
54. Racine E, Amaram R, Seidler M, et al. Media coverage of the persistent vegetative state and end-of-life decision-making. Neurology. 2008;71:1027–32.
55. Riechers 2nd RG, Ramage A, Brown W, et al. Physician knowledge of the Glasgow Coma Scale. J Neurotrauma. 2005;22:1327–34.
56. Rinkel GJ, Algra A. Long-term outcomes of patients with aneurysmal subarachnoid hemorrhage. Lancet Neurol. 2011;10:349–56.
57. Rost NS, Smith EE, Chang Y, et al. Prediction of functional outcome in patients with primary intracerebral hemorrhage: the FUNC score. Stroke. 2008;39: 2304–9.

58. Rush C. The history of the Glasgow Coma Scale: an interview with professor Bryan Jennett. Interview by Carole Rush. Int J Trauma Nurs. 1997;3:114–8.
59. Rutledge R, Lentz CW, Fakhry S, et al. Appropriate use of the Glasgow Coma Scale in intubated patients: a linear regression prediction of the Glasgow verbal score from the Glasgow eye and motor scores. J Trauma Inj Infect Crit Care. 1996;41:514–22.
60. Schiff ND, Giacino JT, Kalmar K, Vet al. Behavioral improvements with thalamic stimulation after severe traumatic brain injury. Nature. 2007;448:600–3.
61. Segatore M, Way C. The Glasgow Coma Scale: time for change. Heart Lung. 1992;21:548–57.
62. Silverman D. Cerebral death: the history of the syndrome and its identification. Ann Intern Med. 1971;74:1003–115.
63. Silverman D, Masland RL, Saunders MG, et al. Irreversible coma associated with electrocerebral silence. Neurology. 1970;20:525–33.
64. Snyder BD, Ramirez-Lassepas M, Lippert DM. Neurologic status and prognosis after cardiopulmonary arrest: I. A retrospective study. Neurology. 1977;27:807–11.
65. Starmark JE, Stalhammar D, Holmgren E. The Reaction Level Scale (RLS85). Manual and guidelines. Acta Neurochir (Wien). 1988;91:12–20.
66. Starmark JE, Stalhammar D, Holmgren E, et al. A comparison of the Glasgow Coma Scale and the Reaction Level Scale (RLS85). J Neurosurg. 1988;69:699–706.
67. Stocchetti N, Pagan F, Calappi E, et al. Inaccurate early assessment of neurological severity in head injury. J Neurotrauma. 2004;21:1131–40.
68. Sugiura K, Muraoka K, Chishiki T, et al. The Edinburgh-2 coma scale: a new scale for assessing impaired consciousness. Neurosurgery. 1983;12:411–5.
69. Taylor CJ, Robertson F, Brealey D, et al. Outcome in poor grade subarachnoid hemorrhage patients treated with acute endovascular coiling of aneurysms and aggressive intensive care. Neurocrit Care. 2011;14: 341–7.
70. Teasdale GM, Jennett B. Assessment and prognosis of coma after head injury. Acta Neurochir. 1976;34: 45–55.
71. Teasdale GM, Pettigrew LEL, Wilson JLT, et al. Analyzing outcome of treatment of severe head injury: a review and update on advancing the use of the Glasgow Outcome Scale. J Neurotrauma. 1998;15:587–97.
72. Testa C, Andreoli A, Arista A, et al. Overall results in 304 consecutive patients with acute spontaneous subarachnoid hemorrhage. Surg Neurol. 1985;24: 377–85.
73. The Multi-Society Task Force on PVS. Medical aspects of the persistent vegetative state (first of two parts). N Engl J Med. 1994;330:1499–508.
74. The Multi-Society Task Force on PVS. Medical aspects of the persistent vegetative state (second of two parts). N Engl J Med. 1994;330:1572–9.
75. Tuhrim S, Dambrosia JM, Price TR, et al. Prediction of intracerebral hemorrhage survival. Ann Neurol. 1988;24:258–63.
76. Tuhrim S, Dambrosia JM, Price TR, et al. Intracerebral hemorrhage: external validation and extension of a model for prediction of 30-day survival. Ann Neurol. 1991;29:658–63.
77. Tuhrim S, Horowitz DR, Sacher M, et al.Volume of ventricular blood is an important determinant of outcome in supratentorial intracerebral hemorrhage. Crit Care Med. 1999;27:617–21.
78. Wardlaw JM, Easton VJ, Statham P. Which CT features help predict outcome after head injury? J Neurol Neurosurg Psychiatry. 2002;72:188–92.
79. Weir RU, Marcellus ML, Do HM, et al. Aneurysmal subarachnoid hemorrhage in patients with Hunt and Hess Grade 4 or 5: treatment using the Guglielmi detachable coil system. AJNR Am J Neuroradiol. 2003;24:585–90.
80. Whisnant JP, Sacco SE, O'Fallon WM, et al. Referral bias in aneurysmal subarachnoid hemorrhage. J Neurosurg. 1993;78:726–32.
81. Wijdicks EFM. The neurologist and the Harvard criteria for brain death. Neurology. 2003;61:970–6.
82. Wijdicks EFM. The transatlantic divide over brain death determination and the debate. Brain 2012;135: 1321–31.
83. Wijdicks EFM, Bamlet WR, Maramattom BV, et al. Validation of a new coma scale: the FOUR score. Ann Neurol. 2005;58:585–93.
84. Wijdicks EFM, Cranford R. Clinical diagnosis of impaired consciousness in adults. Mayo Clin Proc. 2005;80:1037–46.
85. Wijdicks EFM, Hijdra A, Young G, et al. Practice parameter: prediction of outcome in comatose survivors after cardiopulmonary resuscitation (an evidence-based review): report of the quality standards subcommittee of the American Academy of Neurology. Neurology. 2006;67:203–10.
86. Wijdicks EFM, Varelas PN, Gronseth GS, et al. There is no reversible brain death. Crit Care Med. 2011;39:2204–5.
87. Wijdicks EFM. From clinical judgment to odds: a history of prognostication in anoxic-ischemic coma. Resuscitation 2012, published on line.
88. Willoughby JO, Leach BG. Relation of neurologic findings after cardiac arrest to outcome. Br Med J. 1974;3:437–9.
89. Yamamoto T, Katayama Y, Kobayashi K, et al. Deep brain stimulation for the treatment of vegetative state. Eur J Neurosci. 2010;32:1145–51.
90. Young WB, Lee KP, Pessin MS, et al. Prognostic significance of ventricular blood in supratentorial hemorrhage: a volumetric study. Neurology. 1990;40: 616–9.

8 First Studies in Bioethics

E.F.M. Wijdicks, *Famous First Papers for the Neurointensivist*,
DOI 10.1007/978-1-4614-3182-4_8, © Springer Science+Business Media New York 2013

Short Historical Note 59

LIVING WILL

The Title of the Paper

Kutner L. Due process of euthanasia: the living will, a proposal. Indiana Law J. 1969;44:539–54.

The Paper and the Times

The benefits of aggressive medical management became of interest in the late 1960s, possibly as a consequence of improved access to more sophisticated care, and the general sense that medicine could provide a cure—at least considerable improvement—to many illnesses. Active discontinuation of life support was grossly interpreted as "euthanasia" and illegal, with the potential for indictment for first-degree murder. Before the 1970s no legal document existed that would inform physicians about what a patient would wanted when catastrophically ill [11].

Planning in advance while competent and not terminally ill would become a major departure from the traditional approach—making decisions when they were needed—and different from who would make them—the patient or the physician. These directives could be used when the time came. It was argued that when individuals become patients, they would be unable to make medical decisions and someone else would have to make the decisions. It would make perfect sense to designate someone who is trusted.

In the United States, these discussions became further intensified after the Cruzan and Quinlan persistent vegetative state cases. The Quinlan case launched the end-of-life movement in the United States.

The Details of the Paper

For the first time, Kutner describes a proposal for what he calls a "living will" (Fig. 8.1). After an introduction describing suicide and euthanasia, aiding and abetting, he proposes solutions for patients to make decisions before they become ill. Kutner called it a living will as a "declaration determining the termination of life," "a testament permitting death," "declaration for bodily autonomy," "declaration for ending treatment," and "body trust." The document would provide an individual solution "if bodily state becomes completely vegetated and it is certain that he cannot regain his mental and physical capacities, medical treatment shall cease." He suggested having the document notarized and attested to by at least two witnesses who would confirm that the person was of "sound mind and acted on his own free will." The individual's personal physician or spouse would then keep a copy of the document, with a lawyer or other confidant having an original copy. He also suggested that each individual case should be referred to a hospital committee that would then consider the circumstances under which the document was made. Kutner also felt that at anytime, the individual could revoke the document. Kutner's principle was that "the patient had the ultimate right to decide what is to be done with him and may not irrevocably confer authority on someone else." He identified problems with mental illness and felt that if the patient became mentally ill, the court could find him or her incompetent and appoint a guardian. He also specifically pointed out that although the patient is determining the type of medical treatment, the living will is not used as a means to direct the doctor to terminate the patient's life, and the document does not authorize euthanasia.

Kutner summarized it as follows:

> the living will is analogous to a revocable or conditional trust with the patient's body as the res, the patient as the beneficiary and grantor and the doctor and hospital as the trusties. The doctor is given authority to act as the trustee of the patient's body by virtue of the patient's consent to treatment. He is obligated to exercise due care and it subject to liability for negligence. The patient is free at any time to revoke the trust. From another perspective, the patient in giving consent to treatment is limiting the authority the doctor and other medical persons may exercise over his body. The patient has the ultimate right to decide what is to be done with him and may not irrevocably confer authority on somebody else. The patient may not be compelled to undergo treatment contrary to his will. He should not be compelled to take certain drugs, receive inoculations or therapy or undergo surgery without his express assent. At any point he may stop treatment or he may change physicians.

COMMENTS

DUE PROCESS OF EUTHANASIA: THE LIVING WILL, A PROPOSAL

LUIS KUTNER†

"She asked me to do it," explained Robert Waskin, a young college student, after he had fatally shot his cancer-striken mother while she lay in her hospital room. The Grand Jury of Cook County, Illinois, dispassionately returned an indictment of murder in the first degree.[1] The story became headline news, and euthanasia became the subject of editorial comment on radio and television talk shows.

> After a trial of one week, Robert Waskin was freed by a jury that deliberated only forty minutes before determining that he was temporarily insane when he shot his mother three times. The jury further found that he was no longer insane. The foreman of the jury commented: 'He knew he shot his mother. That was not disputed, but the prosecution failed to show he was of sound mind when he did it.' Robert Waskin is quoted as he prepared to pick up the threads of a nearly shattered life: 'The moral issue of euthanasia . . . was not taken up at the trial, and it should have been faced squarely. Some day it will have to be.'[2]

Fig. 8.1 Title page

The Message and Acceptance

Over time, the living will became known as an advance directive. Legally, living wills or advance directives fall under the Patient Self Determination Act (PSDA 1990). The act requires hospitals to give patients written notice regarding advance health care directives applicable to the state. The PSDA also includes patient rights: the right to facilitate their own health care decisions, the right to accept or refuse medical treatment, and the right to make an advance health care directive. Facilities must inquire as to whether the patient already has an advance health care directive and make note of this in the patient's medical records.

Three types of directives are known. First, the *living will* gives specific direction on health care or appoints an agent or proxy to make decisions on the patient's behalf in the event of terminal illness [22, 24]. A living will should inform surrogate decision makers of any wishes to withhold or withdraw treatment in situations at the end of life [25, 26, 28].

Second, *a durable power of attorney for health care* authorizes another person to make decisions on the patient's behalf even though the patient may not be terminally ill. Third, a mental *health declaration* provides specific direction or designates a proxy to make decisions about intrusive mental health treatment [5].

Advance directives commonly have statements that would indicate that there is an incurable, irreversible illness, and often, a vegetative state is implied. In the United States, state legislatures passed laws in support of a living will in every state in the Union, but still a low percentage of Americans do complete a living will [1, 9, 29].

The ambiguity of the language used has been a major criticism, as is whether the person who signs the document fully understands the potential implications. Generally, the presence of an advance directive in some way helps physicians and families to understand the patient's wishes and is a basis for further discussion about the level of care provided [27].

The situation in the United States seems legally settled, although none of it will resolve controversies in bioethics that surface once a while. The situation in countries other than the United States is no less complicated. No living will legislation exists in Italy and Germany. In the United Kingdom, a court order is needed to withdraw nutrition and hydration from the patient.

Short Historical Note 60

LIMITING THE LEVEL OF CARE

The Title of the Paper

Tagge GF, Adler D, Bryan-Brown CW, Shoemaker WC. Relationship of therapy to prognosis in critically ill patients. Crit Care Med. 1974;2:61–3.
Rabkin MT, Gillerman G, Rice NR. Orders not to resuscitate. N Engl J Med. 1976;295:364–6.

The Paper and the Times

In the late 1950s when patients with acute brain injury could be maintained on a ventilator, discussions emerged that questioned the reality of pushing extraordinary procedures to maintain life. When patients were fully aware of their condition, they could reject further interventions such as hemodialysis or even resuscitation, but the futility discussion here pertained to unconscious patients. Beecher called it the "agonizing death watch" of the family.

Key to Beecher's article addressing the futility of hopelessly injured patients (Fig. 8.2) was a symposium on ethics on medical progress that addressed the futility of care [4]. Hospital administrators were on the sidelines but understood that costly procedures in hopeless cases could or should be avoided.

The level of support in intensive care units (ICUs) remained optimal for the vast majority of patients. Patients were admitted to ICUs simply to provide the best care and the best opportunity for survival. Prognostication in ICUs and critical assessment of success of intervention were always on the mind of physicians but rarely put into workable categories.

Very few articles appeared that would question the possibility that for some patients, care in the ICU would be in vain. "Saving lives" and thus "full-court press," "do everything you can, doctor" were mantras of the 1950s and 1960s. Medicine, and in particular intensive care medicine, was about the best in medical care with the best-trained physicians and the best chance to survive a disorder spiraling out of control. The paper from Mount Sinai School of Medicine in New York addressed these issues. They introduced their paper with the following sentence:

> This difficulty in determining appropriate patients for intensive care is in part due to the fact that insufficient medical data of predictive failure has been accumulated; but it is also in some instances due to the illogical desire to preserve spark of life long after any reasonable hope for survival as a whole person has vanished.

Similarly, orders not to resuscitate the patient were virtually nonexistent before 1970, although practices were unknown. Although the 1974 Quinlan case was about withdrawal of care in prolonged unconsciousness, it clearly identified the start of a medical era that would include a do-not-resuscitate (DNR) order as an option. How to go about DNR orders was largely unknown, and both articles clearly spelled out the criteria and circumstances (Fig. 8.3 and Fig. 8.4) when these orders would be appropriate.

The Details of the Paper

Tagge et al.'s paper placed patients in the ICU in several categories of level of care. Their classification system had been in use for 2 years, and the authors felt it to be very helpful in determining therapeutic plans in their patients. The following categories were proposed:

> Category I – Maximal therapeutic effort without reservation.
> Category II – Maximal therapeutic effort without reservation for a given period (usually 24 hours) and obligatory reassessment at that time with reclassification if indicated.
> Category III – No active or specific therapy (transfusions, antibiotics) to be initiated. Conservative, passive medical care replaces heroic measures (volume ventilators, cardiac pacemakers) already in use are continued but not initiated de novo. No emergency resuscitation will be initiated. Particular attention is given to comfort, including oxygen therapy for shortness of breath, intravenous fluids to prevent excessive thirst, and analgesics for relief of pain. If the patient improves, he is a candidate for reclassification.
> Category IV – All therapy will be stopped and life support assistance will be discontinued.

Fig. 8.2 Beecher's editorial

SPECIAL ARTICLE

ETHICAL PROBLEMS CREATED BY THE HOPELESSLY UNCONSCIOUS PATIENT*

HENRY K. BEECHER, M.D.

Vex not his ghost: O, let him pass! he hates him
That would upon the rack of this tough world
Stretch him out longer. *King Lear*, v. iii

THE following remarks are limited to the single situation of the *unconscious* and irretrievably injured man who is kept "alive" only by extraordinary means. Four very different kinds of questions arise from this situation:

Under what circumstances, if ever, shall extraordinary means of support be terminated, with death to follow?

From the earliest times the moment of death has been recognized as the time the heartbeat ceased. Is there adequate evidence now that the "moment of death" should be advanced to coincide with brain death while the heart continues to beat?

When, if ever, and under what circumstances is it right to use for transplantation the tissues and organs of a hopelessly unconscious patient?

In failing (so far) to accept irretrievable coma as a true indication of death, society condones the discard of the tissues and organs of the hopelessly unconscious patient when they could be used to restore the otherwise hopelessly ill but still salvageable individual. Can society afford such waste?

This matter is pertinent to the ever-broadening experimentation in the transplantation of tissues and organs, which has already led to the use of organs of hopelessly unconscious patients while their hearts were still beating. The ethics of such a step have been questioned. There is, therefore, some urgency to face up to the problems mentioned.

The moment of death can have legal importance,† but the criteria by which death is established must depend upon medical evidence. Granted that there

*Presented at a symposium on "The Ethical Aspects of Experimentation on Human Subjects," held under the Auspices of the American Academy of Arts and Sciences, November 3 and 4, 1967.

From the Anaesthesia Laboratory of Harvard Medical School at the Massachusetts General Hospital (address reprint requests to Dr. Beecher at the Department of Anaesthesia, Massachusetts General Hospital, Boston, Mass. 02114).

†*And theological as well:* "Extreme Unction would certainly not be valid [after death], for the recipient would certainly not be a man any more," an indispensable condition for receiving the sacraments.[1]

Relationship of therapy to prognosis in critically ill patients

GARTH F. TAGGE, MD; DIANE ADLER, RN, MS; CHRISTOPHER W. BRYAN-BROWN, MD; WILLIAM C. SHOEMAKER, MD

A prognostic classification system was developed to help define overall therapeutic goals in critically ill patients with rapidly changing clinical status, in order: a) to force the conscious decision as to use or omission of heroic measures (including cardiopulmonary resuscitation); b) to promote dialogue between the primary physician, ICU staff and the family with respect to the treatment goals and likelihood of success; c) to prevent confusion in those charged with the overall care of the ICU; d) to encourage the development of a treatment plan based on a frequent reassessment of the patient which does not ask the ICU staff to render extraordinary care to a patient who has no reasonable hope for survival as a person; e) to minimize the medical legal risks; f) to dignify the entire ICU operation for the patient, his family, and the staff; and most importantly, g) to guarantee continual reassessment of each individual case with respect to the goals of treatment and the determination of that point in time when treatment should be stopped, when the goals are no longer attainable.

Intensive care provides maximal support to the critically ill patient in his fight for life by assembling a highly competent staff in sufficient numbers to provide adequate surveillance and treatment in a suitable physical environment. This endeavor has proven fruitful and is therefore endorsed by every segment of the medical profession.

However, our experiences indicate that scientific advances in this field have in some instances outstripped our ability to recognize which critically ill patients qualify for intensive care by virtue of a reasonable expectancy of recovery as a whole person. This difficulty in determining appropriate patients for intensive care is in part due to the fact that insufficient medical data of predictive value has been accumulated; but it is also in some instances due to the illogical desire to preserve a spark of life long after any reasonable hope of survival as a whole person has vanished. These experiences suggest the need for the development of a system of categorization which would relate the intensity of treatment to the patient's prognosis; such classification to be subject to repeated revisions dictated by the

Fig. 8.3 Title page

ORDERS NOT TO RESUSCITATE

MITCHELL T. RABKIN, M.D., GERALD GILLERMAN, J.D., AND NANCY R. RICE, J.D.

MEDICAL opinions on the inappropriateness of cardiopulmonary resuscitation of certain patients are now openly discussed, as acknowledged by the New Jersey Supreme Court in its recent Quinlan decision. As early as 1974 the AMA proposed that decisions not to resuscitate be formally entered in patients' progress notes and communicated to all attending staff.* There has been little open discussion, however, of the process by which a decision not to resuscitate is formulated. Within a single institution, practices may vary among physicians, in part from the lack of a clearly articulated hospital policy.

An apparent need for hospital definitions of the process by which decisions not to resuscitate should be made led to the development of the following statement, which is proposed as a policy statement for hospitals concerned with regulating the process whereby Orders Not to Resuscitate may be considered and then implemented. It was developed by us out of discussions held over the past six months in the Law and Ethics Working Group of the Faculty Seminar on the Analysis of Health and Medical Practices, an activity of the Center for the Analysis of Health Practices of the Harvard School of Public Health. We are indebted to the other members of the Working Group for their useful and constructive criticism.

Having witnessed impressive medical developments over the past 25 years, the health-care community is now confronted with complex questions arising from interplay of two such developments, technologic advances and the increased emphasis on the patient's role in decisions concerning his own health care. There is a growing concern that it may be inappropriate to apply technologic capabilities to the fullest extent in all cases and without limitation. Moreover, increased awareness of the rights of patients to be treated in accordance with their own decisions and expectations means that the use of heroic measures to sustain life can be justified only by adherence to the dictates of both sound medical practice and the patient's right to elect or decline the benefits of medical technology.

Both as a standard of medical care and as a statement of philosophy, it is the general policy of hospitals to act affirmatively to preserve the life of all patients, including persons who suffer from irreversible terminal illness. It is essential that all hospital staff understand this policy and act accordingly.

As a matter of policy hospitals also respect the competent patient's informed acceptance or rejection of treatment, including cardiopulmonary resuscitation, and recognize that in certain cases, the unwanted use of heroic measures on a patient irreversibly and irreparably terminally ill might be both medically unsound and so contrary to the patient's wishes or expectations as not to be justified.

To ensure adherence to each of these policies, we have prepared this statement to guide a hospital in the

Address reprint requests to Dr. Rabkin at the Beth Israel Hospital, 330 Brookline Ave., Boston, MA 02215.

*Standards for cardiopulmonary resuscitation (CPR) and emergency cardiac care (ECC). V. Medicolegal considerations and recommendations. JAMA 227:Suppl:864-866, 1974.

Fig. 8.4 Title page

The authors further elaborated on the categories. New patients would be automatically assumed to be in category I. Category II was for patients whose chance for survival were slim, but when members of the ICU team still felt uncertain, maximal therapy would be continued. Patients would be treated aggressively for an additional 24 h, and the situation would then have to be readdressed. Category III was for mostly deteriorating patients despite maximal measures. The authors suggested that to designate a patient category III, the estimated chances of survival would have to be in the order of magnitude of 1 in 100,000. They also stated that "a Category III designation would require a common agreement among the physicians and nursing staff that there was no reason to continue to pursue aggressive care." Category IV would be for patients who nearly fulfilled the clinical criteria of brain death, but also, "the conscious decision is made to relinquish a life which no longer has meaning." Category IV would include active withdrawal of mechanical ventilation.

The paper by Rabkin et al. clearly stated that patients who are irreversibly and irreparably ill and death was imminent, the appropriateness of cardiopulmonary resuscitation (CPR) could be discussed and reconsidered by the patient's physician. However, it also could be raised by the patient or by family members. Most of the criteria concerned patients who were basically dying and CPR would interrupt the dying process. The paper also highlighted that it would be inappropriate to introduce a DNR order in a competent patient who may not be able to cope with it psychologically. The paper emphasized that when competent patients decide on a DNR order, family members cannot override it. Competence was defined as "to rest on the test of whether the patient understands the relevant risk and alternatives, and whether the resulting decisions reflected deliberate choice by the patient." The authors suggested to document a summary of staff discussion, the patient's competence, and the patient's decision to inform appropriate family members, although a verbal order was also considered appropriate.

The Message and Acceptance

Rabkin et al.'s paper was soon followed by a report from an ad hoc subcommittee of the critical care committee of Massachusetts General Hospital that further elaborated on these categorizations and changed them into class A to D [26]. Although none of these classification systems are currently in use, their principles are. Patients are admitted to ICUs with the assumption that they will receive comprehensive care. Palliative care will be provided if there is no hope for a recovery or if advance directives have clearly identified patient's wishes [16].

In 1983, a President's Commission for the Study of Ethical Problems in Medicine published "Deciding to Forego Life Sustaining Treatment" and summarized levels of care into "heroic" or "ordinary" and treatment into "withholding" or "withdrawing." The document elaborated on the proportionality of treatment and also emphasized no ethical difference between stopping therapy and failing to initiate therapy. In a similar vein, administration of pain medication could hasten death but was justified as long as the purpose was palliation—also known as the double effect. The committee accepted that surrogates or proxy could express wishes for de-escalating care.

Over the years, a considerable body of work has appeared that described the practice of withdrawal of care and emergence of the concept of a "shared decision model," where physicians, the patient, and the proxy would decide on the best approach [7, 12–21, 23, 25, 26, 28, 30].

These discussions are now well known to a new generation of intensivists. Paternalism (doctor knows best) now contrasts itself with autonomy (the patient knows best). Patients and family preferences would gradually become better known, and one study would find that patients and their family would value quality of life over survival. Judging how this quality of life would be became a great challenge for intensivists and now neurointensivists. In one study, about 40% of patients said they would not choose ICU care if it meant they would become a burden to the family, adding another level of complexity to the determination of the level of care [10].

DNR orders in ICUs are commonplace. Over time, DNR orders may have impacted admission to the ICU, but still, a considerable portion of patients in the ICU may have a DNR written and are provided the best possible care. There has been a concern that level of care and DNR orders are correlated. In other words, the DNR could lead to less attentiveness of the physician and less aggressive care. The reason to provide DNR orders are now far more lenient and could involve the probability of survival (older age or prior comorbidity) rather than DNR orders in a dying patient.

Patients are resuscitated unless it is explicitly directed otherwise. A DNR directive is justified when quality of life is anticipated to be very poor or when a severely disabled state or persistent vegetative state is expected. Families most often say that their loved one "would not want to live as a vegetable in a nursing home." What they mean is not always clear, but there is a sense that being totally dependent on others with no happiness and just misery is not an acceptable outlook. Some surveys in ICUs suggest few families would want resuscitation in elderly debilitated patients [8, 23].

The DNR order implies withholding CPR, but all other treatment continues. When DNR is discussed, family members and the patient should understand that CPR implies chest compression and multiple drugs next to placement on a mechanical ventilator, which is a complicated procedure and is successful in only one-third of patients, maybe even fewer.

CPR, despite known questionable long-term outcomes, is more successful in the general ICU. In our study in the neurosciences ICU, CPR was performed in 21 patients but only 33% had return of pulse and blood pressure. As expected, CPR in deteriorating neurologic patients is mostly unsuccessful.

Several position statements about limiting level of care by major academies and societies have appeared over time [2, 3].

One historical overview stated:

> After 25 yrs of DNR orders, it remains reasonable to presume consent and attempt resuscitation for people who have an unexpected cardiopulmonary arrest or for whom resuscitation may have physiologic effect and for whom no information is available at the time as to their wishes (or those of their surrogate). However, it is not reasonable to continue to rely on such a presumption without promptly and actively seeking to clarify the patient's (or surrogate's) wishes. The DNR order, then, remains an inducement to seek the informed patient's directive [6].

References

1. Alexander GJ. Time for a new law on health care advance directives. Hastings Center Law J. 1991;42:755–78.
2. American Academy of Neurology Ethics and Humanities Subcommittee. Palliative care in neurology. Neurology. 1996;46:870–2.
3. Anonymous. Withholding and withdrawing life-sustaining therapy. This Official Statement of the American Thoracic Society was adopted by the ATS Board of Directors, March 1991. Am Rev Respir Dis. 1991;144:726–31.
4. Beecher HK. Ethical problems created by the hopelessly unconscious patient. N Engl J Med. 1968;278:1425–30.
5. Berger JT, DeRenzo EG, Schwartz J. Surrogate decision making: reconciling ethical theory and clinical practice. Ann Intern Med. 2008;149:48–53.
6. Burns JP, Edwards J, Johnson J, et al. Do-not-resuscitate order after 25 years. Crit Care Med. 2003;31:1543–50.
7. Carlet J, Thijs LG, Antonelli M, et al. Challenges in end-of-life care in the ICU. Statement of the 5th international consensus conference in critical care: Brussels, Belgium, April 2003. Intensive Care Med. 2004;30:770–84.
8. Christakis NA, Asch DA. Biases in how physicians choose to withdraw life support. Lancet. 1993;342:642–6.
9. Cugliari AM, Miller T, Sobal J. Factors promoting completion of advance directives in the hospital. Arch Intern Med. 1995;155:1893–8.
10. Danis M, Patrick DL, Southerland LI, et al. Patient's and family preferences for medical intensive care. JAMA. 1988;260:797–802.
11. Eisendrath S, Jonsen A. The living will – help or hindrance? JAMA. 1983;249:2054–8.
12. Gillon R. Ethics need principles-four can encompass the rest-and the respect for autonomy should be 'first among equals'. J Med Ethics. 2003;29:307–12.
13. Helft PR, Siegler M, Lantos J. The rise and fall of the futility movement. N Engl J Med. 2000;343:293–6.
14. Levy MM. End-of-life care in the intensive care unit: can we do better? Crit Care Med. 2001;29(2 Suppl):N56–61.

15. Lt N. Advance directives and the concept of competence: are they a moral barrier to resuscitation? J Physiol Pharmacol. 2007;58 suppl 5:477–84.
16. Luce JM, White DB. History of ethics and law in the intensive care unit. Crit Care Clin. 2009;25:220–37.
17. Manara AR, Pittman JA, Braddon FE. Reasons for withdrawing treatment in patients receiving intensive care. Anaesthesia. 1998;53:523–8.
18. Mariner WK. Rationing health care and the need for credible scarcity: why Americans can't say no. Am J Public Health. 1995;85:1439–45.
19. Muller JH. Shades of blue: the negotiation of limited codes by medical residents. Soc Sci Med. 1992;34:885–98.
20. Nyman DJ, Sprung CL. End-of-life decision making in the intensive care unit. Intensive Care Med. 2000;26:1414–20.
21. Perkins HS. Controlling death: the false promise of advance directives. Ann Intern Med. 2007;147:51–7.
22. Pollack S. A new approach to advance directives. Crit Care Med. 2000;28:3146–8.
23. Robinson EM. An ethical analysis of cardiopulmonary resuscitation for elders in acute care. AACN Clin Issues. 2002;13:132–44.
24. Samuels A. The advance directive (or living will). Med Sci Law. 1996;36:2–8.
25. Silverman HJ, Vinicky JK, Gasner MR. Advance directives: implications for critical care. Crit Care Med. 1992;20:1027–31.
26. Smedira NG, Evans BH, Grais LS, et al. Withholding and withdrawal of life support from the critically ill. N Engl J Med. 1990;322:309–15.
27. SUPPORT Investigators. A controlled trial to improve care for seriously ill hospitalized patients: the Study to Understand Prognoses and Preferences for Outcomes and Risks of Treatments (SUPPORT). JAMA. 1995;274:1591–8.
28. Truog RD, Campbell ML, Curtis JR, et al. Recommendations for end-of-life care in the intensive care unit: a consensus statement by the American college of critical care medicine. Crit Care Med. 2008;36:953–63.
29. White ML, Fletcher JC. The patient self determination act: on balance more help than hindrance. JAMA. 1991;266:410–2.
30. Wunsch H, Harrison DA, Harvey S, et al. End-of-life decisions: a cohort study of the withdrawal of all active treatment in intensive care units in the United Kingdom. Intensive Care Med. 2005;31:823–31.

Index

E.F.M. Wijdicks, *Famous First Papers for the Neurointensivist*,
DOI 10.1007/978-1-4614-3182-4,

MIX
Papier aus verantwortungsvollen Quellen
Paper from responsible sources
FSC® C105338

If you have any concerns about our products,
you can contact us on
ProductSafety@springernature.com

In case Publisher is established outside the EU,
the EU authorized representative is:
Springer Nature Customer Service Center GmbH
Europaplatz 3, 69115 Heidelberg, Germany

Printed by Libri Plureos GmbH
in Hamburg, Germany